Research Methods
for Nurses

Research Methods for Nurses

Winona B. Ackerman, R.N., Ph.D.
Department of Nursing
East Carolina University

Paul R. Lohnes, Ed.D.
Department of Educational Psychology
State University of New York at Buffalo

McGraw-Hill Book Company

New York   St. Louis   San Francisco   Auckland   Bogotá   Guatemala   Hamburg
Johannesburg   Lisbon   London   Madrid   Mexico   Montreal   New Delhi
Panama   Paris   San Juan   São Paulo   Singapore   Sydney   Tokyo   Toronto

This book was set in Times Roman by John C. Meyer & Son, Inc. The editors were
Laura A. Dysart and Abe Krieger; the cover was designed by Robin Hessel;
the production supervisor was Jeanne Skahan. The drawings were done by VIP Graphics.
Fairfield Graphics was printer and binder.

RESEARCH METHODS FOR NURSES

2 3 4 5 6 7 8 9 0   F G F G   8 9 8 7 6 5 4 3 2 1

Library of Congress Cataloging in Publication Data

Ackerman, Winona B
  Research methods for nurses.

  Includes index.
  1. Nursing—Research.   I. Lohnes, Paul R., joint author.   II.   Title.
[DNLM: 1.   Research—Methods.   2.   Nursing.   WT20.5 A182r]
RT81.5.A28   610.73'072   80-16720
ISBN 0-07-000182-0

To our mothers
Ivy B. Hulse
and Helen Lohnes,
with our love
and gratitude

Contents

Preface

Change is a way of life to offspring of the twentieth century who have experienced it in professional practice as well as in other aspects of daily life. Change has often been brought about deliberately in an effort to integrate new knowledge that has resulted from research. Nurses have been asked to become "change agents" in nursing practice and in society, yet we may fail to recognize that science changes, too. In reality the scientific process as we have seen it applied to nursing is only slightly older than the formal statement of the nursing process. If the research process is a changing entity, what will be the style of nursing research for the 1980s?

The authors believe that most nursing research is social research and that we are on the verge of a breakthrough in social research. The new style will involve causal modeling as the basis for human policy decisions. It will develop provisional generalizations through applying modern statistics to data collected from ever-widening circles of replications, rather than relying on inferences based on (usually faulty) assumptions or randomly drawn samples.

The new style will represent a radical departure for persons schooled in the Gauss-Fisher tradition of inferential statistics. Those with very long vision, however, may recognize it as the continuation of a trend in nursing research that was given its direction by Quetelet, Nightingale, Galton, and Pearson. Fisher departed from this tradition in a brilliant way that is only appropriate when the subjects of a study can be selected randomly or assigned randomly to treatments. Such samples are not usually feasible in nursing studies. Thus, the book offers an alternative to traditional nursing research texts.

We know that most nurses are first of all clinical practitioners whose main research interest is in understanding research performed by others, but we believe that many more nurses should *do* research as well as understand it and talk about it. Therefore, we have aimed to be intelligible to professional registered nurses, whatever their background of education or experience.

Causal modeling addresses not only one independent variable, but all the variables that contribute substantially to the outcome being studied. This research style demands computer data processing. To that end, we have included FORTRAN code for a simple program that our readers will be able to run without the aid of computer scientists. We think that no other approach to data processing is now worthwhile.

Although we have emphasized a practical process approach, we have not neglected philosophical issues. We discuss theory, models, and causation early in the book, and move steadily toward the goal of building strong theory through developing the ability to provide and defend causal analyses. The general organization of the book is that of theoretical chapters, each followed immediately by a chapter on practical application. We have tried to relate nursing research to the larger context of scientific research (medical, biological, physical, social, psychological) while providing ample nursing examples and making some suggestions regarding techniques that are not customarily used in nursing studies, but could be. We have deliberately left out materials such as taxonomies of research that have often been included in texts without clearly relating them to statistical or clinical theory.

The inclusion of some lesser-known aspects of nursing history has also been deliberate. We display a pervasive interest in Nightingale and Semmelweis because the research attitude they exemplify is one we want to foster among nurses. We want to encourage nurses to believe in themselves as members of a profession that is only beginning to realize its potential for enhancing health, and to recognize that enduring progress must be rooted in sound theory.

To avoid a confusion of pronouns, this book consistently refers to the nurse as *she*. We acknowledge the many men who are also active and successful in nursing practice and do not intend to exclude them through the use of the more traditional pronoun.

Finally, we attend to good writing. Although some may scoff at teaching what ought to have been taught earlier, educational theory tells us that educators should attend to needs, not to our opinions about them.

We thank our families, friends, and colleagues too numerous to name for their support and assistance. We are especially grateful to Nancy Myers for her excellent labors in the preparation of our manuscript, and also thank Mildred Young and Dian C. Jensen for less arduous but similarly excellent manuscript work. The State University of New York at Buffalo generously supported us with computer time, library services, and other assistance.

Winona B. Ackerman
Paul R. Lohnes

Research Methods
for Nurses

Chapter 1

Nurses and Research

Today's nurses feel a strong need for greater professional accord. How can the desired recreation of the profession be achieved? How was the profession created in the first place?

Florence Nightingale forged nursing into a profession by blending altruistic, militaristic, feminist, and scientific elements that were right for nursing in her day. Persons with influence over the profession captured part of her vision, lost part, and prolonged certain parts beyond the times they fit. Today's nurses need to know how their core values and beliefs about nursing are to be constructed and consolidated.

JUSTIFYING NURSING'S NORMS

Who or what shall be the authority for the renewed profession of nursing? By what processes do we ascribe authority? Roth (1957) listed these ways of knowing:

1 Intuition (a glimpse of "truth" through unconscious effort)
2 Authority, tradition, custom
3 Chance (accidental personal experience)
4 Trial and error (deliberate personal experience)
5 Generalization from experience
6 Logic, deduction, syllogistic reasoning, or a formal argument with a major and minor premise and a conclusion

   7   Inductive reasoning, in which a conclusion is arrived at by relating particulars, especially numerous observations
   8   Research, scientific inquiry, or a structured and systematic investigation designed to answer a question, throw light on a theory, or solve a problem (quoted by Henderson, 1967)

It is immediately apparent that Roth's categories overlap. How can we separate intuition from chance? Or trial and error from custom? Isn't generalization from experience very close to inductive reasoning? Can either induction or deduction be distinguished from scientific inquiry?

   It is worthwhile to make a distinction between the origins of a theoretical proposition about nursing and the justification of that proposition. We think that any of Roth's eight sources of knowledge can describe the origins of propositions about nursing, and all have. Propositions arise in our minds in such a variety of ways and arrive with such different forces and pressures behind them that it is impossible to be definitive about the origins of knowledge. For example, although we are in the habit of subsuming technology under science, new technology often originates as a picture—a vision—in the mind's eye of an inventive person (Ferguson, 1977). While there appears to be ample room in nursing for this kind of inventing or envisioning, such activity cannot be claimed by science any more than by art.

   Carper (1978) elucidated four fundamental patterns of knowing in nursing that she called aesthetics (art), personal knowledge (state of being), ethics (values), and empirics (science). If all these ways of knowing are needed and accepted in nursing, what is the special value of science? We think it is that science is both a product and a process, and as a process it offers the best hope of investigating all four components. Yes, we think that values can be investigated (Ginzberg, 1961), as can aesthetics and possibly personal knowledge, when sufficiently creative investigators tackle them. Belief in the ability of science to investigate itself and correct its own errors is, of course, one of the main principles of a philosophy of science. Only the meek and unwary are uncritical about propositions they are asked to believe and act upon. Alert, aggressive thinkers realize that nominated propositions have to be tested somehow. Furthermore, since circumstances change with the passage of time, even propositions which once pass a suitable test for validity cannot be viewed as justified for all time. Especially in the professions which trade upon propositions about human behavior there is need for continual skepticism about the current justifiability of basic propositions on which professional practices are based. An endless cycle of replication of tests of knowledge is the fate of any human services profession such as nursing, and this implies the continual reconstruction of knowledge. Research can be entirely exploratory, but this text will emphasize the ways in which research can validate theoretical propositions about nursing and thus contribute to the justification of nursing's norms.

   Harman (1972) has pointed out that over the centuries revolutions have tended to remove areas of contention from the jurisdiction of traditional ecclesiastic authority and subject those areas to scientific research. Farberow (1963) wrote an interesting book called *Taboo Topics*, which documents the movement of sex, ESP, and other topics previously taboo for research into scientific respectability. Alex Comfort wrote a marvelously prescient novel, *Come Out to Play* (1961), in which he predicted the development of group therapy methods of sexual counseling and sexual behavior modification as they have recently emerged from a matrix of research on human sexual behavior. Although we live in a scientific age and nursing leaders have urged greater emphasis on research, science has barely touched the core of nursing practice. In fact, nurses are not entirely sure what that core is.

With regard to that core, Luke Smith (1966) and others (Conant, 1967) have observed that nursing takes place at the most extreme point of tension between the scientific, rational world as it exists today and the humanistic, feeling world, the two worlds discussed by C. P. Snow. What is best for a person in the long run may hurt most in the short run. The nurse must help the patient to endure this dilemma and, if possible, to make sense of it. This tension between absolutely rational, bare-bones fact and what is humanely desirable exists for the nurse in research just as in other areas of practice. As Gortner (1973) commented, it is the force of our scientific reasoning that gives meaning to the phenomena we observe; and it is our capability as professionals to be sensitive to human needs, and to act on behalf of those needs, that affords us contact with the real world.

Nurses are often taught research lore by experts from other fields who have dedicated themselves to the traditional Western view that the classic experiment is the noblest form of science. In the classic experiment the sine qua non is random assignment of subjects to different treatments (one of which may be a placebo, or control for no treatment). Under ideal conditions the randomized treatments are administered in a laboratory setting in which all possible influences other than the treatment variable on the outcome measure are carefully held constant. Even randomly assigned subjects may be especially sensitive to a treatment in much the same way that one patient may be hypersensitive to a medication which most persons can take safely. Random assignment, however, eliminates subject sensitivity to treatment as an explanation of systematic differences among treatments.

A teaching emphasis on experimental method may put the novice nurse researcher in a schizophrenic world. On the one hand, she must be enough at home in the artificial, laboratory world to read research reports that emanate from it and to make ethical decisions concerning a possible role in collecting experimental data for others. On the other hand, in her own complex, delicately balanced, real-life world, the nurse needs quite different research methods and a different research style.

A major premise of this text is that what may be best in the physics or physiology laboratory is not necessarily appropriate or effective for research on whole humans in the complex situations in which nursing care is provided. We hold that each nursing situation is so unique, complicated by so many situational variables, and so transient that the classic experimental method is unlikely to be either practical or reasonable as the usual method for research on nursing. We hope to be persuasive about methods which we believe are practical and reasonable.

Research, when defined as systematic problem solving, is hardly new to nurses. Table 1-1 shows three manifestations of problem solving in nursing. Nursing is commonly described as the application of the nursing process (Yura and Walsh, 1973), the elements of which are listed in the left-hand column. These in turn are described in terms of problem solving and presented as in the middle column of the table. In the right-hand column appear elements of the problem-oriented charting system espoused in recent years by both medicine and nursing (Walter et al., 1976). Presumably most, if not all, nurses have considered problem solving from the perspectives of both nursing process and problem-oriented records. This book will attempt to provide a broader look from the perspective of scientific method. We hope it will further illuminate the nurse's practice, whether that practice be clinical, administrative, educative, investigative, or a combination.

Q: A very difficult nursing problem is how to talk to terminally ill patients about their prognoses. What theoretical ideas are useful guides to policy about this? What research could be done that might produce useful knowledge in this area?

Table 1-1   The Relationship of the Nursing Process and Problem-oriented Charting to Scientific Methodology

Nursing process	Scientific method	Problem-oriented charting system
	Problem finding	
Assessment	1 Gather information 2 Examine information 3 Interpret information	Data base
	4 Identify the problem 5 State the problem	Problem list
	Problem solving	
Plan	1 Develop alternatives 2 Make a decision 3 Decide on a plan of action	Plan
Intervention Evaluation Revision	4 Execute the plan 5 Evaluate the results 6 Redefine change	Progress notes

Source: The Western Pennsylvania Regional Medical Program and the University of Pittsburgh School of Nursing.

ORIENTATION TO THE RESEARCH PROCESS

Our book is organized around a commonly accepted view of the research process as extending from defining a problem through reporting the study of that problem. In the long run, however, reporting a study of one problem does not provide a final, definitive answer any more than does establishing a nursing care plan or making a patient's problem list. Care plans and problem-oriented records both involve continual evaluation and revision. Science, too, demands continual evaluation and new statements of problems. It is often said that the best research study is a fertile one that generates more questions than it puts to rest. In science the "patient" never gets well! That is, the problems never disappear entirely, but are replaced by the need to replicate on an increasing scale, in different settings, with different types of subjects, or by stating new but related problems.

The thin slice of science we call a research study is thought of as a complete entity more because of our psychological need for beginnings and endings than for any other reason. Perhaps it is more accurate to think of research as a spiral in which each cycle involves a more complete understanding of the problem, and any cycle, part of a cycle, or multiple cycles are activities that may appropriately be called "research." Heidgerken (1971) emphasized that the research process is neither unified nor sequential. Thus it is necessary to keep the research goal clearly in mind in order to prevent the many twists and turns from being disorienting.

Thinking of research goals in terms of what must be reported at the end of a study may help the researcher to keep her bearings. Table 1-2 displays a chart which has been helpful to some nurses who are planning studies. If all the questions are considered thoughtfully, recognizing that of course they cannot be fully answered at first, facing the final report is less likely to strike terror into the faint-hearted (as which of us is not when facing a blank page in a typewriter). The chart may help the investigator to avoid some of the congenital research maladies that are often incurred at the stage of conception. All the items on the chart, as well as puzzling issues of interpretation of data analyses and the justification of generalizations, will be taken up fully in later chapters. Table 1-2 is placed here as an overview and advance organizer. While it shows some of the skills you can hope to acquire, it is not intended to be a guide to the actual writing of a report. That help is provided in other chapters. Figure 1-1, in turn, shows a typical flow of a graduate student's research study, from start to finish. The flowpoints and checkpoints are similar for any research, although the adviser may be called a principal investigator, project director, or senior researcher, instead of "adviser."

In summary, this introductory chapter has suggested that norms for the nursing profession may be articulated by diverse authorities on the basis of diverse ways of knowing, but the testing of proposed norms, the establishment of validity for theoretical propositions, and the ultimate justification of the fundamental knowledge of the profession are dependent in large part upon nursing

Table 1-2   Considerations To Be Covered by the Proposal

1 *Problem:* What do I want to know?
2 *Purpose:* What is the goal? Why am I doing this study?
3 *Review of related literature* (often a separate section): What is the context of knowledge in which I examine the problem?
4 *Hypothesis(es)* or questions to be answered: What do I expect to find?
5 *Assumptions:* What do I accept on evidence or faith? What will I *not* test?
6 *Definition of terms:* What do I mean by _____? Using my definition, could another professional measure it?
7 *Procedure or methods:* How will I find out?
8 *Limitations and setting:* Where will I collect data? What are my criteria for selecting the locale?
9 *Data analysis, statistics, and tables:* What can I compare? How can I make a comparison?
10 *Selection of sample:* Which cases can I compare?
11 *Instruments* (tools, log): What will I measure with? When will I make my measurements?
12 *Identification of researcher(s), agency permission, human subjects clearance, members of project committee, staff, etc.:* What other odds and ends must be included?

research. The classic randomized experiment and all the laboratory and statistical lore that surround it are not likely to be of much use in nursing research. It remains for our book to propose and demonstrate other research methods which can provide the needed approach to scientific problem solving in nursing. The point of view espoused here emphasizes the natural evolution of knowledge and the importance of continual replication of tests of knowledge that lead to repair and reconstruction of nursing theory.

Q: What is an example of a nursing norm? Where do you suppose it came from? How could research justify or challenge this norm?

REFERENCES

Carper, Barbara A.: Fundamental patterns of knowing in nursing. *Advances in Nursing Science*, 1978, *1*(1).

Comfort, Alex: *Come out to play*, 1961. New York: Crown, 1975, American edition.

Conant, Lucy: A search for resolution of existing problems in nursing. *Nursing Research*, 1967, *16*(2), 114–117.

Falardeau, Jean: The role of the nurse in a changing society. *Canadian Nurse*, 1962, *58* (March).

Farberow, Norman L.: *Taboo topics*. New York: Atherton, 1963.

Ferguson, Eugene S.: The mind's eye: Nonverbal thought in technology. *Science*, 1977, *197*(4308).

Ginzberg, Eli (Ed.): *Values and ideals of American youth*. New York: Columbia, 1961.

Gortner, Susan R.: The relations of scientists with professional and sponsoring organizations and with society. In *Issues in research*. Report of American Nurses' Association Council of Nurse Researchers Program Meeting, August 1973.

Harman, Willis: The new Copernican revolution. In Robert Theobald (Ed.), *Futures conditional*. Indianapolis: Bobbs-Merrill, 1972.

Heidgerken, Loretta E.: The research process. *Canadian Nurse*, 1971 (May).

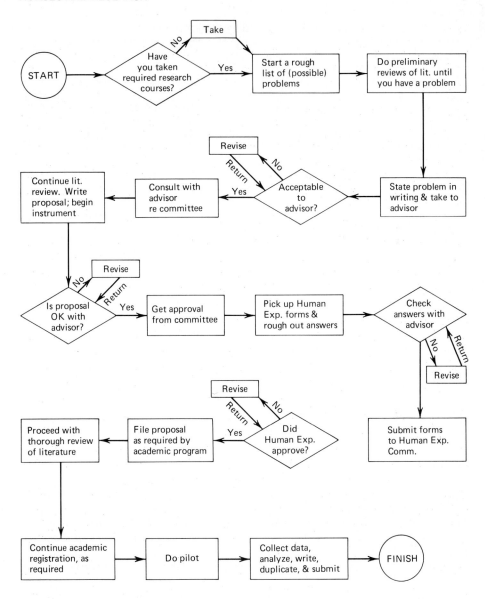

Henderson, Virginia: *Nature of nursing*. New York: Macmillan, 1967.

Roth, Julius A.: Ritual and magic in the control of contagion. *American Sociological Review*, 1957, *22* (June). Quoted by Virginia Henderson in *Nature of nursing*.

Smith, Luke M.: The system—Barriers to quality nursing. In Jeannette R. Folta and Edith S. Deck, *A sociological framework for patient care*. New York: Wiley, 1966.

Uprichard, Muriel: Ferment in nursing. *International Nursing Review*, 1969, *16*(3).

Walter, Judith, Geraldine Pardee, and Doris Molbo: *Dynamics of problem oriented approaches*. Philadelphia: Lippincott, 1976.

Yura, Helen, and Mary B. Walsh: *The nursing process*. New York: Appleton, 1973.

Chapter 2

What Problems Can Be Solved by Research?

Patient-oriented nurses may sometimes find it difficult to be interested in philosophy of science, and this seems natural enough. Pure philosophy and the theories that stem from it have been thoroughly depersonalized, and in their lack of human interest they are at the opposite end of an interpersonal spectrum from the world in which the nurse lives and works. Yet, paradoxically, the personal, specific, particular-case aspects must be removed before theory can be generalized to future situations. Thus it seems appropriate to seek some understanding of the relationships among philosophy, theory, science, logic, research, and application in professional practice.

What are these relationships? A full answer is beyond the scope of this book and beyond the authors' capabilities, but we can seek to make some path through the forest. Bear in mind as we pursue our shortcut that those who take a direct route miss the pleasure of meandering through the woods roundabout and getting directions from the natives. Probably all of us who work in a profession which draws support for its beliefs and practices from natural sciences owe it to ourselves to read regularly and widely in the many popularizations of their work which scientists make available, as well as in the philosophy of science. While our personal altruism and sense of responsibility may be derived from allegiance we give to religious or humanistic ideologies that predate modern scientific thought, we all share a professional intellectualism which is solidly rooted in contemporary scientific ideas. We do need to know our roots!

PROBLEMS IN GENERAL

A reasonable place to begin is with the word *philosophy*. Of course you know some basic meanings for this word, but we hold with the counselor who advises using "one good dictionary or three" (Offutt, 1978), because the richness of meanings the dictionary associates with important words like this one can stimulate broader insights. We commend to your attention these tags from the definition in *The American Heritage Dictionary*, along with our comments:

1 *"Pursuit of wisdom by intellectual means"* reminds us that in the Middle Ages theology and philosophy were the two distinctly separated, more or less equal authorities, with theology holding sway over spiritual matters and philosophy over intellectual matters. Remember what we said in Chapter 1 concerning the historical movement of topics of inquiry from ecclesiastic authority into the domain of science, and consider the dramatic contemporary example of research into the question of whether there is life after death (*Newsweek*, 1978). Without taking sides in the controversy over adequacy of methods, we observe that prior to the mid-twentieth century, most people in Western civilization would have regarded even raising the question as the occasion of sin, and thus a spiritual matter, rather than as a legitimate expression of scientific (intellectual) curiosity. This tag also gives us the opportunity to assert to our readers that nurses have the solemn obligation to be and act like intellectuals, exactly to the extent that they want to be seen and treated seriously as professionals. A hallmark of a profession is that its members are truly intellectuals. Leadership and authority belong only to those who are actively, aggressively intelligent and inquiring.

2 *"Inquiry into the nature of things based on logical reasoning rather than empirical methods"* can be a confusing definition for nurses because the medical meaning of the word *empirical* may be uppermost in our minds. In medicine, empirical has a negative connotation, suggesting practice guided only by experience rather than by theory. In modern philosophy of science empirical has a positive connotation, namely that knowledge is derived from systematic comparison. Of these two meanings of empiricism, we shall always imply the respectable rather than the derogatory one. Still, this tag suggests correctly that philosophic inquiry uses a different method than does empirical or scientific inquiry, and of course this book is more concerned with the method of science than with the method of philosophy. However, in the end we will find that it takes the method of philosophy to figure out the implications of scientific findings.

3 *"The critique and analysis of fundamental beliefs"* foreshadow some difficulty in integrating two notions about theory, one of which is that scientific theory deals only with issues of fact, while philosophy deals especially with issues of value. We are left with a modern duality of knowledge similar to that which prevailed in the Middle Ages, except that science has now taken over the metaphysical issues which used to belong to philosophy and philosophy is now closer to theology. We do not like this change. It seems preferable to regard fact and value as constantly interacting aspects of one world of general experience, just as the real and the ideal are constantly interacting and inseparable parts of a professional nursing practice.

4 *"The investigation of natural phenomena and its systematization in theory and experiment"* hark back to a day when philosophy and science were not yet differentiated. This historical definition of philosophy is now more accurately a definition of natural science.

5 *"The synthesis of all learning"* is pretty grandiose, but perhaps we have to strive for goals we know cannot be achieved. All these meanings for philosophy are in use, and they all have some relevance to the research enterprise.

Theoretical Propositions

The report of a study should hang together logically, and the conceptual-theoretical skeleton it hangs on should be exposed carefully in the written review of literature related to the study. If you think out the purposes of empirical research on nursing, we are convinced you will decide that consideration of theory in each research report is very worthwhile. Reputedly it was Keynes who remarked that people who feel no need of philosophy are sure to be relying on some outmoded philosophy (Fischer, 1971). An unwary researcher may subscribe to either a feeble theory or a defunct philosophy in interpreting her research findings if she fails to examine her footing adequately. A truly lazy researcher may choose simply to report the facts and defer interpretation of them to someone else. Chances are she will not like the interpretation that someone else puts on her findings when she sees it in print, but she will deserve the frustration she then feels. We really cannot relegate to someone else the responsibility (and the pleasure) of puzzling out the meaning of experience, even when we are impressed with the research we have done to record and analyze experience. Facts are tools with which beliefs and practices can be reconstructed. When, as researchers, we make new facts available we should not shun the task of reconstruction they energize.

Some leaders in the field of nursing will disagree with the emphasis we place on theorizing, perhaps because they feel that right now the greatest need is for more reliable facts about nursing situations and practices. We *do* want to encourage empirical research, which after all is simply the collection of facts in the first instance (although we emphasize that analysis of the relationships among facts is also part of the research process), but we are aware that large collections of facts sometimes fail to make much impact on practice because they are not theorized about. One of us is a psychologist, and it has been noted that psychology is a field in which researched facts often seem to be "wasted."

As Bakan has noted, "The yield of new and significant information concerning the human psyche is relatively small in comparison with the enormous resources being expended" (1969, p. xii).

In physiology, a tragic example of inadequate theorizing leading to wasted observations is provided by the case of knowledge about the circulation of blood. The Greek Herophilus, who lived from 460 to 370 B.C., was a leading anatomist who actually dissected to death some 200 prisoners (Watson, 1856). He must have observed arterial, venous, and cardiac pulsations, but he failed to discover that blood circulates. It was left for Harvey, some 20 centuries later, to think of an adequate explanation—the concept of circulation—which was comparatively easy to demonstrate, once postulated.

It is commonly asserted that the purpose of research is to test theory, but that is only part of it. This statement can be fleshed out with Merton's declaration that research may clarify theory, reformulate theory, deflect a theory, or initiate a new theory, and, furthermore, that these consequences may follow from any part of the research process (Beshers, 1957). Thus, Watson and Crick built a model that reformulated existing theory about the structure of the DNA molecule. By contrast, descriptive surveys may end with the production of hypotheses to be tested later. It is worth asking yourself in the planning stages of research exactly how the findings of your study will relate to nursing theory.

Many writers have noted the special problem nurses have when they attempt to identify a theoretical framework at the beginning of a study. This has been attributed to a lack of special nursing theory. It seems to us that the problem lies not so much in a lack of theory as in a superabundance of theoretical propositions relevant to nursing which may, however, be difficult to integrate into a single general framework. The settings in which nursing care is delivered are so complex that a wide variety of generalizations apply at one point or another. Theorists who seek prescriptive theory for nursing may ultimately find that little progress can be made until the context in which nursing care is delivered is greatly simplified. Can outcomes of nursing care be predicted and eventually prescribed only when variation in settings is minimal? An affirmative answer is supported by literature about the Loeb Center, Benedictine Center, and other locations where the excellence of care has been praised and where a precondition of this excellence has been careful screening of patients before admission. While the laboratory is too artificially simple a setting for most nursing research, the typical care situation may be too lavish to permit accurate and complete measurement of the relevant variables. Thus, innovations such as primary nursing that simplify the context of nursing care may improve care directly and also enhance researchability in care settings.

To read more about prescriptive theory or other nursing theories refer to Riehl and Roy (1974), whose book explicates conceptual models for nursing extremely well. Meanwhile, we urge that in the planning stage of research an effort should be made to indicate how the intended findings will relate to one or several expressed theoretical propositions, even if it is not possible to sketch a complete theory to which the findings will relate.

Q: State a theoretical proposition about some aspect of nursing (e.g., practice, recruitment, education, retention, career patterns, administration). What are some parts of the theoretical framework which might surround this proposition?

Constructs, Models, Hypotheses

What we term a theoretical framework, which would consist of a set of logically interconnected propositions, Riehl calls a conceptual model. The concepts of theory, framework, and model clearly overlap. *Concept* itself is variously defined as: (1) "an idea, especially a generalized idea of a class of objects; a thought; general notion" (*Webster's*, 1968); (2) "a concrete or abstract idea; a hypothetical construct; a building block of a full-blown theory" (Reynolds, 1971); (3) "a general idea or understanding, especially one derived from specific instances or occurrences" (*American Heritage*, 1970). These definitions of a concept are unsatisfactory for our needs because they fail to discriminate one type of building block—which is an idea of an entity, force, or process (a "something")—from another type of building block—which is an idea of how one something influences or is influenced by or merely related to another something. We prefer to use the more exact term *construct* for an idea of an entity, force, or process, and to avoid the less exact *concept*. We use the term *theoretical proposition* for an idea of the influences or relationships between two constructs or among several constructs. A construct usually represents something that cannot be heard, seen, felt, tasted, or touched, and for this reason cannot be measured directly. Why bother with such ephemera when the world is so full of real things that must be dealt with? Well, constructs may designate classes of experiences which are "real" enough, such as pain, clinical shock, depression, hypothesized hormones and enzymes—the list goes on and on. The great utility of constructs is that they summarize many discrete experiences of something.

Constructs are building blocks for theoretical propositions. In turn, propositions can sometimes be interrelated to create a theory, or a theoretical framework. Why is it so important to lay out the theoretical (conceptual) framework in specific detail?

It is important to be specific because all speaking and writing are based on assumptions and hypotheses that are sometimes openly displayed, sometimes deliberately hidden, and perhaps even more often unrecognized, unacknowledged, and often inconsistent with one another—in short, a hodgepodge. In everyday life we can convey our own messages as plainly or as secretively as we choose; or we can remain wavering in ambiguity, not knowing our own position from one moment to the next. Even in the work situation a hodgepodge of illogicality often provides the basis of thought and action. Think for a moment about problems of unidentified expectations that a busy staff nurse may encounter in a patient care unit where the RN role is not fully agreed upon. A physician who believes that nurses exist only to help physicians may order a nurse to take a patient to an examining room on a different care unit and to remain there and assist with a physical examination. If she refuses, she may be viewed as insubordinate. If she complies, her head nurse may complain that she is neglecting responsibilities on the unit to which she is assigned. The nurse (who views herself as an autonomous professional) may feel that she is capable of making appropriate priority decisions for herself. In turn, someone higher up in nursing service may clarify matters by formally censuring the nurse for violating established policy. But the difficulty arose because of different expectations—differences in the frames of reference of the persons involved. The expression *frame of reference* implies a manner of thinking and speaking that is common to a particular discipline or background and points to accepted philosophy or theory.

In scientific endeavors the outcome of only a few trials, selected cases, or representative samples may affect the lives of thousands or millions. Scientists should therefore be extremely thorough in stating their problems in a manner that is not only understandable, but nigh impossible to misunderstand. The scientific ideal is clarity, definitude, and exactness. Scientific writers attempt to get the reader on the right track from the outset, so that by the time the problem is presented there is no place else to go but straight ahead. Part of the effort to get the reader on the track is setting up the conceptual (theoretical) framework to make sure that the reader is coming from the same place and going in the same direction toward the same goal.

All nurses can recognize the importance of communicative accuracy in all forms of human endeavors because a good share of their working day in any nursing position is spent checking, verifying, clarifying, interpreting, summarizing, and reporting.

We should not accord to frameworks more mystery than they deserve. *Framework* is only a metaphor, even though it is a good one. You can visualize a strong, slender radio tower with no superfluous materials, only functional steel to make the structure withstand the onslaught of wind and temperature changes. Or you can establish your own metaphor and analytical questions to test the firmness of your ideological footing. Are the ground rules clear? Do you know what is out of bounds? Do the arguments in the literature hold water? Is the train of ideas clear? In short, is the conceptual (theoretical) framework logical?

A framework is a skeleton of logically related concepts strong enough to support the hypotheses of the investigation at hand. It integrates or is consistent with the assumptions and may or may not be stated as a formal theory. Thus, in use, conceptual framework may overlap some definitions of philosophy, as well as theoretical framework or model.

We think that the term *model* implies some metaphor for a process or relationship, such as saying that it is machinelike (when it does not reside in a machine) or that it is lifelike (when it does not reside in an organism). Thus a model is a theory stated in metaphorical terms.

Like the outmoded philosophy mentioned earlier, a too-popular model can dominate to the point where we are no longer aware of it. It becomes part of the mental landscape and is not acknowledged for the metaphor it is. Take the organic system model, for example. All sorts of things are compared to an organism that is born, lives, grows, and dies. Organizations and institutions are spoken of as though they had lives of their own and must inevitably proceed through life stages from infancy to adulthood to senility and death. Sometimes the analogy may be historically accurate, but if so it is because people who worked within the organization behaved in certain ways at various times and not because of the genetic nature of some organic entity.

For the ancient Greeks the dominant model was the organic one, just as it seems to be today. But during some of the intervening centuries the machine model dominated Western civilization. Thus, one of the first books on gravity was called *The Mechanism of the Heavens*. The mechanical analogy helped produce that book, but it was a less successful model for authors a generation or two ago who attempted to describe the "machinery" of the human body. To speak of the body as a machine denies procreation, growth, adaptation, and evolution. In short, it is just the opposite of attempting to breathe biologic life into an institution. To compare a person to a machine is to end up speaking of repair, maintenance, replacement, and so on—and, of course, to dream of engineered solutions to problems. Seeing things as like other, quite different things can be stimulating but also dangerous if the inventive perspective becomes fixated.

A model may be a physical construction like Watson and Crick's for DNA, or it may be verbal or mathematical, and thus abstract. (Keep in mind that verbal means written as well as oral.) A mathematical model is stated in symbols according to the conventions of a mathematical system such as algebra, geometry, calculus, or perhaps statistics. A verbal model is built up of construct names related to each other in sentences, and is what we usually expect a nursing theory or theoretical framework for nursing research to be. Thus, whether a researcher considers herself to be working from a model or theoretical or conceptual framework may matter little, so long as it is clear and logical.

Hypotheses are educated guesses about relationships between or among constructs. They are untested theoretical propositions stated as hunches. Our favorite hypothesis is Halley's speculation that the famous comet which now bears his name would appear in 1910 because just such a brilliant phenomenon had appeared in 1682, 1758, and 1834, suggesting to him one entity with a fixed periodicity. Stated as a hypothesis Halley's guess was: If what has been described in the history books is in fact a comet in a 76-year orbit, then it will appear again in 1910. The constructs involved are *comet* and *orbit*. Halley must have been nearly as brilliant as his comet to think of a hypothesis for which the only mathematics was three simple sums ($1682 + 76 = 1758$; $1758 + 76 = 1834$; $1834 + 76 = 1910$) and the only necessary test datum was enthusiastically collected by millions of viewers who cheered the 1910 appearance!

The comet hypothesis demonstrates that it is not necessary for the investigator to manipulate or control one construct in order to get a test. Thus even historians are increasingly stating formal hypotheses to be tested statistically after the appropriate data are recovered from records. But the hypothesis must state how the *if* (controlled or independent) construct and the *then* (dependent) construct are related and make a change in the dependent construct predictable from a known change in the independent construct. (After we introduce the notion of a *variable* in relation to a construct in Chapter 5, we shall be able to place a hypothesis in a more exact relationship to a theoretical proposition.) It is interesting to return to the ways of knowing (Chapter 1) and read them again, this time not as ways of knowing but as ways of hypothesizing. Although most of them are not fully satisfactory as ways of knowing, they may all be creative routes to testable hypotheses.

A hypothesis is a hunch, explicitly or implicitly, about a computable relationship. The comet hypothesis stated that the comet, if it was a comet, would orbit close to the earth once every 76 years. In some nursing studies it may be worthwhile to predict quite loosely, i.e., that half or three-quarters of the cases studied will exhibit a certain common phenomenon. Even when the hypothesis does not explicitly state the arithmetic of the guess, it is still there because of the implicit understanding that the hypothesis will be tested by some statistic that measures the scores obtained against what might have been obtained by chance.

Medical hypotheses, or "rule-outs," may not seem at first to be true hypotheses in this mathematical sense. They are, however, based in large part on the physician's knowledge of the statistical probability of each rule-out (Wulff, 1976), moderated by pattern recognition and causal thinking. Each patient trusts that the physician's diagnosis is based on the right combination of probability, experience, and logic.

Two things are necessary before a hypothesis can be useful. One is a plan for collecting those data which are capable of testing the hypothesis. The other is a method of analysis that yields a convincing test. Some researchers have a strong predilection for a particular mode of analysis, and even decide on design and sample to fit the analysis they intend to use, rather than the other way around. As we have noted elsewhere, an adequate sample size is likely to be the main concern of a consulting statistician. Similarly, we have attempted to point out that there is no one required sequence in which research decisions are made and the research process implemented. Although researchers may test hypotheses according to purely mathematical, statistical models, they may, like diagnosticians, make use of other decision modes in their discussions and conclusions.

Q: Name two constructs which are important to nursing theory and relate them to each other in a sentence that states a researchable hypothesis.

Assumptions and Evaluations

Whether a restricted proposition or a general theory establishes background for a study, a clear statement of the investigator's point of departure must involve acknowledgement of what she is willing to take for granted and not attempt to test. These elements taken for granted are *assumptions*. They can be thought of as the opposite of hypotheses.

Assumptions can be divided into two types which Suchman (1967) calls *value* and *validity*. Validity assumptions are based on tested propositions with relation to some more or less clearly identified framework. The following could be validity assumptions:

Addition of up to 1 part per million of fluoride to a communal water supply prevents dental cavities.

The incidence of chronic obstructive lung disease has been increasing for 100 years.

Note that in order to make a proposition "valid," i.e., to test it and have it pass the test, it is usually necessary that some sort of measurement have taken place. It follows that the study or studies which attest to your validity assumptions should be cited in your own study.

Value assumptions, in contrast, are beliefs about how good or bad, how desirable or undesirable, something is. Some philosophers and theoreticians take the position that questions of value cannot be investigated by scientific methods. Our position is that they can and ought to be for a couple of reasons. One is that awareness of values can help to maximize the investigator's objectivity. Our value positions affect our perceptions of other research (validity assumptions) and influence us in setting priorities for inquiry, in deciding what needs to be known. People with flexible intelligence (open minds) are alert to unsought validities which challenge their values, but this is less likely to happen if they have not identified the value positions from which they begin their research. At the extreme, a study, especially an exploratory one, may turn up information that is contrary to the researcher's expectation. Finding herself in a world different from the one she thought she was in challenges the investigator to reexamine all her assumptions, both value and validity.

Highly prestigious scientists are sometimes benighted with regard to value assumptions, too. Louis Agassiz (1807–1873) was an eclectic scientist who established glacial theory and knew more about fish than anyone else up to that time. He was perhaps a higher-ranking scientist than Charles Darwin (1809–1882) at the time Darwin put forth the theory of evolution, yet Agassiz failed to reexamine his own assumptions in the light of Darwin's new theory. Along with the famous physiologist Claude Bernard and microbiologist Louis Pasteur, Agassiz believed that the species were divinely created and fixed for all time. His failure to reexamine weakened his own work and probably destroyed some of his fame (Mason, 1956). Knowledge is always subject to thoughtful revision. As professional practitioners, nurses should be wary of both resistance to change and premature adoption of what is new. Rational evaluation of the products of science is the unavoidable, though heavy, burden of a profession.

Whitehead said that if you want to know what is truest about a society, you should look for what is not written rather than what is. One nurse did this (Norris, 1973) and found six unjustified value assumptions she could not take for granted even though most nurses appear to. These were propositions such as "Knowledge prevents disease" and "Nursing is patient-centered." Values are usually undocumented, but we urge that they be stated in research writing. Other examples of value assumptions might be:

Society requires a large number of registered nurses.
Human life is always worth saving.
Suffering is to be avoided at all costs.
Medical care is the right of all who can pay for it.

Does the last one make you uncomfortable? American attitudes toward the conditions under which a right to medical care exists have probably been undergoing a substantial shift recently, and thus the final example may no longer be an assumption held by large numbers of Americans. But think of the generations when it was not questioned or identified as a value assumption. That values change with the times is a second reason for a researcher to be explicit about them.

The importance of assumptions is that they are part of the conceptual framework of the investigation whether or not they are recognized and stated. Thus, in the example of studies of attrition from nursing school mentioned earlier, unrecognized value assumptions undoubtedly influenced outcomes by influencing the choice of variables for study. For example, an assumption was made that defects in students rather than archaic educational philosophy caused attrition. Had due consideration been given to such variables as behavior of women in other educational programs of similar length, the effect of school rules on the adjustment of young women to adult sex roles, the monastic stance of nursing schools (as compared with public high schools and colleges), and the power of high school grades as predictors, there might have been fewer studies of dropouts and more progress in explaining and predicting attrition from schools of nursing. Some data were available on the ignored variables, and they could to some extent have been converted into validity assumptions through adequate reviews of literature.

A statement that values cannot be researched by scientific method can only increase dissonance for learners who may know that many "research" grants are awarded to programs whose closest link to research is the final evaluation of the program's effectiveness in implementing a value or values that a grantor currently holds dear. According to *American Heritage*, to evaluate means "(1) to ascertain or fix the worth of, (2) to examine and judge; appraise; estimate." Thus, questions for evaluation of research stem from an assumption of worthwhileness and ask "Did it work?" and "How well?"

Clearly, evaluation can be research, but not all evaluation is research. To qualify it should have the same relationship to theory as any other research study. Cooley and Lohnes (1976) have applied John Dewey's famous theory of valuation (1939) to problems of evaluation in education, and we could similarly apply it to problems of evaluation in nursing. Later in this chapter, when we discuss problems for nursing research, we note the large proportion concerned with some aspect of program evaluation.

Q: What assumptions or values are related to the hypothesis you stated in response to the Q in the previous section?

Testing and Fitting

To what purpose have we discussed philosophy, theory, models, hypotheses, constructs, assumptions? Our purpose has been to illuminate the conceptual tools employed in the principal business of science, which is to answer questions about causes of natural phenomena. This is done indirectly by checking out measurements taken (data) to see how well they fit the hypothesized model. This process is much the same as that used by a tailor or dressmaker in making a suit or dress for someone who is absent. An absent model cannot be measured directly whether it is a human or an abstract hypothetical construct. Although the tailor may have gained considerable confidence from comparing the measurements of the garment with the specifications obtained from the client, he or she is not entirely comfortable until the customer has actually tried it on. The scientist, in contrast, must be content with testing for fit by comparing measurements taken with the "specs" of the model. Such testing for fit is one of the major aspects of statistical inference. We intend to teach you how to test the fit of a model to the reality represented by measurement data.

Testing for fit requires the existence of a theory mature enough that numerical measurements can be predicted from it. More often than otherwise in nursing research, we shall find that immature theory exists from which the general shape of the "garment" can be predicted but not the precise numerical specifications. In this case the data will have to be allowed to specify the precise fit of the theory to nature. We shall then want to speak of *fitting* rather than of *testing*. This is a puzzling distinction, and we hope we can be trusted to make it meaningful by examples used later in this text.

Induction and Deduction

Related to the distinction between fitting and testing is a conventional distinction between inductive and deductive logic. *Induction* is defined as reasoning from the particular to the general (an example of which is fitting the precise numerical values of a theory from the average values of measurements taken on many events). *Deduction* is defined as reasoning from the general to the particular (an example of which is predicting from a mature theory exactly what values measurements of specific events will take, then testing those predictions against the data).

Collecting data in nursing practice situations with the plan of producing theory about nursing practice is regarded as the inductive method in the Baconian tradition. The term *Baconian* refers to Francis Bacon, whose "new" (in 1605) system of discovering truth—new because it departed from the centuries-old system of formal logic stemming from Aristotle—was a fourfold process. Bacon's four steps called for empirical observations, analysis of observed data, inference resulting in hypotheses, and verification of hypotheses through further observation and experiment (Kiernan, 1965). We would point out that this method seems to have three steps that lead to fitting followed by a fourth step that leads to testing. It is a method in which the emphasis is on induction, but it does involve a deduction element in its fourth step. We are not told how one knows what empirical observations to make in the first step, but we suggest that these decisions will usually be based on deductions from previous systematic inquiry or theory. Thus there is a cycling between induction and deduction, and what Bacon did was to place a new emphasis on the importance of induction.

Beginning explicitly with a theory to be tested, on the other hand, is considered a deductive method. In practicing the art of research (and it is an art if it is the creative activity it is usually advertised to be), it is impossible to remain entirely in either the inductive or the deductive mode. The neat distinction between the two may be intellectually satisfying, but to cope with the disorderly movement of knowledge, an investigator will need to keep both her inductive and deductive wits about her, and not necessarily use them in a prescribed sequence. Both observation (induction) and deduction are necessary for any knowledge worth having, said Whitehead (1929).

PROBLEMS FOR NURSING

How can research contribute to the growth of knowledge for nursing? Individual studies can take one of three general approaches: replication, extension, or breakthrough. The beginner may as well forget about breakthrough. Although it is fun to read about serendipitous, accidental discoveries, most of the stories are romantic fiction. Medewar (1975) explored the fiction that Fleming discovered penicillin by accident, and came to the conclusion that he discovered it because he was looking for it. That is, he had known for several decades that such a substance existed. Although in the meantime he carried out other less important investigations, it could be said that he was never not on the lookout for penicillin. The discovery of such a substance had been an ambition of his for years.

Approaches to Nursing Studies

Practical types of studies, then, include replications of past studies in addition to extensions and branches of them. *Replication* is a word that implies exact duplication or reproduction, but not all replications are so exact, nor need they be. Some research writers have carefully classified the types and varieties of replications, but such activity seems unproductive. Reflection suggests that exact duplication of any study involving human beings is not possible. It is not necessary that a study be duplicated exactly, but rather that the replicating investigator carefully record the circumstances under which the new test of the previously warranted theoretical propositions is conducted. Actually, a demonstration that a proposition holds under new and different circumstances can serve to increase the generality of the proposition. Only through replication studies in varied settings will it be possible to ascertain the limits of applicability of any generalization. We should not expect sharply defined boundaries for generalization, such that a proposition holds exactly under certain circumstances and does not apply at all under all other circumstances. Rather, we are likely to see a shading off of validity from circumstances under which a proposition is highly valid, through circumstances under which it is decreasingly valid, to circumstances under which it has almost no validity. The researcher who assists in mapping the contours of validity of a proposition or a network of propositions in varying settings may not make a splashy new generalization available—may not make headlines, as it were—but she can make a solidly valuable contribution to the scientific knowledge of nursing.

We have smuggled into our text the notion that the validity of a proposition or a theoretical framework is not so much a "yes" or "no" issue as it is a matter of degree in relation to the set of circumstances under which the generalization is to be applied. This implies that we shall have to provide you with a method for estimating the degree of validity of a generalization for a particular setting as a numerical quantity that varies between zero and one, never quite reaching either of these logical limits. We do indeed intend to supply such a measure of validity, and we hope you will come to view it as one of the most useful things you learn from us. It is, however, a statistical device and must wait upon your learning some statistical theory.

The other practical type of study for novice researchers involves looking at some established knowledge about nursing and imagining some logical extension of that knowledge, then testing for empirical verification of the extension. Planning this type of study is not routine because it depends upon a flash of insight to point the way to a hypothesis. We do not know how human intelligence accomplishes these leaps of creative thought, so we cannot teach you how to do this. We do know that persons who are fully informed about a problem area are more likely to get such flashes than those who are amateurish in their involvement, and we know that possessing a reservoir of information about how problems have been solved in many fields of science seems to facilitate creative thinking in one's own field. We can also envy some people what is apparently a natural bent for creative thought. What seems certain is that only by trying to imagine extensions of knowledge does one have a chance of creating a new idea, so we recommend the habit of reading research about nursing with an attitude of wondering what else might be true in the light of what has been established. In our dialectic, replication studies are fitting studies while extension studies are testing studies. The former can always be done to good advantage to the profession; the latter can only be done after a bright idea has occurred that deserved to be tested.

Priorities for Research

Three areas for research have been identified as essential to the advancement of nursing and the improvement of health care (Jacox, 1978). They are:

   1   Studies to improve the care of people with existing health impairments
   2   Studies to develop preventive methods designed to reduce the occurrence of illness, complications, and disability
   3   Studies to identify vulnerable groups

The American Nurses' Association (ANA) Commission on Nursing Research identified these areas with the hope of influencing funding sources to make more support available for these kinds of studies as well as to influence nurses to conduct them. There can be no question that the three areas outlined by the commission are legitimate concerns for nurses. Stated as generally as they are, however, they could just as legitimately be areas of concern for almost any other kind of health worker, professional, or citizens' group. This lack of precision leads to two questions the nurse should ask herself concerning any specific problem in these areas. First, is some facet of the nurse's unique knowledge (language, philosophy, theory, or practice) being put to use in the investigation (Fox, 1964)? In other words, is the study really a nursing study? Second, is the proposed study exclusively a nursing study? As we and others have pointed out (Ackerman, 1976; Brown, 1974; Dickoff and James, 1975), research is typically a team enterprise, both in the here and now and in the context of scientific history, because through the review of literature we relate our problems to previously reported studies. Possibly another person or persons representing other disciplines ought to be sharing the responsibility for the proposed research.

Lindeman (1975) asked a panel of nurse administrators, clinicians, educators, and researchers to identify priorities for research directly concerned with patient welfare. The ranking that resulted from her Delphi survey is shown in Table 2-1. (*Delphi* refers to a method which requires repeated surveys of a selected panel of experts, providing them with a report on each survey, until finally the experts have reached a consensus on the issues or until a preset number of surveys have been completed. See Chapter 6.) Lindeman's priorities, like the ANA's, emphasize patient care as the core function of nursing. This appropriate emphasis may be compared with the lack of focus in nursing research in recent decades, when a great many studies, perhaps too many, had to do with psychological or sociological characteristics of nurses, with nursing education, and with the socialization of student nurses (inducting them into the

Table 2-1   Items Identified by Nursing Experts for Highest Research Priority because of Potential Impact on Patient Welfare

Rank	Research item
1	Determine valid and reliable indicators of quality care.
2	Identify interventions* that are most effective in reducing psychological stress of patients.
3	Find effective means to implement and evaluate change in practice.
4	Find means of enhancing the quality of life for the aged in institutions.
5	Develop a set of physical and psychological assessment procedures that provide information necessary for nursing intervention and improved patient care.
6	Identify interventions that are effective in reducing stress in patients who have a terminal disease.
7	Clarify the patients' rights and decision-making role in their own health care.
8	Study nursing interventions for the management of pain.
9	Define and evaluate an expanded role for the nurse in patient care.
10	Increase the application of research findings in practice.
11	Find means to educate the public to better use of health care systems.
12	Locate factors contributing to education for self-care of patients with chronic diseases.
13	Compare individualized care planning with standard practices in terms of impact on patients' recovery rates, understanding of illness, and self-care abilities.
14	Assess ways of improving hospital patient safety.
15	Determine effective interventions for reducing respiratory and circulatory complications in surgical patients.

*The term *interventions* in all priorities refers to nursing interventions exclusively.
Source: Lindeman, 1975.

culture of the profession). An appropriate emphasis on patient care issues in the planning of nursing research, however, must not be allowed to blind us to the continued need for research on recruitment, nursing education, career development and career patterns of nurses, and professional acculturation. All these areas which are of concern to nursing leadership must also be of concern to nursing researchers. Still, patient care is the heart of the matter.

Program Evaluation

Frequent use in all the lists of research topics of words such as evaluate, assess, improve, prevent, intervene suggests that a central problem in nursing today is program evaluation. *Improve* implies knowing that something would work; *prevent* implies avoiding a situation known to be bad or undesirable; *intervene* implies knowing how to turn around a deteriorating situation. None of these initiatives would be rational without prior evaluation results. In fact, an opportunity for evaluation research is automatically created whenever professional intelligence leads to the design of a new or modified program or treatment policy. That many programs and policies are accepted on trust or are not evaluated for shortage of resources just shows again what we all know, that we do not live in an ideal world. It may be that expanded understanding of evaluation methods will encourage nursing leaders to sponsor and participate in more evaluation studies. It is a pressing reality that the federal government is now reluctant to fund any innovative program which does not include some provision for evaluation. One of our ambitions for this text is that it provide you with some definite, useful paradigms for evaluation research.

Expanded List of Nursing Problems

We would expand the list of problem areas for nursing research to include:

1   Program evaluation
2   Any aspect of clinical practice
3   Administration of nursing
4   Education of nurses
5   Professional organizations and the "charter" of the profession
6   Career patterns of nurses (Astin and Myint, 1971)
7   Interpersonal relations with clients, families, other nurses, other professionals, other staff
8   Roles, functions, tasks of nurses
9   Psychological and sociological characteristics of nurses (Raskin et al., 1965; Roe, 1956)
10   History of nursing and biography of nurses

Remember that current events are history by the time they can be written down, and in that sense *all* research on nursing is historical. Wolfle (1964) asked why social scientists fail to study the processes and effects of major and foreseeable social changes more thoroughly *while those changes are happening*. The same could be asked of nurses.

In summary, this chapter has stressed that nurses ought to be intellectuals who are thoughtful about the beliefs and practices of their profession, and who know how those ideas and norms are rooted in scientific knowledge. Constructs have been shown to be the building blocks of theoretical propositions, which are then integrated into theoretical frameworks. Mature research tests the validity of extensions of knowledge phrased as hypotheses. Exploratory research fits established propositions in detail to new settings and determines their degree of validity. The interpretation of new empirical knowledge is always a challenge and a responsibility. Researchers have to be explicit about their assumptions and values as part of the act of interpretation. No rigid boundaries can be placed around nursing research, but the core problems are surely centered on patient care; beyond that, all aspects of nursing pose legitimate and important research problems. These include career issues, professional issues, human relations issues, and especially evaluation of nursing programs and policies.

Q: What is a patient care issue that could be the basis for a research project? Why is it important? What is already known about it? What needs to be discovered?

REFERENCES

Abdellah, Faye G., and Eugene Levine: *Better patient care through nursing research.* New York: Macmillan, 1965.

Ackerman, Winona B.: The place of research in the master's program. *Nursing Outlook*, 1976, *24*(12).

American heritage dictionary of the English language, William Morris (Ed.). New York: American Heritage and Houghton Mifflin, 1970.

Astin, Helen S., and Thelma Myint: Career development of young women during the post-high school years. *Journal of Counseling Psychology*, 1971, *18*(4).

Bakan, David: *On method: Toward a reconstruction of psychological investigation.* San Francisco: Jossey-Bass, 1969.

Beshers, James M.: Models and theory construction. *American Sociological Review*, 1957, *22*(32).

Brown, Esther Lucile: Keynote speech, American Nurses' Association Convention, 1974. Reported by M. Elizabeth Carnegie in an editorial: Toward more clinical research in nursing. *Nursing Research*, 1974, *23*(5).

Butterfield, Herbert: *The origins of modern science.* New York: Free Press, 1957.

Conant, James: *Science and common sense.* New Haven: Yale, 1951.

Cooley, William W., and Paul R. Lohnes: *Evaluation research in education.* New York: Irvington, 1976.

Dickoff, James, and Patricia James: Theory development in nursing. In Phyllis J. Verhonick (Ed.), *Nursing research I.* Boston: Little, Brown, 1975.

Fischer, David Hackett: *Historians' fallacies: Toward a logic of historical thought.* London: Routledge, 1971.

Fox, David J.: A proposed model for identifying research areas in nursing. *Nursing Research*, 1964, *13*(1).

Gillispie, Charles Coulton (Ed.): *Dictionary of scientific biography.* New York: Scribner, 1970.

Jacox, Ada: Interview. *The American Nurse*, 1978, *10*(5).

Kiernan, Thomas: *Who's who in the history of philosophy*. New York: Philosophical Library, 1965.

Lindeman, C. A.: Nursing practice research: What's it all about? *Journal of Nursing Administration*, 1975a, *5*(6).

————: Priorities in clinical nursing research. *Nursing Outlook*, 1975b, *23*(11), 693–698.

Linstone, Harold A., and Murray Turoff: *The Delphi method*. London: Addison-Wesley, 1975.

Living with dying. *Newsweek*, 1978, *91*(18).

Mason, Stephen F.: *A history of the sciences*. New York: Macmillan, 1956.

Medewar, Peter: Scientific method in science and medicine. *Perspectives of Biology and Medicine*, 1975, *18*.

Merton, Robert: Quoted in James M. Beshers, 1957.

Morton, Leslie T. (Ed.): *A medical bibliography*. London: Andre Deutsch, 1943.

Norris, Catherine M.: Delusions that trap nurses. *Nursing Outlook*, 1973, *21*(1).

Offutt, Andrew J.: Stand out! *Writer's Digest*, 1978, *58*(7).

Raskin, A., J. K. Boruchow, and R. Colob: Concept of task versus person orientation in nursing. *Journal of Applied Psychology*, 1965, *49*, 182–187.

Reynolds, Paul Davidson: *A primer in theory construction*. Indianapolis: Bobbs-Merrill, 1971.

Riehl, Joan P., and Callista Roy: *Conceptual models for nursing practice*. New York: Appleton-Century-Crofts, 1974.

Roe, Anne: *The psychology of occupations*. New York: Wiley, 1956.

Shils, Edward A.: Primordial, personal, sacred, and civil ties. *British Journal of Sociology*, 1957, *8*.

Sinclair, William J.: *Semmelweis: His life and his doctrine*. Manchester: University Press, 1909.

Suchman, Edward: *Evaluative research*. New York: Russell Sage, 1967.

Watson, James: *The double helix*. New York: Atheneum, 1968.

Watson, John: *The medical profession in ancient times*. New York: New York Academy of Medicine, 1856.

Webster's new twentieth century dictionary of the English language. Cleveland: World Publishing, 1968.

Whitehead, Alfred North: The organization of thought. In *The aims of education*. New York: Macmillan, 1929.

Wolfle, Dale: Lost opportunities. *Science*, 1964, *143*, 999.

Wulff, Henrik R.: *Rational diagnosis and treatment*. Philadelphia: Lippincott, 1976.

Chapter 3

How Can You Define a Research Problem?

PROFESSIONAL EXPERIENCE

Whitehead (1929) described science as a river with two sources, the practical and the theoretical. Both of these sources are disorderly, but the practical one, in particular, seems a turbulent flux of perceptions, sensations, emotions. How can the nurse arrest one small part of this flux and impose some order on it?

Personal Experience

Since defining a research problem is a creative act and creative acts have not been successfully dissected, we cannot describe exactly how to do it. But if the nurse begins to pay extra attention to the things that are not "right" in nursing practice and to jot down a list of them, she may soon have a considerable number of problems, some of which may be researchable. At least one psychologist (Bakan, 1969) has called for a more systematic place in the research enterprise for the thought and experience of the investigator. In the meantime, personal experience should neither be ignored nor used to the exclusion of the cumulative professional experience that is reported in nursing and related literatures. Sources of ideas for studies include:

1 Research priorities identified by nursing organizations as noted in Chapter 2.

2 Specific categories of clients. (In a nursing service organized around medical specialties, how is the patient who is admitted for eye surgery affected by being placed in a general surgical ward? If poverty is a culture, what are the implications for patient teaching?)

3 Characteristics of facilities in which nursing care is provided. (How do problems differ in hospitals, clinics, offices, homes, ambulatory, and industrial settings?)

4 Therapeutic procedures. (What is the best technique for encouraging deep breathing after surgery? Does it principally involve a person, a mechanism, preoperative teaching, the patient's personality, or a plan that integrates several variables?)

5 Consideration of "healthy" rather than ill persons. (How might the nursing process apply to subclinical problems such as pain, cold sores, stiff neck, menstrual cramps, flatulence?)

6 "Recommendations for further study" in published and unpublished reports, especially graduate student projects, theses, dissertations that are available in university libraries or described in compendiums such as *Dissertation Abstracts*. (These can be found in the reference section of university libraries; see also *International Nursing Review*, *Nursing Outlook*, *Nursing Research*, and other professional journals.)

7 Ideas developed through talking with other health workers or clients. (Ambulance drivers, physical therapists, nutritionists, dentists, physicians—all these and others may recognize problems with nursing implications.)

8 Challenges to what has been. (Can you imagine the reception co-workers may have given to the first introduction of the idea of a wet-towel "bath"? Yet any problem connected with patient comfort and cleanliness is certainly appropriate for a nurse to study.)

Feasibility of the Study

We mention feasibility at this point mostly to suggest postponing consideration of it. By feasible we mean, "capable of being utilized or dealt with successfully; suitable" (*American Heritage*). Thus the questions of available time, money, help, and interest all enter in. But the investigator should not allow her own fears or colleagues' premature questions of "How?" to dissuade her even before the problem or question for study has been fully conceptualized. In turn, when our advice is sought, we should remember principles of therapeutic interviewing and avoid dousing delicate not-quite-born ideas with cold water.

Some research writers have listed additional questions which we believe are unnecessarily discouraging. For example, "Is the problem important?" This strikes us as a crystal-ball kind of question. The history of science is replete with examples of inventive "crackpots" like Mendel, who frittered their time away according to the mores of their era, but whose judgment was suddenly vindicated when commercial interests or new fashions in scientific thought discovered them. If the researcher finds the problem within her interest and resources, someone else's opinion of its relative worth may be spurious. The wet-towel bath may have been such a problem. Surely if there was anything nurses already knew how to do, it was to give a bed bath. Was another method needed? Possibly so, since clients report that the newer method provides greater comfort than the traditional one.

Similarly, the question, "What need will be met by the solution of the problem?" also violates the first ideal of science—finding out for the sake of knowing. It may be within a funder's right to ask, but it seems to complicate matters unnecessarily at the point where a novice researcher is trying to achieve conceptual clarity about the problem and method. She may not care yet whether she is doing *basic research* (finding out for the sake of knowing) or *applied research* (finding out for the sake of solving a problem). Incidentally, in this book you will not find any attempt to classify research further than this distinction between basic and applied. We agree with Wolfle (1959) that a short list is sufficient. Most classifications violate the rules of scientific categorization (mutually exclusive, exhaustive) their authors purport to live by.

Additional discussion of feasibility appears in Chapter 5.

LITERATURE REVIEW

Once the general problem area has been selected, it becomes necessary to state the specific problem in a researchable way. Even before that, however, it is necessary to decide whether the problem is merely one the individual nurse is ignorant about, or one that genuinely requires further investigation. In other words, does the problem exist only in the gap between what is known and what is put into practice (Ketefian, 1975; Notter, 1973) or is new knowledge actually needed?

Preliminary Review

A preliminary review of literature can help the investigator to make this decision. For references to helpful literature, consult such indexes as *Cumulative Index to Nursing and Allied Health Literature, International Nursing Index, Index Medicus*, and perhaps also more general indexes such as *Reader's Guide*. (Balanced background articles appear surprisingly often in the better lay journals. Thus Norman Cousins' "Anatomy of an Illness" appeared in *Saturday Review* as well as *The New England Journal of Medicine*.) Notice how much has been written on your subject area in the past few years, and read enough articles to get an idea of what is known. How many articles should you read? Who can say? Obviously you will continue to search so long as you continue to find articles that are of sufficient use or interest to hold your attention. If a real demon has you, you may be caught for the rest of your life.

Possible sources of appropriate literature are:

National Library of Medicine sources including *International Nursing Index, Index Medicus*, and perhaps MEDLARS computer search
Cumulative Index to Nursing and Allied Health Literature

NHPIC (National Health Planning Information Center), Nursing Compo-
nent (P.O. Box 1600, Prince George's Plaza branch, Hyattsville, Maryland 20788,
telephone (301) 927-6410)
New York Times Index
Dissertation Abstracts
Reader's Guide to Periodical Literature
Research news and abstracts in nursing journals
References from appropriate articles
Specialized bibliographies compiled by librarians or others
Reference librarians
Colleagues
Government document collections

Whether or not you pause in your literature review, what you need most is a
one-sentence statement, preferably a question, that expresses what you intend
to find out. Krathwohl (1965) advocates drawing a mental circle around the
problem, thinking not only in terms of what it includes, but also what is clearly
outside it. This seems a good test. Can a colleague read your problem statement
and understand clearly what you intend to find out as well as what you will not be
concerned with?

Asking a colleague to read your problem statement suggests that you will
not be working totally alone on your research. Although we find it convenient to
speak of "the investigator," we have already noted that every study is, in one
sense or another, a team effort. Thus your team may include coinvestigators
from other fields or disciplines, or advisors who represent your funding source,
employing agency, or academic program. Every investigator needs at least one
person to turn to for reasonably objective and articulate suggestions concerning
omissions and errors in research activity as well as optimal organization and
clarity of the final report. One adviser may not be enough.

Theoretical Propositions

Either before, after, or during the writing of the one-sentence problem statement, it will be necessary to develop some background for the problem.
Guidelines for development of research proposals may variously call for rationale, purpose, objectives, or justification. Although these are not identical, all
state the purpose of the study, describe the hoped-for outcome, and answer the
question, "Why?" (see Table 1-2). The immediate candid answer may be that it is
required in a program of study, or that it will advance you professionally. Try
again: "Why *this* study rather than some other?"

The review of literature must finally clarify any lingering questions about the
conceptual framework of the study in the minds of both the investigator and her
readers. We have already noted that the review of literature is likely to be a
continuing process, and this is a paradox. How can a researcher identify a
conceptual or theoretical "skeleton" on which to hang the review of literature
before she has reviewed the literature? How can she know which literature to
review until she has identified the context of theory in which she intends to

review? Thus there may be considerable trial and error in the early phases of a literature review. We know of no way to avoid this. We have already taken the position that thought is economical when compared with other steps in the research process or with actual experience. The safest place to make false starts seems to be the library.

During the early stages of the literature review you will conceptualize your problem more clearly and refine your statement of it. Ellis (1973) said that asking the research question is the most important and most difficult task of any investigator. You should state and restate it until you are entirely sure it expresses your query in the most direct way possible.

It is likely that our readers may have a rather widely varying orientation to nursing theory. Some will have had one or more graduate or undergraduate courses in nursing theory, others will have knowledge absorbed from their professional reading or continuing education courses, while some may be unaware that the topic is now so sophisticated that a few nurses are making entire careers in the development of nursing theory. Those who lack this awareness should do some reading in books such as Riehl and Roy (1974) and Stevens (1979). Such reading may help to identify clues to theories you have already relied on. In Chapter 2 we pointed out the danger of clinging to feeble theory. To avoid that danger, look for theoretical implications in your earliest jottings. Such innocent-looking words as *family*, *need*, *role*, *crisis* implicate volumes of theory. Perhaps you have relied on more than one theory. If so, are they compatible? Which is the more comprehensive? Will you discard one completely or attempt to fit them together? Will you decide they are all inadequate and search for another existing theory or attempt to build a model of your own? In any event, the final construction must be logically unassailable, clearly stated, and accommodate appropriate research literature.

A fascinating historical example of a researcher who had an overabundance of theories to deal with was Semmelweis. In attempting to identify the cause of puerperal fever with certainty, he had to deal with in excess of 30 speculations put forth by more or less prestigious scientists and medical practitioners of the day. Sinclair (1909) said that Semmelweis devoted all his time to the study of the malady in the library, in the dead house, and at the bedside. Had the review-of-literature convention been better established and Semmelweis disliked writing a little less, he might have written a formal review, and the book he finally published would have been stronger for containing more literature citations and less personal emotion. Table 3-1 gives a trail of ideas Semmelweis might ideally have used in a review of literature that could have saved time, harassment, and even patients' lives and his very sanity.

Shils (1957) pointed out that the growth of knowledge is a disorderly movement, full of instances of things known but overlooked, unexpected emergencies, and rediscoveries of long-known facts which in the time of their original discovery had no fitting articulation. Although a single research project is often compared to a link in a chain, "chain" is not an adequate analogy. The scientific endeavor is not a neat, sequential, longitudinally connected series of indepen-

**Table 3-1   Trail of Ideas for a Post Hoc Review of Related Literature for
Semmelweis' *Aetologie***

ca. 350 B.C.	Aristotle proposed the idea of spontaneous generation.
1546	Fracastoro put forth a germ theory of infection, recognized typhus and the contagiousness of tuberculosis.
1774	Thomas Kirkland wrote a treatise on puerperal fever (London).
1795	Alexander Gordon published a paper on the epidemic of puerperal fever in Aberdeen, Scotland.
1822	Marie Humbert Bernard Gaspard studied pyemia by injecting putrid fluids (pus, vaccine, lymph, blood, bile, urine, saliva, carbonic acid, sulfuretted hydrogen) into dogs, sheep, foxes, and pigs.
1835–1836	Agostino Bassi demonstrated that parasites cause a disease of silkworms.
1836	Theodor Schwann concluded that alcoholic fermentation is the work of a live organism.
1838	Pierre Francois Olive Bayer inoculated a donkey with pus from a patient with glanders, thus transferring the infection.
1840	Friedrich Gustav Jacob Henle showed that contagia and miasma could not be separated because carriers of disease were living materials that colonized the host body.

Source: Dictionary of scientific biography, and Leslie T. Morton (Ed.), *A medical bibliography*. London: Andre Deutsch, 1943 and 1970.

dent links. It is more like a piece of chain mail—that flexible armor composed of overlapping loops of chain, possibly connected in several directions—but in our analogy a ragged piece full of holes, raw edges, and loose ends (Ackerman, 1976). A breakthrough, once it occurs, can invariably be traced backward, suggesting that it was an idea whose time had almost come and was waiting only for a brilliant mind or minds to bring it to its culmination.

The importance of locating even the simplest of problems within an adequate framework probably cannot be overemphasized. Sociologists have discussed "kindergarten" theories that are too weak and immature to hold the weight that is imposed on them (Parsons, 1966; Znaniecki, 1954). This happened quite obviously two or three decades ago with regard to nursing education. There were numerous studies of student nurse attrition based only on the personalities of students, with no attention to admission practices, the climate of the school, how the withdrawal rates compared with those of females in other professional schools or other programs of similar duration, whether the dropouts were failures or whether they went on to greater satisfaction and success in better accord with their personal goals. As Dorothy Canfield Fisher remarked, one idea can be worth a million facts. We cannot afford to connect ideas hastily or unmindfully, thus risking short-circuiting or overlooking brilliant possibilities.

Once the review of literature has set the problem in an ample context, it is time to consider your expectations concerning the answer to the research question. If you were including your question in a classroom test, you would write the answer key before obtaining the students' answers. In much the same fashion you will state your expectations, including details of how much, how many, in what direction, so that the answers can be checked later against this expectation.

Research outcomes differ from the test analogy in that if they do not match, it will be the questioner who is wrong, rather than the world "out there." The expectations you have written, if sufficiently specific to be compared later with the actual data, are hypotheses. If they are more general, concerning areas where you will look for clues, they can only be called subproblems or subquestions, rather than hypotheses.

Reading the Literature

You have a piece of literature in hand. What do you do with it? This is not a facetious question. Some reviewers, realizing they cannot fully analyze each report they locate on the spot, think first of getting a photocopy which can be read later at home. Other reviewers laboriously note 12 or 15 points of analysis for each article. We think that both these "just in case" approaches waste time and effort. Adler and Van Doren (1972) give advice they say is applicable to anything worth reading. They describe four levels of reading, one of which they call *inspectional*. It is characterized by a process of systematic skimming, or prereading, in which the reader pays close attention to the title page, preface, table of contents, index, publisher's blurb, pivotal chapters or paragraphs, epilogue (summary), and final pages (paragraphs). They speak mostly of books, but the same approach is effective for briefer materials. Articles sometimes include abstracts, specially illustrated quotes or other blurbs (rather than table of contents or index) to which the principles apply. This process of inspectional reading can be accomplished in a short time and can help to identify those special resources you intend to return to and read more analytically.

Adler and Van Doren also have some suggestions for analytical reading. The various kinds of reading necessary to produce an adequate review of literature should not be slighted. Carnegie (1975) has admonished readers about the frequency with which articles lacking adequate reviews of literature are submitted for possible publication in *Nursing Research*. Experience also suggests that reviews are often inadequate in planning for the solution of curriculum, administrative, and other practice problems. Thus the need to produce adequate reviews can hardly be overemphasized for any nurse, regardless of her research orientation.

We hasten to add other approaches to the review, some form of which are probably necessary. Making bibliography cards for resources you want to cite or to relocate later is one approach. Ideally, each card lists author, title, name, and date of publication in the same form they might be listed for the reference section at the back of your research report. This form should be established early and followed meticulously. Probably inexperienced writers will insist on learning some things from experience, just as we did and do. But remember that we told you how wise it is to adhere closely to your stylebook from the earliest moment.

Some writers apparently prefer notebooks to cards, and we ourselves use a combination. For detailed discussions of all aspects of organizing your reading and writing see Barzun and Graff (1970).

It is our prejudice that overusing the photocopy method can destroy its effectiveness. Since copies cannot help until they have been run through one's thought processes, those who carry home piles of photocopies may simply be postponing their troubles. Although it is sometimes helpful to have a photocopy which you can read, re-read, underline, and return to as often as necessary, we think copying should only follow inspectional reading. A second approach to analytical reading is to take notes. We think each person will develop a unique system, and that the only iron-clad rule in note taking is to write on one side of the paper only. This permits flexibility such as cutting the notes apart, filing them according to the portion of your report in which you expect to use them, clipping them together with similar ideas from other sources, and so on. After all, the review is a story of ideas and their testing, not of dates or researchers.

Suppose that some literature has been reviewed and a brief background of the study has been written. Reviewing continues, but the researcher does not feel ready to write an adequate review of related literature. Probably she should continue writing, anyway. The best way to know what you are going to say in an adequate review may be to start saying it. What is wanted is not a mere catalog listing of all the investigations that have been carried out, but an organized and congruent account of articulated ideas that have been affirmed or refuted. In other words, organize what is known and not known about your special problem. Adequate citations must be provided, but the ideas are of more concern than names of investigators. It is better to avoid a weak chronological approach such as "In 1965, Jones found . . ., then in 1970 Smith found . . . and in 1973. . . ." Organizers such as "Among those who refuted the idea of . . ." can be of benefit.

A neatly organized presentation is not likely to happen on the first attempt. Abortive attempts, however, can move the writer toward a final, polished presentation and can contribute meanwhile to efficient reading. The reviewer progresses with the review by prodigious reading and thinking, sifting, sorting, integrating, summarizing, synthesizing, and relating to existing theory.

Q: In response to the Q in Chapter 2 you stated a theoretical proposition. Conduct a library search for references bearing on this proposition and report what you find and how you find it.

Q: Find a literature review in a nursing book, journal, or thesis or dissertation, and make a report on the references employed. Check in your library to see which of the references are available locally.

REFERENCES

Ackerman, Winona B.: The place of research in the master's program. *Nursing Outlook*, 1976, *24*(12).

Adler, Mortimer J., and Charles Van Doren: *How to read a book*. New York: Simon and Schuster, 1972.

Bakan, David: *On method: Toward a reconstruction of psychological investigation*. San Francisco: Jossey-Bass, 1969.

Barzun, Jacques, and Henry F. Graff: *The modern researcher*. New York: Harcourt Brace Jovanovich, 1957 and 1970.

Carnegie, M. Elizabeth: A serious omission. Editorial in *Nursing Research*, 1975, *24* (March–April), 83.

Cousins, Norman: Anatomy of an illness. *Saturday Review*, 1977 (May 28).

Ellis, Rosemary: Asking the research question. In *Issues in research*, Report of the American Nurses' Association Council of Nurse Researchers Program Meeting, August 1973.

Fisher, Dorothy Canfield: Quoted by Mary R. Parkman in *High adventurers*. New York: Century, 1920.

Ketefian, Shake: Application of selected nursing research findings into nursing practice. *Nursing Research*, 1975, *24*, 89–92.

Krathwohl, David R.: *How to prepare a research proposal*. Syracuse, N.Y.: Syracuse University, 1965.

Notter, Lucille E.: The editor's report. *Nursing Research*, 1973, *22*, 3.

Parsons, Talcott: *Societies*. Englewood Cliffs, N.J.: Prentice-Hall, 1966.

Riehl, Joan P., and Callista Roy: *Conceptual models for nursing practice*. New York: Appleton-Century-Crofts, 1974.

Shils, Edward A.: Primordial, personal, sacred, and civil ties. *British Journal of Sociology*, 1957, *8*, 130–145.

Sinclair, William J.: *Semmelweis: His life and his doctrine*. Manchester: University Press, 1909.

Stevens, Barbara J.: *Nursing theory*. Boston: Little, Brown, 1979.

Whitehead, Alfred North: The organization of thought. In *The aims of education*. New York: Macmillan, 1929.

Wolfle, Dale: Taxonomy of research. *Science*, 1959, *130*, 1163.

Znaniecki, Florian: Basic problems of contemporary society. *American Sociological Review*, 1954, *19*(5).

Chapter 4

How Is Research Funded?

Viewing research as a team effort is consistent with the funding situation, too, in which funders are experts at distributing money according to their own criteria, and some members of the research team are so specialized in their money-obtaining efforts that they are willing to call themselves grantsmen. This, in turn, has given rise to a group of specialists who go about teaching would-be grant recipients the secrets of obtaining grants. Happily, though, most of these secrets are available at the cost of patient effort.

WHO FUNDS

Who are the givers? Funders can be classified in a variety of ways: by whether they distribute public or private money, by the size of their annual giving, by the time of year in which they accept proposals, by the kinds of projects they fund and how actively they solicit proposals, and so on. Perhaps the most immediately useful classification for the first-time seeker of funds should be in terms of whom the funder is trying to help. Thus, the people most interested in trying to help you, the beginning researcher, may be fairly near to you. Look first close to home where there may be modest funds available through educational, honor, alumni, and service organizations, local branches of professional associations, local government, private foundations concerned with the local area, or local chapters of volunteer agencies.

If there is no money available from these sources, there ought to be. If we believe in the research effort, we can aid it not only by doing, reporting, disseminating, or using research, but also by underwriting it—that is, by encouraging organizations to which we belong to make small grants available to deserving applicants and by doing our share in reviewing grant applications from an informed point of view. When you feel ready, you may want to write to granters who are listed in the *Federal Register* and offer yourself as a field reader for proposals they receive. From the perspective of cultivating research support, then, we do a kind of professional service when we ask for research funds, because we call attention to the need and cause organizations to deliberate concerning their response.

The more local your search, the less likely that there is an organized list of possible sources. Even a large university which regularly prints news about research funding may overlook sources that make small grants of less than $2000 or $3000. Ultimately, dissemination of research news at a university is probably aimed at how much money can be brought into the university, not how many researchers can be helped. Yet, $200 or $300 may mean the difference between getting started and not getting started on a first exploratory project. Funders, like universities, may prefer to deal in larger sums. The difficulty is not merely that funders have no feeling for "small potatoes." It may cost the funder as much to give away $350 as $35,000. Thus, if the funder gives $3500 to each of 10 recipients, it may cost 10 times as much as giving $35,000 to 1 recipient. As individuals, we customarily judge the charitable causes to which we give according to how much of their money goes into direct services and research support, and how little into administrative costs. As givers to the funders, we in effect have told them to favor fund-seekers who ask for a lot rather than a little. Thus, we share in funding concerns in several ways and therefore have a stake in seeing to it that research funds are used properly.

An additional reason for the modest researcher to look close to home is that a request for funding must put the project activity into context for the funding agency. The farther away this agency is, the more elaborate the proposal must be in terms of describing your geographic area and community, your agency, and the cooperation and support you can count on. For a small project, a proposal to strangers can easily become too costly in terms of effort to be practical.

For that matter, any proposal for any size project to any funder involves the risk of an investment out of proportion to the return, particularly since more proposals are rejected than are funded. Thus, fund seeking may only be practical if it is conceived of as an effort to learn a process that will be of future use.

WHERE TO APPLY

The following is a list of resources the energetic seeker can use in the pursuit of funds.

General sources include:

White, Virginia P.: *Grants: How to find out about them and what to do next*. New York: Plenum, 1975.

The Grantsmanship Center News, The Grantsmanship Center, 1015 West Olympic Boulevard, Los Angeles, California 90015, $15 per year (six issues).

For information about federal grants see:

Catalog of Federal Domestic Assistance, Office of Management and Budget (published annually, updated periodically).

Federal Register, U.S. General Services Administration (published weekdays).

These two resources can be used to augment each other. The *Catalog*, since it is published annually, gets out of date between publications. The *Register* should be followed for up-to-date information about rules, regulations, and final decisions concerning programs listed in the *Catalog*. Both publications are available from the Government Printing Office, Washington, D.C. 20402 (*Catalog*, $18; *Federal Register*, $50 per year), and from libraries in agencies, universities, and regional government document repositories.

Any librarian should be able to help locate these resources on the shelves of the home library or some other one. If your institution has a research office, be sure to seek advice there, too.

For information about private foundations see:

About Foundations, published by The Foundation Center, available from Columbia University Press, 136 S. Broadway, Irvington-on-Hudson, New York 10533, $3. A guide to starting a search for grants, describes sources of information available in The Foundation Center's national and regional collections.

Foundation Directory, compiled quadrennially by The Foundation Center, available from Columbia University Press (above), $35 per year with four semi-annual supplements. This widely distributed directory lists those nonprofit, nongovernmental foundations which make grants of at least $50,000 per year or have assets of at least $1 million. Each foundation listing includes name and address, purpose, activities, assets, limitations, expenditures, and names of donor, officers, trustees, and directors of the foundation. Entries are cross-indexed by field of interest, names of donors, trustees, and administrators. The current edition lists 2533 foundations. The supplements list foundations by state, for which recent fiscal data are available on microfiche. (Each fiche costs $3 and can be ordered from the Center's New York office, address as listed above.)

Foundation Center Sourcebook, published by The Foundation Center, available from Columbia University Press, 1975–1976, vols. I and II, $65 per volume. Includes national and major regional foundations with assets of $10 million or more. Lists all grants made in year of record plus statements of policies, application procedures, and recent fiscal data.

Foundation News, published bimonthly by The Council on Foundations, 888 7th Avenue, New York, New York 10019, $20 per year.

Foundation Grants Index, compiled annually by The Foundation Center, available from Columbia University Press, $15. An annual index of grants listed in the *Foundation News* insert. Lists current grants of at least $5000. Lists foundations alphabetically by state and cross-indexes by recipient name and subject.

Foundation Center materials are available in at least one major library in at least 40 states.

HOW TO WRITE THE REQUEST FOR FUNDS

The onerous burden on reviewers of reading numerous extensive proposals destined for nonfunding has led to the increased use of preproposals and abstracts of proposals (Malasanos, 1976). In the Appendix at the end of this chapter we provide an example of one approach that proposal writers have used in order to achieve clarity and to be certain that they have stated their intentions. As previously suggested, short digests may function either as a way to organize a longer narrative or as an abstract of an already completed document. Either way, they may aid in the achievement of clarity and efficient use of time. For the proposer, however, these briefer documents may save little except postage. If the proposer intends to seek funds until she finds them, she must sooner or later write a full-scale proposal. The sooner the better, since it is often more difficult to write a clear, accurate, persuasive document in a strictly limited number of words, paragraphs, or pages than in a longer form. Probably the best way to produce an adequate short proposal is, as the word suggests, to abstract it from a more complete document.

This more complete document will vary according to the guidelines of the prospective funder or preferences of academic or other advisers, but certain elements are generally included:

1   Introduction: the statement of the problem against the background of review of relevant literature and theory
2   Specific aims: statement of the objectives including hypothesis(es) to be tested or the subquestions to be explored
3   Methods of procedure: specification of population, sampling, design, instrumentation, data collection and analysis
4   Justification: a summary of the significance of the work to knowledge in general and the funding agency in particular; the method of disseminating information or applying results
5   Facilities available, collaboration, appendix: buildings, equipment, personnel, budget, time schedule, human subjects clearance

If the funder provides instructions or application keys, they should be followed closely. According to Dr. Fearn, the U.S. Office of Education receives many proposals that clearly do not meet the criteria outlined by the agency, as though the requester had not read the criteria set forth. She suggests that it is useless to try to force a proposal that clearly does not fit. If it does fit, then it may be helpful to use headings or number keys that show plainly which criterion a specific section of the proposal addresses. (See the Appendix, The New York Education Department Mini-Proposal from Cantalician Center at the end of this chapter.) Such keys may prevent harried reviewers from overlooking something important. Gortner (1971) emphasized that the proposal should be pre-reviewed by one or more respected colleagues whose research experience has been in the proposed subject area or who are particularly knowledgeable about design and methods. Again, your local research office may be helpful. It is also expected and perhaps necessary to become personally acquainted with funders at professional conferences, or through visits and phone calls. This is not for the purpose of attempting to exert influence, but to obtain all the information, hints, clarification, news about changes and about other research that may help you to prepare a forward-looking document. It is acceptable to ask a proposed funder for a preliminary review of an early draft, although it will not always be provided.

In the funding proposal it seems wise to avoid unexplained jargon. In general, we agree with Carlyle that it would be "Wholly a blessed time: when jargon might abate . . . and genuine speech begin." (Then all of us—even the sporadic reader—could read the sports pages when we felt like it!) The special reason for a lucid, jargon-free presentation is to avoid turning off reviewers who are likely to be highly literate, but may be uninformed about certain professional slang. It may be wise, however, to use some of the same language the reviewing agency has used in its guidelines. The purpose here is not to be obsequious, but simply to avoid introducing doubt or confusion. Incidentally, you are not "writing a grant." You may be writing a grant proposal, funding proposal, or request for funds.

It will have been a good idea if, in scouting the local scene, the applicant has asked potential sources if they know of other interested persons. This may have led to partnerships or cooperative arrangements in either seeking or granting funds. One of the criteria that agencies use is whether the researcher is clearly qualified to carry out the investigation. Their judgment is made principally on the applicant's research experience. Thus, a team with at least one prestigious name may be the only sensible arrangement for obtaining funding.

As the trail leads onward, the seeker may be helped by knowing that, in general, private foundations are more innovative and flexible than government agencies (Rockefeller, 1973), even though government agencies fund by far the largest proportion (probably more than 90 percent) of research. That is, private foundations consciously attempt to support new ideas and projects in which federal or other government agencies are not yet involved.

A search for funds carried to this point will have revealed the importance of the broad definition of research given previously. A large proportion of available funds are not for research in the strict, narrow sense of the word. This is recognized in the use of the phrase *research and development*. Frequently, the only research connection is the evaluation of a program.

If you have responded to a request for funding proposals (RFP) and failed to obtain funding, you may want to ask why. If your proposal was not recommended for funding or was not funded, federal funding agencies are obligated to explain why not. Some private agencies will also provide this information, although they are under no obligation to do so.

Q: Ask around your faculty to borrow a research funding proposal, and write a brief analysis of it. Would you have funded it? Why?

REFERENCES

Carnegie, M. Elizabeth: Financial assistance for nursing research—Past and present. *Nursing Research*, 1975, *24*(3), 163.

Eaves, G. N.: Who reads your project grant application at the National Institutes of Health? *Federation Proceedings*, 1972, *31* (January–February), 2–9.

Gortner, Susan: Research grant applications: What they are not and should be. *Nursing Research*, 1971, *20*(4), 292–295.

Krathwohl, David R.: *How to prepare a research proposal*. Syracuse, N.Y.: Syracuse University, 1965.

Malasanos, L. J.: Research Q and A: What is the preproposal? *Nursing Research*, 1976, *25*(3), 223–224.

Rockefeller, Jeannette E.: Philanthrophy and research today. In *Issues in research*. Selected papers from the American Nurses' Association Council of Nurse Researchers, 1973.

APPENDIX: Example of a Funding Proposal
Submitted to the New York State Education
Department (Note the use of a nurse consultant and the
numbers directing the reviewer to key sections of the
proposal.)

The University of The State of New York
THE STATE EDUCATION DEPARTMENT
Division of ESC General Program Planning
Albany, New York 12234

NYSED Mini-Project Program Application
1977–1978

Name of applicant (school or school dist.) _____Cantalician Center for Learning_____
Address _____3233 Main Street—Buffalo, New York 14214_____
Title of project _____Cardiovascular Fitness for the Severely Mentally Retarded_____
   No. of students to be involved: K-6 __25__ 7-12 __25__ Public ___ Nonpublic __X__
   Check one: Rural _____ Suburban _____ Urban ____X____
Project dates: From _____September 1, 1977_____ to _____June 30, 1978_____
                                    Final reports due June 30, 1978
Person preparing proposal __Susan Zippiroli__ Title _____Curriculum Coordinator_____
Address __3233 Main Street—Buffalo, New York 14214__ Telephone __(716)833-5353__
Building administrator __Sister Raphael Marie, CSSF__ Title __Executive Director__
_____January 13, 1977_____   _____
               Date   Signature, chief school administrator
If applicant is other than a public school:
_____   _____
               Date   Signature, chief public school officer

Submit __8__ copies of this proposal to your regional or city OEP representative by January
14, 1977. Do *not* submit directly to State Education Department.

                                          Tom Maloney
                                          School 72
             SEND TO: 71 Lorraine Avenue
                                     Buffalo, New York 14220

Each proposal must complete the following sections:

Limit	1 Statement of need	6 Budget page
to	2 Description of problem	
two	3 Statement of objectives	
pages	4 Solution proposed (including activities)	
	5 Evaluation design strategy	

Mini-Project Program Application—1977–1978

1 STATEMENT OF NEED. Describe the gap between the present state and the desired state. The local educational need for this project should be substantiated.

To our knowledge, no one knows much about the cardiovascular fitness of the severely mentally retarded. At the Cantalician Center for Learning, however, we do know that a large number of our students are overweight and lead very sedentary lives. Consequently, we think it is very likely that many are already characterized by less than optimal cardiovascular conditions and that even more are headed that way. If they are, we have no practical, low-risk program in which we can intervene and change this pattern. We believe that the following are needed:

1 Better knowledge of the cardiovascular condition of our population
2 An effective, practical, low-risk program that will provide the foundations for long-term cardiovascular health

2 DESCRIPTION OF PROBLEM. Describe the particular problem which this project will attempt to solve. (Please note that the problem should be capable of being solved in 1 year.)

This project addresses two related problems: (1) What is the cardiovascular status of our severely mentally retarded population? and (2) Will a practical, low-risk cardiovascular training program, adapted to the individual needs of a severely mentally retarded population, result in enhanced cardiovascular fitness?

The first problem involves testing each student at the center for *resting heart pulse rate* and for *maximal attainable heart rate* and then comparing various age and sex groups.

The second involves planning an adapted cardiovascular training program for the severely mentally retarded, training teachers how to use the program, implementing it with a cross section of our center's population, and studying both its processes and results.

3 STATEMENT OF OBJECTIVES. Who, what, when, how described in specific, behavioral terms.

(1) A measure of resting heart pulse rate and of maximal attainable heart rate will be recorded for each student at the center. Averages for given age and sex groups will be determined and compared to normative data. (2) Students' postprogram mean resting heart pulse rate will be significantly *lower* than their preprogram mean resting heart pulse rate. (3) At the program's conclusion a significantly greater number of students will fall within the 70 to 85 percent maximal attainable heart rate range than was true at the program's beginning. (4) Students will develop a liking for the program as evidenced by initiating the activity, persisting in the exercises, and expressing a willingness to participate. (5) Program carryover at home will be evidenced by an increase in the number of days systematic exercise takes place at home and by an increase in the length of exercise periods taking place at home.

4 SOLUTION PROPOSED.   Include the activities you will conduct to satisfy the
stated objectives. Be sure to justify items in the budget and vice versa.

(1) All students involved in the program will undergo a physical examination before
starting the program to guarantee their health. (2) A resting heart pulse rate and a
maximal attainable pulse rate will be recorded for all students at the center. These will
be done under the direction of a consultant from the Buffalo Cardiology Associates.
This information will be charted according to age and sex groupings. (3) The five
teachers involved in the program will attend a workshop given by a cardiologist and a
registered nurse. They will explain the physical aspects of such a program. (4) The five
teachers will set up a schedule whereby the 50 students in the program will receive the
exercise program 45 minutes a day, 3 days per week. (5) The activities will include
warming up, exercise, and cooling down. The exercises may include walking, jogging,
running, and jumping rope. (6) On a regular basis, evaluations will be made and the
results charted. The teachers will meet each month to compare results and to plan and
modify the program. (7) Three workshops with the parents, teachers, and consultants
will be held. These will take the form of instruction, demonstration, and explanation of
the importance of carryover. The parents will be asked to chart the number of times the
students exercise at home. (8) Posttesting will be done at the end of the year.

5 EVALUATION DESIGN.   Indicate what evaluative measures you will use to determine how successfully the stated objectives will be met. List standard tests to be
used, if any, or indicate how you plan to develop your own evaluative instrument.
Provision should be made for the collection of baseline data.

Objective 1: Pre-post measures on all students will be taken. Evidence of this will be
signed statements by the center's director and by the evaluator. Filed copies of the
results will be available on request. *Objective 2:* A pre-post test of significance will be
performed using a correlated t with alpha set at .05. *Objective 3:* A simple chi-square
test of differences will be performed with alpha set at .05. *Objective 4:* Because the
students at the Cantalician Center are severely mentally retarded, we cannot rely on
their ability to state whether or not they like the program. Therefore we will chart, for
each session, the students' positive participation. For the purposes of the grant, we will
define positive participation as the willingness to exercise and persistence in the
exercise until the end of the session. The positive participation will be summarized
graphically, and success will be indicated by an ascending linear trend. *Objective 5:*
Parents will be asked to keep records of the amount of systematic exercise undertaken
at home. The frequency and length of exercise over the program will be summarized
graphically with its criterion of success being an ascending linear trend. Additional pre-
post group comparisons will be made and reported.

NYSED Mini-Project Program Budget—1977–1978

Title of project ___Cardiovascular Fitness for the Severely Mentally Retarded___ Project no. ___**6**___

Mailing address ___ Telephone ___(716)833-5353___

Project dates ___September 1, 1977___ to ___June 30, 1978___ LEA (City or BOCES) ___Cantalician center___ Region or city ___Buffalo___

Activity code no.	Item	Quantity/hours/ rates	Amount budgeted, $	Purchase order no.
Professional salaries: 210	Teacher/Coordinator	60 hours @ $9.50/hour	570.00	
	Teachers (4)	51 hours/ea @ $7.50/hour	1530.00	
			2100.00	
Nonprofessional salaries: 215				
Other expenses: 240.d	5 Stop watches	Est. $35/ea	175.00	
	Paper supplies for parents and teachers for charting, etc.		50.00	
Travel: 250.2				
Contracted services: 250.3	Consultant—Cardiologist	2 full days @ $100/day	200.00	
	Consultant—Registered nurse	8½ days @ $50/day	425.00	
Equipment rental: 260.3				
Fringe benefits: 310	F.I.C.A. @ 5.85% of Cat. 210 ($2,100 = $122.85)		122.85	
Minor remodeling: 1220.3				
Equipment purchase: 1230				
Total			3072.85	

(Signature here indicates approval)

Title and signature of applicant ___ Curriculum coord.,___ Date ___ January 13, 1977___

Signature of applicant's chief school officer ___ Date ___

Signature of public school's chief school officer (if nonpublic applicant) ___ Date ___ January 13, 1977___

Signature of district superintendent (BOCES) ___ Date ___

or Superintendent (city) ___ Date ___

(Signature after typewritten name, please)

43

Florence Nightingale

In Victorian England there grew and flourished an amazing woman who has long been recognized as nursing's greatest heroine, but who has yet to be fully recognized for her pioneering greatness in two other roles, as social scientist and as feminist. We are particularly interested in her innovative, visionary endeavors to demonstrate the importance of social statistics throughout the public and parliamentary debates on pressing social issues of her times.

Florence Nightingale (1820–1910) was a failure according to the standards of the homebound women of her day, the standards of present-day career women, and her own standards of perfection. In addition, she made her parents feel like failures. They had raised a brilliant, graceful, pretty daughter who looked to the outside world much like any other old maid in an era when young women were doomed to the awful fate of waiting helplessly, sometimes through an entire lifetime, for an offer of marriage that might never come. In spite of these attitudes, she returned from the Crimean War to find herself the most admired Englishwoman of the day, more popular than the Queen herself. In 1856, Charles Darwin exclaimed, "What woman ever took so high a position as she does now!" (Darwin, 1915). At the time of her christening, Florence was as peculiar a first name for a girl as her sister's name of Parthenope. It was because of Florence Nightingale herself that the name became a standard one. Among the first to use it were Dr. Samuel Gridley Howe and his wife, Julia Ward, who were so impressed by the young Miss Nightingale that they named their firstborn after her a decade before the Crimean War (Richards, 1935).

Her fame continues and is sufficiently well deserved, although not only for the reasons that have long been so well known. Most people think only of her war service and of the two appellations "angel of mercy" and "the lady with the lamp." The lady with the lamp was the supervisor of 4 miles of beds, working early and late with her lamp, the mover of others, the rational and efficient administrator, relying on organizational systems. The angel of mercy, on the other hand, gave personal, direct care to individuals, sharing in suffering even unto death, and was expressive rather than instrumental, emphasizing personalities rather than organizational systems. Florence Nightingale was both, but she was also a pioneering social statistician.

During her life she exchanged letters and maintained personal contact with a wide circle of people, not the least of whom were her own relatives in a large clan of cultivated, wealthy, socially prominent, and active people. These included both men and women, but the women were only too often "ladies" like her own mother and sister, who had frequent fits of fainting and hysterics and to whom entertainment was the chief business of life. Their views of the maverick Florence were colored by her refusal to reinforce their affected behavior. One young woman asked of another in a letter, "Seriously, don't you think Flo is a bit cracked?" (Woodham-Smith, 1952).

Quite a contrasting set of assessments were provided by the men who worked and socialized with her. Even the suggestion that she had dozens of male friends who could properly be called *her* friends rather than merely friends of male relatives is sufficient to bring into question the ascetic, hermetic view of Florence Nightingale. Above all, she was subject to an excess of human passion and feeling that she was not always able to control. She went to almost every extreme of feeling, narrowly escaping suicide and insanity, and wavering for years before making a final decision not to marry. Her life story could be viewed as an example of the problem of integrating strong feelings and outstanding intelligence through a long life span. She herself asked, in her *Cassandra*, "Why have women passion, intellect and moral activity—these three—and a place in society where no one of these can be exercised?" (Housman, n.d.).

During her childhood, she knew two men who were to have a significant effect on her future. One was her nephew Shore, heir to both the Nightingale estates because Florence had no brother. Shore was only a few days old when she, at age 11, began taking care of him. The enormous family clan of nearly two dozen aunts and uncles and 27 first cousins recognized the special devotion between Flo and Shore, and their relationship was so important for so many years that she can hardly be said to have been childless. When she wrote "Minding Baby" in *Notes on Nursing*, she must have included much that she learned from caring for Shore. As he grew up, Shore returned often for visits and once to be nursed by Flo when he had measles. Decades later, in 1873, when she temporarily gave up her own work to look after her failing and nearly blind mother and to settle the painful details centering around her father's death, Florence wrote that the affection she had lavished on Shore was a thousandfold repaid during this time, and that his good sense and consideration were her comfort.

The first adult male in Flo's life, of course, was her father. He was rich, cultivated, at leisure. He loved oddities and jokes, and himself taught his two daughters Greek, Latin, German, French, Italian, philosophy, and history. They learned music and drawing from a governess (Woodham-Smith, 1951, p. 13). Woodham-Smith said that Flo and her father were deeply in sympathy, that both had the same regard for accuracy, the same cast of mind at once humorous and gloomy, and the same passion for abstract speculation. Though he did not come to it easily, her father eventually provided her with an annual allowance of £500 so that she could live independently of the family. She proved perennially unable to live within this allowance, probably because she did not consider it important to do so, since she was able enough to administer institutions within their budgets. At any rate, her father rescued her again and again, and finally bought a permanent home for her. They remained close friends for as long as he lived, frequently engaging in discussions of metaphysics. After Mr. Nightingale's death, Richard Monckton Milnes wrote to her: "His reverent love for you was inexpressibly touching" (Woodham-Smith, 1951, p. 332).

That Richard Monckton Milnes should still have been writing to her is a circumstance almost beyond the grasp of modern Americans. He had proposed marriage when they were both young adults, and had waited 9 years before accepting her refusal as final. He was no colorless Milquetoast, relegated to the company of women. He was wealthy, handsome, of a high social class, a member in turn of both houses of Parliament, and the finest wit in London, according to Henry Adams (Pearl, 1955). He was responsible for the collection and publication of the first edition of the collected poems of Keats, and his personal charm extended even to a method of calming animals. He taught the method to Florence, and she practiced it on a long procession of pets ranging from her owl Athena, to chameleons in Egypt, to her many cats (Woodham-Smith, 1951, p. 34), and perhaps even to the military horse she rode so spectacularly in Turkey (Cook, 1942).

By her own admission, Florence adored Richard Monckton Milnes. Though he may have been the first man who wanted to marry her, he was not the last. The list included her cousin, Henry Nicholson; Sir Harry Verney, who finally married her sister; Benjamin Jowett, a celebrated Oxford fellow and tutor, and perhaps others who knew better than to ask, or who were already married. Monckton Milnes was unquestionably the one she would have chosen, had she wished to marry. She refused him because his life-style was too much like her mother's social merry-go-round, and Florence had known since age 17 that she had a greater mission in life than to become another Victorian wife. (In 1837 she experienced the voice of God calling her to service.) He married another woman, but continued to write to Florence on all the important occasions of her life. When she sailed for Turkey, she carried with her three personal letters, including one from Monckton Milnes. While she was away, he was active on the committee that collected the Nightingale Fund, which ultimately enabled her to start the first Nightingale nursing school at St. Thomas Hospital in London.

Besides the letter from Monckton Milnes, one of the letters she carried was a long-sought blessing from her mother, who had previously opposed Florence's professional ambitions. The third was from Father Manning, a Roman Catholic priest whom she had met in Rome during the winter of 1847–1848 when he was still an Anglican archdeacon. It was said of him that, like Newman, he was such a powerful preacher that he could fill St. Mary's even on a weekday. His strong personality proved a help to her on several occasions, as will be seen below.

After years of frustrated attempts to get training as a nurse, of secretly reading books of information about hospitals, of giving up plan after plan to further her own preparation in order to perform a "duty" for some relative, Florence had finally taken a position as an administrator at the Hospital for Poor Gentlewomen on Harley Street. Although it was hard work, it was hardly a job in the modern sense. She received no pay. Because of her youthful appearance, the hospital board stipulated that she must bring a matron with her, and Florence had to pay this matron out of her personal allowance. But she did have authority, she did a good job, and she readied her skills and reputation to take on her huge responsibility in the war. In the course of her work on Harley Street, she ran across a young Irish Catholic girl who was being forced into prostitution. Unable to obtain help or action from civil authorities, Miss Nightingale turned to Manning. He acted overnight in placing the girl safely in a convent school.

Pleased with Manning's decisive action, and attracted by the sisterhoods and other good works of the Church, she studied the Catholic faith seriously. Historians record two versions of her position with regard to the Church. One version says that she tried to join the Church, but was refused because she lacked comprehension of the Catholic idea of submission (Woodham-Smith, 1951). The other says that Manning tried to convert her (Nash, 1927). In either event, he recruited nuns to go with her to Turkey as nurses, and it was understood that they were to obey her instructions as to the place of religious observance within the care setting. Of the 38 nurses who went with Miss Nightingale, 10 were Roman Catholic sisters, 14 were Anglican Catholic sisters, and 14 were nurses who, Mary Clarke said, were of no particular religion, unless the worship of Bacchus should be revived (Woodham-Smith, 1951, p. 86).

Sir Sidney Herbert and his wife, Liz, were personal friends of Florence's; she met them in Rome the same year she met Manning. The Herberts were religious people who felt the responsibility of their wealth and position, and had been waiting in the wings to help Florence find appropriate occupation as soon as this could be done without splitting the Nightingale family asunder. They felt concern over her family's reluctance to permit her sufficient freedom to find the work she felt called to do. Sir Sidney knew that she was an inveterate collector of pamphlets, returns, and statistics, and he obtained for her many of the government reports that she read over the years. He knew the extent of the knowledge she had gleaned and knew, too, of every hospital visit she had made. (Shortly after the war, she was able to tell a royal commission that she had visited all the hospitals in London, Dublin, Edinburgh, Paris, and Berlin, and many in other parts of Germany and in Lyons, Rome, Alexandria, Constantinople; the war hospitals of the French and Sardinians; some of the naval and military hospitals in England; and had studied at the Institution of Protestant Deaconesses at

Kaiserswerth on the Rhine, and with the Sisters of Charity in Paris.) Sir Sidney also knew of every occasion when she had taken over some large household during an emergency and set it in order, and he knew the outcome of the nursing experiences she had had.

When Herbert asked Florence to go to the Crimea, he was following his usual policy of appointing the best person he could find and letting that person organize the task without interference. The Nightingale appointment was almost beyond his authority as Secretary at War—the British bureaucracy of the day also accommodated a Secretary *for* War—and he probably risked his political future in making the appointment, it was so shocking an innovation.

Florence and Sir Sidney kept up a double correspondence during the war years—personal letters in addition to her official reports and his formal replies. She wanted to justify his confidence in her, but most of all the two appear to have been extremely close in their humanitarian desire to improve the lot of the British soldier. She was haunted by the thousands of men she had seen die, not from wounds, but from cholera, typhus, and dysentery brought on by the unsanitary conditions of barracks life, by inadequate food and clothing, and by poisonous liquor. She called herself the mother of 18,000 and said, ". . . nine thousand of my children are lying, from causes which might have been prevented, in their forgotten graves" (Cook, 1942, I, p. 314). During the first 7 months of the Crimean campaign, the mortality rate from disease alone exceeded the mortality rate of the Great Plague of London, or of a typical epidemic of cholera. At Sebastopol, the disease mortality was seven times the number felled by the enemy, but no one before Florence Nightingale thought to count it.

She did not believe a man ought to have to die alone, and during the awful winter of 1854–1855, she estimated that she witnessed 2000 deaths. After the war, she was unable to eat or sleep normally. It is easy to scoff at the way she kept herself and nearly everyone else convinced for years that she was actually dying, as she would gladly have done, but it is more difficult to explain what is to be done with such an excessive burden of emotion. She was unable to forget, and this inability led in the postwar years to an interest in sanitary reform and prevention of illness that superseded her interest in hospital nursing. Sir Sidney understood and shared her feelings. She said he had the quickest perception of anyone she had ever known, and she called him a better conversationalist than Macauley. Sir Sidney lived for only 5 years after the war, during which time they worked together almost daily, and to which time she referred for the rest of her life as her "heaven on earth."

In his turn, he announced to the world in his famous speech at Willis' Rooms in 1855, at the kickoff of the Nightingale Fund collection, that she was "a woman of genius." More privately he wrote to her, "I never intend to tell you how much I owe you for all your help . . ." (Cook, 1942, I, p. 312).

Dr. Sutherland was another of her distinguished acquaintances. He was an expert on sanitation and had been a member of the commission sent to investigate the hospitals and camps at Scutari. She said the commission saved the lives of what was left of the British Army, when they found, among other things, that a large part of the water supply for one hospital had been flowing through the carcass of a dead horse. By correcting this and worse circumstances, they effectively lowered mortality rates from 42 to 2 percent. Thus it was natural that Miss Nightingale should nominate Sutherland to be a member of the postwar Royal Sanitary Commission on the Health of the British Army. What went beyond expectation was that he should give up his own career to become, as various writers have suggested, "her slave."

She complained that he spent too much time digging in his garden, that he took too many vacations, that he was too facetious. Perhaps they argued about his grouse shooting, since she believed that wild birds ought to be protected (Wolstenholme, 1970). She accused him of childishness, looseness of thought, and carelessness with her papers ["Sutherland took my copy of the Army Medical Schools report and now he can't find it," (Woodham-Smith, 1951, p. 288)]. In a manner reminiscent of a melodramatic scene from one of the operas she loved so much in her youth (Strachey, 1918; Sullivan, 1963), they occasionally sat in separate rooms and sent notes back and forth, rather than conversing face to face.

Why did he put up with it all? Not because he was really a slave; he never lost his independence or his judgment. He must have known that Captain Galton avoided the note writing method of communication by simply letting Miss Nightingale know he did not like to communicate that way. But Sutherland must also have known, as her personal physician, that her debility was so real that she found it tiring to get out of bed and dress, or to talk in loud tones. He knew that the source of her debility was her war experience, regardless of how others might judge its nature. He knew firsthand what she had been through, and he knew the prodigious amount of work she was still doing. He judged her "the most gifted creature God ever made," and he protected her all he could, even though he treated her in an apparently comradely fashion, addressing his notes and letters to "Respected enemy," "Dear howling epileptic friend," and the like.

When their disagreements resulted in too much tension, he sent his wife to ease matters. The two women were close friends, sharing religious convictions as well as nicknames for Sutherland ("the baby"). He disagreed vehemently with some of the ideas she put forth in her manuscript on religious thought, although he tried to avoid telling her so, because, as he wrote to her aunt, ". . . in our own work we have enough difference of opinion to make it desirable not to have more" (Woodham-Smith, 1951, p. 240).

She thought Sutherland was wrong about her book until Monckton Milnes, Sir John McNeill, Benjamin Jowett, John Stuart Mill, and the historian Froude all independently found it badly organized. Mill differed only in thinking that it ought to be published in any case, and we can agree with him now, since she never found time to rewrite it. In informal communication, she called the book "stuff," and wrote that she was so sick of it by the time she finished it that she had lost "all discrimination about the ensemble and the form," and confessed to a friend that she herself was unable to read it (Nash, 1927, p. 50).

Although she never worked as continuously with McNeill as she did with

Herbert, Sutherland, and Farr, Sir John McNeill was one of her "cabinet" of trusted advisers, and the one for whose intellectual power and judgment she had the highest respect (Cook, 1942, I, p. 367). She had met him in the Crimea where he (along with Colonel Tullouch) had made a report on the Army Commissariat, which had set off considerable hubbub in official circles. After better reception had been won for the report, she wrote a letter of congratulation to Tullouch and McNeill, and McNeill said, in his reply:

> There is no one . . . whose testimony I could value so highly. . . . Her favourable opinion is very precious to me, not only because she knew more and was intellec- tually more capable of forming a correct judgment than any one else who visited that strange scene, but because of my regard and affection for her . . . (Cook, 1942, I, p. 339).

He encouraged her in the work she did after the war, saying, "The Nation is grateful to you for what you did at Scutari, but . . . [that] . . . was a trifle compared with the good you are doing now" (Cook, 1942, I, p. 262).

Dr. Farr was a member of the postwar Sanitary Commission as expert in the beginning science of statistics. His special contributions included his ready access to the columns of *Lancet*, and his continual reminders, during the years when she was obsessed with army reform, of the importance of establishing a nursing school. Farr had a ready wit, too, and was apparently able to make her laugh. Although he joked about it, he shared her enthusiasm for statistics as the "most important science in the world" (Cook, 1942, II, p. 238). Quetelet, the Belgian astronomer, meteorologist, and statistician, was their mutual friend, and she valued Quetelet's book, *Social Physics*, as a religious work, because to her statistical inquiry provided a means of discovering the laws of God (Cook, 1942, I, pp. 429, 480).

When she asked Farr in 1869 to destroy all her letters to him because she thought she was dying, he protested that it was sacrilege to destroy so much of wit and wisdom, but he complied. Letters of his that survive show something about their comfortable relationship. One contains his joke that a new reading of the sixth commandment showed that it really said, "Thou shalt not take tea," and that such a translation presented a difficulty of serious magnitude for her (Cope, 1958, p. 102). Her love for facts, columns of figures, and tables was well known, and Farr once wrote that he had a gift for her which she was bound to like, since it was in the shape of tables (Woodham-Smith, 1951, p. 23).

Even though both Farr and Jowett destroyed their letters as she instructed them to do, 12,000 Nightingale letters still survive, along with 200 books, pamph- lets, and articles, most of them produced when she felt too weak to get out of bed. She was more a thinker than a writer, disliking to rewrite or polish her efforts. Jowett once warned her that she must make style a duty, if she wanted her work to last, but he also understood that she had so many ideas and such a large output of fresh material that she had no time or energy left for rewriting. Furthermore, she had no desire to be remembered after her lifetime, and although she was ready enough to use her pen as an influence in her postwar career of "driving

Governments'' (Housman, n.d.), she seems to have lacked the confidence or perception that her ideas could be influential even after her death.

The list of her acquaintances could be extended much farther, showing a dimension of her life that is not suggested by either the angel or the lamp. Perhaps it ought to include Arthur Hugh Clough, who already had considerable fame as a poet before he became Florence Nightingale's aide. Yet, during the years he worked for her, he successfully remained in the background as he evidently desired to do, taken for granted by the Nightingale biographers. The one man in her later life who was more than a colleague was Benjamin Jowett.

Jowett, master of Balliol College at Oxford and a Greek scholar, was also a man of tremendous comprehension and perhaps understood Florence Nightingale as no one else did. He had criticized the organization of her paper on religious thought, but it served to introduce them. He considered her a true mystic and urged her to write on mysticism in everyday life. She never found the energy to do it, yet knowing that she accepted his judgment concerning her mysticism adds to the understanding of her personality. Adds, that is, if we remember that it is twentieth-century Americans who deviate from the mainstream of humanity in placing an inestimably low value on mystical gifts (Benedict, 1934, chapter VIII). If we can accept with William James that mystical ability is indeed a special gift, then we can add this dimension to the already recognized deep and broad dimensions of her psyche.

When Jowett and Nightingale worked together, it was she helping him in projects of his that were separate from her more usual work. However, he was sympathetic toward the difficulties she encountered in her efforts to bring about sanitary reform and evidently understood what Herbert's death meant to her. Jowett was delighted with her criticisms of children's literature and with her suggestions concerning his Greek translations, and wrote that he was always stealing from her. He urged her to marry him, and though she would not, they remained good friends for decades, exchanging letters and visits.

Why would so many busy, intelligent men spend so much time and effort working with Florence Nightingale, sometimes to the neglect of their own careers, their leisure, perhaps even at cost to health and life itself? They may sometimes have asked themselves this question, but they evidently found her so stimulating—intellectually, emotionally, sexually, or in all these ways—that they stayed on to enjoy their opportunity as worth what it cost them. She was variously seen as a second mother, companion, friend, soulmate, coworker, commander-in-chief, genius, wit, beloved woman, sometimes even "the bird," and, by military men who disliked change, "that damned nuisance." But it must have humbled the intellectual and attractive men she worked with after the war and reminded them of their relative significance to realize that she was less impressed by them than by the memory of her dead soldiers. All told, she was herself a dazzling individual who stands out even in any centuries-long, millions-wide appraisal of humanity.

What were her accomplishments? Preeminently she was a reformer, and most of her accomplishments were prompted by her concern for the welfare of the British soldier. It was her intense desire for sanitary reform for the Army that led her to invent biostatistics and her pictorial method of presentation—the shaded and colored squares, circles, and wedges she used to present her data (Kopf, 1916–1917). Her advocacy for a university chair of applied statistics (Pearson, 1890) and the hungry way she gathered and used data earned her the nickname of "the passionate statistician."

The long years of effort she devoted to Indian sanitary reform were an outgrowth of her recognition that improved conditions for the Army were dependent on improved sanitation in the locales where the troops were stationed. Her accurate, detailed, and clear reports were known to several successive prime ministers, to other cabinet ministers, and to members of Parliament. She also sent papers to the International Statistical Congresses of 1858, 1860, and 1863, and to the Social Science Congress in Dublin in 1860. Poring over the facts made her a greater authority on India than anyone else, so that she was for years the unofficial consultant to every official associated with Indian efforts. Her concern for improved hospital construction, soldiers' reading rooms, and banking facilities were likewise direct outgrowths of her caring about the soldiers.

Although it was nursing that took her to the Crimea where she saw the soldier's fate, nursing was always a secondary interest after her experience in the war. She sometimes felt guilty that she had given up active nursing herself at such an early date, but both McNeill and Jowett assured her that the reform work she was doing was even more important.

Her work within nursing also involved reform. Nurses existed before her, but most were either nuns or drunks. Nuns were also doing military nursing with both the French and Russian Armies before Nightingale went to the Crimea. But it was Florence Nightingale who made nursing a skilled, paid occupation for women who wanted or needed to work and who might now live decently without retreating to a cloister. Thus it is particularly ironic that she was never paid for her war or postwar work. Nurses sometimes scoff at Florence Nightingale as belonging to an era long past, whose minor accomplishments were overblown, and who would be lost in the acute-care hospital where so many modern nurses function. Much has been made of her slowness to accept modern scientific ideas such as the germ theory and the principle of inoculation. Yet, nosocomial infections, for example, illustrate that new technology has not outdated the basic hygiene Nightingale espoused.

Some of Florence Nightingale's writing, particularly *Notes on Nursing*, is so simple as to seem trivial unless we reflect on the conditions of everyday life in most contemporary homes in England and, no doubt, in America as well. Scovil (1927) said there is more knowledge of health in the poorest homes today than in the most luxurious mid-nineteenth century homes, and that the kind of advice Nightingale gave was simply not available in any printed source until she wrote her classic *Notes*. In "Minding Baby" (Seymer, 1964, p. 220), Nightingale gave an example of the kind of ignorant practices she was opposing:

> . . . mothers boasted that *their* "children's feet had never been touched by water; nor any part of them but faces and hands," that somebody's "child had had its feet washed, and it never lived to grow up."

Today's higher standard of living did not automatically accompany industrialization without human, individual, tiring effort toward teaching, learning, inventing, creating. Perhaps no one person has made more difference in family living during both health and illness than Florence Nightingale.

Surely Florence Nightingale would not work in a modern hospital long before she would be issuing dramatic statistical and pictorial reports showing that one-third or more of the cases were suffering from complications and accidents related to overuse of alcohol, mismanagement of chronic diseases such as diabetes, and lack of adequate nutrition and hygiene. One feels certain that her approach to all the functions of nursing would be to get the facts, record them accurately, analyze them carefully, interpret them intelligently, and implement new ideas creatively.

Nightingale has significance for all modern women in her assertion of her right to place a nonsexual goal first in her life, and then to live by it for the remainder of her 90 years. She was one of the first respectable career women. In recognizing that her own orientation was not for every woman, she was more than a feminist. Her advice to women stands unimproved upon:

> I would earnestly ask my sister to keep clear of both the jargons now current everywhere (for they *are* equally jargons); of the jargon, namely . . . which urges women to do all that men do . . . merely because men do it, and without regard to whether this *is* the best that women can do; and of the jargon which urges women to do nothing that men do, merely because they are women. . . . Surely woman should bring the best she has, *whatever* that is, to the work of God's world. . . . (1859)

It is a shame that Nightingale's own writings, as well as all the standard biographies, are out of print and difficult to obtain. Harvard University graciously permitted us to browse in its copy of her famous 1858 report on matters affecting the health, efficiency, and hospital administration of the British Army. This thick document is in many surface respects a typical government report: paperbound, full of tables and appendixes, and literally stuffed with facts. Upon starting to read, however, one quickly senses that it is an unusual government document indeed. There is a rigorous, disciplined logic to the argument, but also a passionate drawing of morals from the progression of facts. It is clear that no committee produced the volume. It speaks with one eloquent voice of a shambles, compounded by incompetence and indifference, that resulted in unspeakable waste of soldiers' lives in the Crimean War. It analyzes the reasons for the debacle and tells forthrightly and forcibly what the future policies and practices should be. We have chosen to quote a few passages with the hope that they will give you a taste of the real Nightingale. We also present an excerpt from one of her pie diagrams, because Nightingale is credited with its invention.

> The amount of sickness which prevailed during these campaigns was enormous. During the whole Peninsular War from 1808 to 1814, the proportion of sick to 100 strength varied from 9.4 to 33; the mean percentage being about 21. . . . But, during the seven months in the Crimea, from October 1854 to April 1855 inclusive, the percentage of sick to strength varied from 24 to 51; the average being actually during the whole seven months nearly 39 per cent. (p. 5)

Table I-1   Annual Rate of Mortality Percent in the Army of the East and in the English Male Population of Ages 15–45

Class of diseases	Deaths annually to 100 living	
	Army of the East	English male population
Zymotic diseases	18.7	.2
Constitutional diseases	.3	.4
Local diseases	.9	.3
Violent deaths	3.0	.1
All causes	22.9	1.0

Source: Nightingale, 1858, p. 314.

This result I have obtained from an examination of the statistics . . . No attempt has hitherto been made to arrive at this fact, though it is obviously most important. (p. 6)

There was nothing new to history in the sanitary results of our campaign. . . . Let us not deny them, but let us set to work to ascertain what is the education, what the organization, what the system of Medical and other Departments, which will prevent the recurrence of such a fearful loss of life? (p. 146)

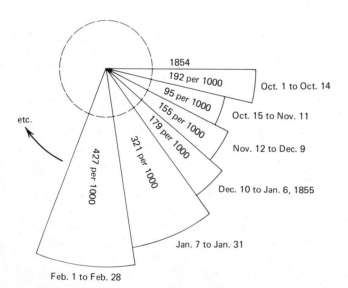

Figure I-1   Diagram representing the mortality in the hospitals at Scutari and Kulali, from October 1, 1854 to September 30, 1855. The area within the dashed circumference represents the average annual mortality in the military hospitals near London = 20.9 per 1000. The solid wedges measured from the center represent by their area the mortality per 1000 of sick treated at Scutari and Kulali. (*Excerpts from a pie diagram in Nightingale, 1858.*)

But what shall we say when we see the proportion in which the Army in the East suffered from Zymotic disease, compared to that in which the Civil Population suffers at home? and the utter insignificance into which sink the Deaths from Wounds of an Army in the field, even when engaged in constant warfare, compared with the deaths from Zymotic disease? (p. 314) [This rhetorical question refers to Table I-1.]

It is unquestionable, and our experience of the way in which, in Civil life, mortality can be, and has been reduced, need hardly be referred to,—it is unquestionable that the mortality and sickness of the Army in peace may be reduced to one-half, at most, of its present excessive amount. . . . The main end of Statistics should not be to inform the Government as to how many men have died, but to enable immediate steps to be taken to prevent the extension of disease and mortality. (p. 329)

REFERENCES

Benedict, Ruth: *Patterns of culture*. Boston: Houghton Mifflin, 1934.

Cook, Sir Edward: *The life of Florence Nightingale*. 2 Vols. New York: Macmillan, 1942.

Cope, Zachary: *Florence Nightingale and the doctors*. Philadelphia: Lippincott, 1958.

Darwin, Emma: *A century of family letters: 1792–1896*. New York, 1915.

Gilgannon, Mary: *The Sisters of Mercy as Crimean War nurses*. Ann Arbor, Mich.: University Microfilms, 1962.

Housman, Lawrence: In H. J. Massingham and Hugh Massingham (Eds.), *The great Victorians*. London: Ivor Nicholson & Watson, n.d.

James, William: *The varieties of religious experience*. London: Longmans, 1922.

Kopf, E. W.: Florence Nightingale as statistician. *American Statistical Association Journal*, 1916–17, *XV*.

Nash, Rosalind: *A short life of Florence Nightingale*. New York: Macmillan, 1927.

Nightingale, Florence: *Notes on matters affecting the health, efficiency, and hospital administration of the British Army, founded chiefly on the experience of the late war*. London: Harrison, 1858.

———: *Notes on nursing*. Philadelphia: Lippincott, 1947. (Reprint of 1859 edition.)

Pearl, Cyril: *The girl with the swansdown seat*. Indianapolis: Bobbs-Merrill, 1955.

Pearson, Karl: *Life, letters and labours of Francis Galton*. London: Cambridge University Press, 1890–1914. vol. II.

Richards, Laura, E.: Letters of Florence Nightingale. *Yale Review*, 1935, *24*, 326–348.

Scovil, E. R.: Florence Nightingale: Notes on nursing. *American Journal of Nursing*, 1927, *27*, 355–357.

Seymer, Lucy: *Selected writings of Florence Nightingale*. New York: Macmillan, 1964.

Strachey, Lytton: *Eminent Victorians*. London: Chatto & Windus, 1918.

Sullivan, Howard A.: *The Florence Nightingale collection at Wayne State University*. Detroit: Wayne State University, 1963.

Whittaker, Elvi, and Virginia Olesen: The faces of Florence Nightingale: Functions of the heroine legend in an occupational sub-culture. *Human Organization*, 1964, *23*, 123–130.

Wolstenholme, G. E. W.: Florence Nightingale: New lamps for old. *Proceedings of the Royal Society of Medicine*, 1970, *63*, 1282–1288.

Woodham-Smith, Cecil: *Florence Nightingale*. New York: McGraw-Hill, 1951.

———: Florence Nightingale revealed. *American Journal of Nursing*, 1952, *52*, 570–572.

How Are Variables Measured?

Planning how and where to make measurements is the link between thinking about a problem and doing empirical research on that problem. (We classify library research, historical research, consulting experts, applications of deductive logic, and informal observations of situations involving the problem within the general category of thinking about the problem.) In this chapter we deal with planning *how* to take measurements in general nursing research. The next chapter involves you in planning a specific research project of your own, and becomes more specific about a variety of measurement procedures you might use. Chapter 7 deals with planning *where* to make measurements in a general way (sometimes called *sampling theory*) and is followed by a chapter which challenges you to make a sampling plan for your own research project. Upon completion of these four chapters you should be well informed about how research interests are translated into actual research data collections.

CONSTRUCTS, VARIABLES, VARIATES

Constructs are the building blocks of nursing theory. A *construct* is an *idea of a class* of forces, processes, or entities. *Theoretical propositions* are sentences which assert relationships between constructs. Thus *environment*, *genotype*, and *phenotype* are construct names, and the sentence "The genotype and the environment interact to produce the phenotype" is a theoretical proposition. A more useful proposition, the tests and consequences of which are more obvious, is, "Different environments interacting with a fixed genotype will produce different phenotypes." This proposition has inspired studies on identical twins separated by adoption into different families. Another testable and useful proposition is, "Different genotypes interacting with a fixed environment will yield different phenotypes." This proposition leads to research on children from different parents placed in the same foster home, as well as research on differences among fraternal twins raised by their own parents. Constructs such as these are abstract and unreal in the sense that they denote classes of events and not single events. Each event may be unique in many ways, but a construct is an idea of something a group of events has in common. Each family situation is unique in many respects, yet the idea of childrearing environment is necessary to distinguish what homes provide to children *as a class of forces* from what genes provide to children as a class of forces. The characteristics genes provide are different for every child (except between identical twins), but it is helpful to name the idea of a class of forces based on genes as the genotype. Research on a home can reveal only imperfectly and incompletely the characteristics of the childrearing environment it provides. Study of the anatomy and physiological-psychological functioning of a person can support inferences about that person's genotype only imperfectly and incompletely.

Constructs are ideas in the thoughts of men and women. To do empirical research it is necessary to find a way to take measurements on observed events which can stand in for a construct. A device created by analysis of research data to stand in for a construct is called a *variable*. For example, when human twin births occur, a series of measurements on the blood, saliva, and afterbirth make it possible to create the variable *zygosity*, which takes one of the values *identical* or *fraternal* for each twin pair, as a proxy for the construct of *genotype fixity* (present or absent). This construct is usually named *monozygosity* and valued 1 for identical twins and 0 for fraternal twins. The variable has an operational definition provided by a rule for scoring it from a series of measurements on blood, saliva, and possibly placental tissue. The variable may carry the same name as the construct it represents, but the two must not be confused. The construct is an idea which probably has a somewhat fuzzy denotation and a host of attached connotations, or surplus meanings. The variable stands for the construct only approximately, and usually fallibly. Even when elaborate blood, saliva, and placental data are summarized in an estimate of zygosity, some errors in scoring the variable are possible, leading to mistaken designation of a single-egg twin pair as a fraternal pair or a two-egg twin pair as an identical pair. Thus the variable only estimates the construct more or less reliably.

A *variate* is a rule for taking a measurement in research. The properties of blood, saliva, and placental tissue samples which are scored as the first step (the data-collection step) of research on twins are the variates out of which the variable zygosity is created. We often speak of the scores on variates as the *raw data* of a research project.

Moving from thought to action, we have constructs which sponsor variables which require variates for their operationalization. Moving from action toward thought, we have the scores assigned to variates (data), out of which analysis creates the scores taken by variables (information), which stand as proxies for the undeterminable magnitudes of constructs (truth). Sampling and measuring yield data. Analysis transforms masses of data to variables and computes relationships among variables, yielding information. Interpretation and conclusion processes evaluate information for possible causal connections among constructs in a realm of ideation, of truth claims, and probably of ideology. In one direction (research planning), our beliefs tell us what it is important to observe, measure, and relate. In the other direction (reconstruction of knowledge), the relationships we analyze from data inform us about what we can afford to believe, if we want to be rational. The early chapters of this text focus on the planning of research, while the later chapters focus on the reconstruction of knowledge. Analysis is the pivot.

Social class can be discussed as an example of the relationships among the terms we are considering. Modern sociology has properly invented and popularized social class as one of its primary constructs for explaining almost anything in Western civilization that interests sociologists. The construct is indeed fuzzy. Everyone likes the idea and everyone talks about everything in relation to social class, but every individual has a unique viewpoint on the meaning of it. This fuzziness and ambiguity of denotation, accompanied by a veritable halo of connotations, is characteristic of all great ideas which we apply to human affairs. Exactly what is meant by intelligence? What is character? What is love?

One does not have to be a Marxist to recognize that most people assume the role expectations that are the birthrights of their parents' social classes, and that these role definitions make behavior patterns somewhat predictable from parental social class. This assumption is involuntary and automatic, coming with the mother's milk, as it were (or sometimes with the alternative infant succorance). Only in adolescence do some youths question the class models they have inherited for belief and behavior, and then a breakthrough to a different class and its model may be won by some. A few hardy youths may even fight through to personal freedom from a class role, or they may find the appearance of freedom in a counterculture role which is really the stigma of a new and growing social class. This last thought suggests to us that the present fuzziness of the social class construct may be the inevitable symptom of a society in transition, a society which is changing so quickly that its intellectuals cannot keep the pace.

We cannot quite agree on what we mean by social class, but we do feel that it should be involved in our social research, including research on nursing. The social class origins of nurses probably affect their attitudes toward patients, toward supervision, and toward career opportunities. The social class origins of patients may strongly influence their personal health habits and their acceptance of nursing.

Persons do not enter research studies as subjects with social class labels attached. A social class variable has to be created from research data to stand for the construct in data analyses. The researcher has to collect data representing the educational achievements, the occupations, the home environments (whether of the subjects themselves or of their parents has to be decided). Then a scoring scheme has to be imposed on the scores for these variates, and possibly other variates as well, to create a social class variable score.

Usually different weights will be given to the different variates that enter the variable. Let's pretend that we know the relative importance ("weight") to social class of levels of education, occupation, and home culture. Thus if X_1 is the educational level of an individual, X_2 her occupational level, and X_3 the cultural level of her home (books, magazines, papers, music, etc.), her social class variable score S might be created by the formula

$$S = .7X_1 + 1.0X_2 + .3X_3 \qquad (1)$$

The choice of variates and weights for them are not plucked from the imagination as ours were in the example, but are issues for research expertise to resolve. Our ambition is for you to acquire at least rudimentary skills in the making of such choices. For the moment we emphasize that the research variable that stands for a theoretical construct is scored from data variates after the fashion of Equation (1).

STANDARDIZING OBSERVATIONS

A crucial rule of research is that all variates must be observed and scored in the same way for all subjects (and all variables must be scored in the same way from the same variates for all subjects). Variates must be based on standardized procedures (ditto for variables). It would not do to ask one subject for self-report on her educational level, then require a second subject to submit school transcripts. Self-report from *all* subjects would be a standardized procedure. Alternatively, school transcripts from *all* subjects would be a standardized procedure. Research methods have to be arbitrary, but they must be uniform.

Here is a possible scoring rule for the educational level variate.

Category	Points
No response or high school dropout	0
High school diploma only	1
Some post-high school education but no degree	2
Two-year college degree (AA, AAS, ADN, etc.)	3
Baccalaureate degree	4
Master's degree	5
Doctorate or equivalent (MD, etc.)	6

Here is another possible scoring rule for the same variate.

Category	Points
No response	0
No baccalaureate degree	1
Baccalaureate degree only	3
Graduate degree(s)	5

And yet another.

Category	Points
No response or high school dropout	0
High school graduate plus anything else	2

Many other ways of scoring the variate "educational level" can be invented. All are arbitrary. Obviously, it is desirable that a good rule be found for the purposes of the research in hand, but the minimal requirement is for a uniform rule. The categories which are set up must be mutually exclusive and exhaustive. That is, each response obtained must fit into one and only one category of the variate.

What is at stake in uniformity of scoring is the objectivity of the research. The rules for collecting data have to be arbitrary, but once they are established the actual data which are collected should depend as little as possible on the subjective perceptions or judgment of the scientist doing the collecting. The reason we like to have electronic machines score protocols wherever possible, rather than using human scorers, is that scoring machines are more likely to treat all protocols in the same way. (A protocol is a record of responses made by a subject, often a test answer sheet or a questionnaire answer sheet.) The hope is that data will give a "true" rather than a subjectively distorted picture of reality to a greater extent if the procedures for collecting and scoring observations are properly standardized. This pious hope still leaves ample opportunity for experts to argue about what constitutes proper standardization.

RELIABILITY

Reliability refers to the correctness or accuracy of scores, in the sense of their reproducibility by repeated measurement acts. A temperature is measured reliably to the extent that repeated acts of measuring the temperature at the same time agree on the readings or "scores" assigned. It is unreliable to the extent that several readings taken at the same time may disagree. Since temperature can undergo quite rapid change, checking the reliability of a temperature measurement procedure requires some quick action to take two or several readings as close together in time as possible. We will see that a suitable technique for estimating the degree of reliability of a measurement is not always easy to contrive, but what we need to be clear about initially is that reliability means the tendency of scores from a measurement procedure to be in agreement when two, several, or many readings are taken on the same subject in such a short period of time that the subject's "true" score would not have changed. The issue is whether scores can be reproduced (or better, the extent to which scores can be reproduced). This aspect of measurement theory could have been termed *reproducibility* to advantage, and we urge you to learn this term as a synonym for reliability.

A measurement procedure can by some chance or accident produce a score for a particular subject which is radically incorrect, and yet be reliable to a high degree when it is applied to a large number of subjects for most of whom a rather accurate score is obtained. Thus the degree of reliability of a measurement in a research study has to be thought of (and possibly computed) in relation to the extent of the errors in the scores for all the subjects. For this reason, reliability is a statistical construct.

We are now dealing with a very important idea, so please think vigorously about this. A statistical construct describes a property of a set of scores. Another statistical construct is *score distribution*, which refers to the set of scores for all subjects. Yet another statistical construct is *average*, which refers to some indicator of the center of a set of scores (more technical detail coming in Chapter 9, in the section on score distributions). Now we have three statistical constructs under discussion: reliability, score distribution, average. They all refer to properties of an entire set of scores, rather than to a property of any single score. If we think of the possibility that the observed score for any subject on a variate X might be partitioned into a "true" score part and an "error" part, so that

$$X = t + e \tag{2}$$

and then think of the distribution of error scores, the e, for all subjects, the average of the absolute values (any negative signs ignored) of the e could represent the extent of unreliability of the measurement procedure as applied to the subjects of the study. By itself this number would be uninformative because its magnitude could only be judged in relation to the magnitude of the average observed score (or alternatively, of the average true score). We could make an index of unreliability by dividing the average absolute error by the average absolute observed score, and the complement of this ratio could serve as an index of the degree of reliability. Actually, there is an extensive literature on reliability which contains a variety of formulas for it and several ways of collecting the data needed to compute according to the formulas. That none of these methods is definitive only testifies to the complexity of the matter. At our stage of study, it is more important to realize that social science measurements are always fallible and to accept that there will be errors in our data than it is to worry about what we do not know about reliability. We can agree to be careful in taking measurements, to try to develop an instinct for sources of errors in measurements and ways to reduce them, and to remember that at best our data will have some "noise" in them that confuses the signals they send us.

A common mistake made in discussions of reliability is attaching the construct to a particular measurement procedure as though the two will hang together in all kinds of studies. Think for a moment about forms to obtain self-reported patient histories. Would you expect the information obtained to be equally reliable from an inner-city clinic, an upper-class private practice, an adolescent care unit, and a geriatric setting? Actually, the reliability with which the measurement procedure operates in one setting can tell us little about how accurately it will operate in a different setting. In general, reliability has to refer to the accuracy of the measurements taken in a specific research setting, not to an innate property of a measurement procedure. It may be reassuring to be able to review evidence that the measurements we plan to use in our research have performed with substantial reliability in other research designs, but there is no guarantee that special circumstances in our research design cannot lead to substandard reliability, and we must be on guard. Similarly, if we are reading a research report in which it is asserted that a measurement "has" a certain reliability index value because that value had been reported from some other research project, we can suspect that the author of the report is either naïve or devious.

It is an amusing fact that all longitudinal survey studies which send questionnaires to the same subjects at intervals have found that noticeable numbers of subjects report their sex differently at different times. Most of these erratic reporters have not had a real sex change; they are simply careless or mischievous in responding to a question for which one might think one could get totally accurate data. When human beings are being interrogated, no totally reliable data can be expected!

The particular standardization of an item can affect the reliability of the item scores. In the previous section we discussed the variable of education level and suggested that self-report on this variate is usually solicited from the subjects, but an alternative standardized procedure would be to require schools and colleges to certify the educational attainments of the subjects. This might seem to be an expensive method which would sometimes be justifiable because of the high reliability that could be expected of it. Such optimism is tempered when we start to think of the things that can go wrong. Schools lose and destroy records. Schools and colleges themselves disappear. Students with different records have identical names. Students change their names and forget to report the names under which their school records exist. And so forth. Nothing is easy in the quest for reliable data.

VALIDITY

Social scientists usually do not know exactly what they are talking about (constructs are fuzzy), and do not know exactly what they are measuring (the variables indicated by a variate are a matter of conjecture or a matter which needs to be researched), but they can be certain that what they are measuring is not exactly what they are talking about. The *validity* of a measurement procedure is an interpretation of what it measures. The evidence to support an interpretation of validity can be inconclusive, confusing, contradictory, complex, and often ignored by persons who want to believe what they want to believe. For reasons good and bad, people will make different inferences about what a measurement means or stands for. We cannot give you simple formulations about validity. They can be found in some books, but they just do not serve. What we can do is testify that the measurements made in social science research in the quest for answers to questions more often than not inspire new questions about what has been measured, and these new questions about the validities of the measurements often elevate the inquiry to a higher level of language and meaning, so that the original questions are transcended. Social science does not solve problems as much as it creates better understandings of them.

The validity of a measurement is explored through its *correlations* with other measurements. Correlation is perhaps the most fundamental statistical construct of this book, and the methods of correlation analysis we shall present are our journeyman's tools for dealing with research data. Chapter 9 treats correlation technically. For now, we need an intuitive grasp of the idea. Two measurements are correlated to the extent that they vary together, so that the scores of one measure tend to be paired with corresponding scores of the other measure. The phrase "tend to be paired" is crucial, because an exact correspondence is a functional, not a correlational, relationship. That is, a one-to-one correspondence between a score on the first measure and a paired score on the second measure indicates that one measure is absolutely dependent on the other, not merely related to it. A perfect functional relation (1.0) is the upper limit which a strong correlation can approach, but will not quite reach. In correlational relationships there is always some indeterminancy regarding what value of the second measurement is paired with each value of the first measurement.

In a functional relation there is always a rule which tells exactly what score of the second variate is paired with each score of the first variate. An example would be bank accounts earning a fixed rate of interest. The interest rate is a rule which allows calculation of exactly what interest payment is due for any amount on deposit. Another example is the linear equation

$$X_2 = bX_1 + c \tag{3}$$

which has the graph shown in Figure 5-1. There is no doubt what value of X_2 is paired with any value of X_1 in such a linear functional relation. (The coefficients b and c would be given precise numerical values to designate a particular linear function. Coefficient b is called the slope coefficient, because it is the tangent of the tilt angle of the line of the equation, and c is the intercept coefficient, because it tells what value X_2 takes when $X_1 = 0$, which is where the graph of the equation intercepts the X_2 axis.) We are interested in linear equations because a similar linear equation is used to express the predictability of X_2 from a known value of

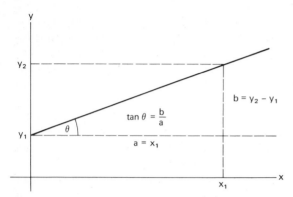

Figure 5-1 Graph of a linear relation.

X_1 in a correlation situation, but the prediction is not perfect. One way of thinking about a correlation is that it tells how close the prediction of a relationship comes to the perfect prediction that would be available for a functional relationship. For example, for human adults height predicts weight to some extent, so that height and weight are correlated variates. The actual weight for a person of any particular height is somewhat indeterminate, however, and only a fallible prediction of weight is available from a known height and the known correlation of the two variates. In contrast, height predicts perfectly the length of a person's shadow (given correction for the source of light). Shadow length is a function of height.

The value of X_2 predicted from a correlation is only an average of all the values X_2 actually takes in pairings with the particular X_1. If the actual X_2 scores that are paired in nature with an X_1 score vary very little around the predicted X_2, the correlation between X_1 and X_2 is strong. If the actual X_2 scores that are paired with an X_1 score in the data distribution vary very much around the predicted X_2, the correlation between X_1 and X_2 is weak. When the X_2 scores that are paired in the data with any particular X_1 score vary around the predicted X_2 just as much as the full set of all X_2 scores (without regard to any particular X_1) vary around the average X_2 score, the correlation is zero, or nonexistent. In short, the correlation between two variates is an index of the extent to which their scores tend to covary, and this covarying tendency of two sets of scores can range from almost none (a nearly zero correlation) to almost perfect (a nearly functional relation).

How does correlation throw light on validity? What it comes down to is that we understand our measurements by the company they do and do not keep. We look to see what other measurements which we already understand are highly correlated with the measurement whose validity we are pondering, and what other understood measurements are almost uncorrelated with the one in hand. In a network of correlations among many variates we seek clues to the validities of one or some measurements which are more of a puzzle to us than are other previously studied elements in the net.

Validity also involves the distinctions among variates, variables, and constructs which we discussed earlier. The validity of a variable is really established by the argument which pairs it with a scientific construct. The validity of a variate is established by the evidence that it is a key element in the operational definition of a variable [i.e., the scoring formula for a variable, as in Equation (1) for a social class variable]. The methods we shall present for operationally defining and theoretically interpreting variables are the ways in which validities are documented. These methods for making variables out of variates and justifying the construct pairings of variables are correlational methods, so we have to teach you to do research on correlations skillfully.

Experience has shown that a particular measurement can contribute usefully to two or more variables. For example, the educational level variate that helps to define a social class variable [as in Equation (1)] may also help to define a variable called *scientist potential*, which stands for the construct in *psychology of careers* of individual differences in capability of becoming a scientist. An operational definition of the scientist potential variable might be

$$P = .5X_1 + .2X_2 + .3X_3 + 1.0X_4 + .7X_5 \tag{4}$$

where X_1 is educational level, X_2 is sex, X_3 is age, X_4 is general intelligence, and X_5 is interest in science. Compare Equations (1) and (4) for the extents to which variate X_1 contributes to variables S and P. Thus it is sensible to speak of the validity of a variable and the validities of a variate.

Physiological variates can have multiple validities, just as psychological variates usually have. Why do nurses take patients' temperatures? There is a construct of fever for which a fever variable can be constructed from several possible indicators, one of which is oral temperature. Do patients' oral temperatures tell enough about how febrile they are? Temperature is an indicator of normal or baseline conditions of the organism, but "You have a fever" or "You have no fever" is an inference. The inference has so often been made carelessly, without proper attention to all the evidence, that clinicians have become chary of using "fever" at all.

Reliability and validity are difficult concepts. Chapter 9, "Observation and the Measurement of Variables," in Kerlinger (1979) provides an excellent and understandable explanation. In fact, this entire book (*Behavioral Research: A Conceptual Approach*) is a lucid and expert presentation of most of the issues raised in our book, and we urge it upon you as a parallel textbook if you have the time now to expand your reading about research. If not, Kerlinger would be a good choice for your next book on this subject.

FEASIBILITY

Many people vaguely distrust social science, and quite a few people actively dislike social science. Such people may not cooperate when they are drawn as subjects in a research sample, and some of them may actively sabotage the work by lying. Passive sabotage by not responding is widespread. Some people are also lazy or selfish, or wisely conservative of their own work, so that even good will toward the project does not lead automatically to good responsiveness. Building rapport with human subjects is an art. If you are going to do research on human subjects you have to be thoughtful and creative about rapport. Maybe the best idea is to approach your subjects with the friendliness, frankness, and respect with which you would like to be approached. We think it is helpful to explain the research to the subjects in a way which engages their intellectual curiosity. The researcher who complains about low response rate and high incidence of missing data probably made little effort to communicate to the subjects the issues and importance of the project. Incidentally, funding agencies are willing to pay stipends to research subjects, and sometimes it is fair and encouraging to offer a stipend for the work requested of them. Taking tests or questionnaires or being interviewed is work.

A special problem that occurs in many nursing studies is that the subjects are ill or in hazard. The fact that the researcher is a nurse with special awareness of the needs of such subjects should lead to wise and humane handling of the problem, but we must remember that the professional status of the researcher is being traded upon in building rapport, and thus a special trust and responsibility are involved. We discuss this again in the final section of this chapter.

Measurement acts, like all acts, are expensive. One must ask in the planning stage whether the data will be worth their cost. It is easy to deceive oneself about what data are going to cost, since some of the effort is one's own or volunteer subjects'. It is also easy to lose sight of some of the coding, scoring, verifying, and organizing operations which must be performed on data before analysis is possible. A flowchart of the work is helpful in the planning stage if the cost-effectiveness of the data is to be weighted intelligently. Once data collection starts, a research design is a trap from which there is no escape short of admission of failure. The feasibility and optimal form of chosen procedures have to be thought out at the planning stage. Time should always be taken to brain-storm the measurement scheme. Is there a better way? What novel methods can be thought of that might work? What clever measurement devices that worked in published research projects could be adopted or adapted to this research?

Pretesting the measurement plan on a small sample of subjects is almost mandatory. This is where the unanticipated "slip twixt cup and lip" can be found before resources have been irretrievably wasted.

The success of research depends on the use of standardized measurement procedures that scale valid variables reliably *and that are practical*.

HUMAN SUBJECTS, RESEARCH ETHICS

In Chapter 1 (Table 1-2) we listed parts of a research prospectus from the "inside out." That is, we gave questions the investigator might ask herself in thinking about and clearly expressing her overall research plan. In Chapter 4 we discussed the prospectus, or proposal, from the point of view of a prospective funder. We have already advocated continuing review by academic and professional colleagues. Now we must discuss the research plan from yet another perspective, that of informed consent of subjects. To nurses in clinical practice, this is not a new concept, but the notion of a review of assurances for informed consent as mandated with regard to research may be new.

Most thoughtful nurses know that many of the forms that patients have signed in the past, giving consent to various diagnostic and surgical procedures, have not truly represented informed consent. In their role of patient advocate many nurses have refused to ask patients to sign such consent forms; some clinical agencies, medical staffs, and ethical physicians have taken the position that it is the responsibility of the physician who intends to perform the procedure to obtain the patient's signature to the consent. This is on the ground that only the physician knows exactly what he or she intends to do and can assure that the consent is truly informed. Physicians are sometimes researchers as well as clinicians, and medical investigators sometimes employ "research nurses." Gray (1975) reported that a research nurse was nearly twice as likely to be the person who explained the study to a subject as were the principal investigator, co-investigator, private physician, or house staff member combined. Regardless of who explains the research and obtains the consent, however, nurses have a moral and professional responsibility to understand any data collection that takes place on human subjects in our domain of practice (ANA *Code*, 1968; Ellis, 1970). In addition to the responsibility, we have a right to the satisfactions derived from true collaboration. When a nurse is the principal investigator, she, of course, assumes total responsibility for informed consent.

Institutions have some powers of their own, and they may require more than HEW demands. In fact, HEW says that institutional committees should "determine the acceptability of the proposal in terms of institutional commitments and regulations, applicable law, standards of professional conduct and practice, and community attitudes" (Gray, 1975). Thus, an institutional review board (IRB) may want to ask whether the research appears to have merit. They are within their rights, even though it can be questioned whether such additional review is effective or efficient use of their personnel. A university, in turn, may demand a certain level of writing in the proposal document itself. Although the same question concerning effectiveness and efficiency can be asked, we are biased in believing that an educational institution's first responsibility is to enforce reasonable standards of human communication, especially (at the present time, at least) reading and writing. The real message, perhaps, is that these IRBs have power in their local realms, and the researcher needs to learn to work with them.

For information on the effects of requiring consent to be written, deceit, and other issues, see Singer, 1978. In general, nurses can feel safe in abiding by the ANA *Code for Nurses* and the *Human Rights Guidelines for Nurses in Clinical and Other Research*.

Q: Name and define a construct (perhaps the one you used in response to the Q in Chapter 2) and list some variates which might be used as research indicators for a variable to stand for the construct. What problems in collecting data by means of these variates might attack the reliability of the variable? What limitations would the variable have on its validity as a research measure of the construct?

Q: Looking at the list of Project TALENT variates in Appendix B, what construct would a variable made by adding together the scores on variates 8 and 9 stand for? What limitations can you see for the validity of this variable?

REFERENCES

American Nurses' Association: *Code for nurses with interpretive statements*. Kansas City, Mo. (2420 Pershing Road, 64108): ANA, 1968.
———: *Human rights guidelines for nurses in clinical and other research*. Kansas City, Mo.: ANA, 1976.
Department of Health, Education, and Welfare: *Research projects involving human subjects*. Washington, D.C.: U.S. DHEW, 1976 (August).
Ellis, Rosemary: The nurse as investigator and member of the research team. *Annals of the New York Academy of Science*, 1970, *169*, 435–441.
Fleming, Juanita W.: Human rights and ethical concerns of scientists. In *Issues in research*, Selected Papers from the American Nurses' Association Council of Nurse Researchers Program Meeting, August, 1973.
Gray, Bradford H.: *Human subjects in medical experimentation*. New York: Wiley, 1975.
Kerlinger, Fred N.: *Behavioral research: A conceptual approach*. New York: Holt, 1979.
Singer, Eleanor: Informed consent: Consequences for response rate and response quality in social surveys. *American Sociological Review*, 1978, *43*, 144–162.

Chapter 6

What Measurements Are Called For by Your Problem?

This chapter provides a critical survey of measurement procedures currently used in the social sciences. It should help you to visualize the possibilities for measuring the variables of your research proposal, although you will have to do further reading on the methods you select.

NAMING YOUR VARIABLES

Before deciding on data-collection methods, an investigator should have reviewed literature, decided on an adequate conceptual framework in which to study the chosen problem, and identified the variables that the literature and personal experience tell her will strongly affect the measurement to be obtained on the criterion (dependent) variable. Thorndike and Hagen (1969) say that measurement always involves three common steps: (1) identifying and defining the quality or attribute to be measured, (2) determining a set of operations by which the attribute may be made manifest and perceivable, and (3) establishing a set of procedures or definitions for translating observations into quantitative statements of degree or amount. These three tasks are subsumed in the concept of operationalization.

The operational definitions the researcher selects or creates for the particular study translate the grand theoretical constructs (variables) into items (variates) that can be counted or measured. Thus they are the means by which the researcher gets back and forth between the practical and theoretical "streams" of science. Phrased another way, operational definitions represent arbitrary dividing lines between the quantitative and qualitative aspects of a study. To some adherents of traditional objective-positive science, this quantified material is all that can be reported. We disagree (to be discussed later in this chapter).

Standard definitions (with citations) should be used whenever possible. If it becomes necessary to create a definition, then a new term should be used rather than one that has previously been used with other meanings. For example, just as we cannot now use the word *rose* to refer to anything other than the familiar flower of that name, we should not attempt to use *primary nursing care* in a new way, now that numerous studies of that phenomenon have been reported. It is understood that technical terms or abstractions used in the problem statement or hypothesis should appear in the same form in the definitions. Thus, one should not define *perceived attitude* and then shift to *perceptions* unless the definitions state that the two terms will be used interchangeably.

METHODS FOR GENERATING DATA IN NURSING RESEARCH

The aim of this chapter is to help the investigator select a method for data collection. To that end we have provided an overview, discussion, examples, and references which we hope will prove stimulating. We have deliberately neglected techniques that fail to take advantage of computer capabilities, such as the construction of Thurstonian scales. We have likewise avoided discussion of Guttman scales, regarding them as evolving from prior, simpler scales, such as the Likert. We have also assumed a relatively small-scale investigation in which the researcher collects her own data. If she does not, she will have to consult training manuals that may go along with the instrument she selects, or, failing that, consult textbooks more specialized than this one.

How is the researcher finally to decide on method? By piloting as many methods as necessary. (We will have more to say about pilots in Chapter 8.)

Although we recognize that researchers sometimes choose method first and then select problems that can be looked at via the method, that approach is not praiseworthy. Over 30 years ago, Maslow (1946) contrasted the means-centered with the problem-centered approach and listed several research defects that are fostered by a premature emphasis on means. These defects included neglect of problems concerning values and an overemphasis on technical virtuosity, quantification for its own sake, scientific orthodoxy, and emphasis on the differences rather than the similarities between scientists and between sciences. Deciding on the means before stating the problem lessens the chance that an investigator may invent a creative way to solve a problem. In other words, choosing the method before the problem tends to discourage creativity in research, and therefore, probably, innovative change in the profession of nursing. Cannell and Kahn (1968) also advocate methodological breadth rather than parochial habit and advise choice of method on the basis of the problem.

Critical Incidents

The critical incident concept developed by Flanagan in 1954 consists of identifying extreme behavior, either effective or ineffective. Identification of critical incidents has been used for a variety of purposes in nursing—to evaluate clinical performance or safety records of nurses and nursing students, to report and record patient behavior, to investigate problems in institutional management, and so on. And, we suspect, it has often been neglected when it might have been useful.

Hardin (1955) interpreted the idea of critical incidents for nursing research, pointing out that it involves reporting what the subjects actually did without attempting to interpret motivation or ability or inability to do otherwise. Thus it is a natural technique for nurses who have practiced factual reporting on nurses' notes. Hardin pointed out that critical incident in itself is a concept, not a method, and that it can be used in combination with various methods and materials such as observation, interview, questionnaire, logs and diaries, or other records. It seems obvious that reliability will be higher if incidents are recorded as soon as possible after they occur, whatever the means used for recording.

The idea of critical incidents is adaptable to various reporters, too. It can be useful in gathering information from individuals concerning their own behavior, from subordinates with respect to their superiors, from superiors with respect to their subordinates, or from peers. It is equally flexible in providing data for initial exploration (piloting) or more refined analysis.

The classic Hagen and Wolff study (1961) gathered information from a variety of hospital personnel concerning nursing leadership behavior in general hospitals. It seems likely that that study has had an effect on attitudes toward roles of nearly every nurse in practice today, whether or not she has heard of the study by name. The Bermosk and Corsini (1973) study gathered written responses concerning nurses' own behavior in situations involving difficult value judgments. Kramer (1974) observed incidents of "reality shock" and wrote her own notes after leaving the arena of observation.

Tests

Tests, in the research context, usually refer to instruments standardized for the measurement of human traits, such as intelligence or authoritarianism. Behavioral scientists have developed many such instruments, some of which can be located through Buros (1974) and Shaw and Wright (1967). Some of these may be available for use only by accredited psychologists, but this does not preclude the possibility of interdisciplinary research. All avenues should be explored.

When the researcher is not successful in finding an appropriate instrument in published materials, she can contact the National Health Planning Information Center (NHPIC) for a computerized search. In response to a phone call or letter the NHPIC will search for any kind of documents relevant to the labels given, and will also refer the inquirer to other sources and clearing houses. [Address: NHPIC, Nursing Information, P.O. Box 1600, Prince George's Plaza branch, Hyattsville, Maryland 20788, telephone (301) 927-6410.]

Interviews

Interviews cannot be considered merely as an alternative to paper-and-pencil questionnaires. Rather, interviewing will be used at all stages of arranging for and performing a study. It is a technique often used in laboratory studies of human subjects and in field studies involving normal human subjects as well as those whose ability to read and write is deficient or impaired. In addition, it is often useful in piloting all sorts of procedures and may, of course, be the main data-gathering method, as with the Clark and Clark Doll Test used for interviewing children (see Table 6-1).

When interview is the principal method for gathering research data, the five discrete steps required in the measurement process (as noted by Cannell and

Table 6-1 An Example of an Interview Schedule

I am going to ask you some questions about these dolls standing in front of you. I want you to play the doll-choosing game by pointing to one of the dolls in response to the questions. Later, I will ask you some questions about other things not concerned with the dolls. I have a list of questions here and I'll be writing your score to see how you do on the game.

1   Which one of these dolls is most like the one you have at home?
2   Which doll would you like to play with? (Which doll would you not like to play with?)
3   Which doll is a nice doll? (Which doll is a bad doll?)
4   Which doll do you like the best? (Which doll do you not like?)
5   Which doll has a nice color? (Which doll does not have a nice color?)
6   Which doll would you invite to your birthday party? (Which doll would you not invite to your birthday party?)
7   Which doll would you want to walk home from school with? (Which doll would you not want to walk home from school with?)
8   Which doll would you like to have for a sister or brother? (Which doll would you not like to have for a sister or brother?)
9   Which doll would you like to have for a best friend? (Which doll would you not like to have for a best friend?)
10 Which doll would you want to have sit by you in school? (Which doll would you not want to have sit next to you in school?)
11 Which doll would you want to have live in a house near you? (Which doll would you not want to have live in a house near you?)
12 Which doll would you want to see and talk to very often? (Which doll would you not want to see and talk to very often?)
13 Which doll would you want to have living in America? (Which doll would you not want to have living in America?)
14 Which doll looks like a white doll?
15 Which doll looks like an Indian doll?
16 Which doll looks most like you?

The rest of the questions don't involve choosing a doll. I just want you to answer each of these questions.

17 Who are the four children in your classroom that are your best friends?
18 Who are the four children in your classroom that you would like to work with on a special class project?
19 Who are the four children in your classroom that you would like to sit next to?
20 If you could have a birthday party, which four children in your classroom would you invite?

Source: From Frances J. Anderson and N. Hamm, Adaptation of Clark and Clark Doll Test and Bogardus Social Distance Scale. In Western Council on Higher Education for Nursing, *Instruments for measuring nursing practice and other health care variables*. Washington, D.C.: DHEW.

Kahn, 1968) are: (1) creating or selecting an interview schedule, (2) conducting the interview, (3) recording the responses, (4) creating a code and set of rules for translating responses into numbers, and (5) coding the responses.

We have already discussed the selection of an instrument. We will not attempt to recapitulate here all that the nurse has already learned about interviewing, either on her own or through the fine presentations by Cannell and Kahn (1968) or Hyman (1954), which an interviewer should study before collecting data by that method.

Never forget that the interviewer is a participant. Some social scientists regard observers as outside the situation they are studying, as distinguished from a participant observer who shares fully in the ongoing activities of the organization. Johnson (1975), however, recognized that all observers are participant members of society who, at the very least, share a natural language and cultural meanings. Johnson and others (Brenner, 1978) deny that the ideal of objectivity can ever be reached, and they reject the term *objective* for *intersubjective* to emphasize that the observer is part of the field of observation. Thus Johnson includes even experimental research, surveys, and field research as modes of participant observation. If anyone present is a participant, then it is obvious how thoroughly an interviewer participates.

Argyle (1978) studied the process of interviewing and noted that error is introduced by uncontrolled interaction between interviewer and respondent, by failure to communicate with shared concepts, by respondent tendency to say "yes" even when "no" may be a truer answer, and by the tendency to give socially desirable answers. Furthermore, he called attention to the importance of finding out whether a respondent has the necessary experience or knowledge to answer a question usefully, and to the necessity of using pilot studies to uncover the language respondents actually use.

The research interviewer should clarify the objectives of the interview before beginning. This involves describing the possible or probable benefits of the research for the individual respondent and for society. This may require a tactful sales pitch, since the benefits will almost always be removed in time, space, and person from the individual respondent. The interviewer should inform the respondent of an estimated length of time required for the interview, should provide her own credentials, and should assure confidentiality of the information she is about to receive.

Respondents have the right to terminate their participation at any time they wish, leading one to ask, "Why should any of them consent to participate at all?" Cannell and Kahn have discussed both intrinsic and instrumental motivation. Intrinsic motivation depends on the fact or hope that the respondent values the experience of the interview and his or her relationship with the interviewer. He or she wants to maintain self-esteem and be perceived by the interviewer as a person who does not violate important social norms in thought or act. This may, in fact, bias the data. Instrumental motivation derives from seeing the research as a worthwhile effort.

The researcher must finally provide the observations or interpretations of them regardless of who actually spoke the words, checked the paper, or experienced certain physiological states. The researcher provides interpretations regardless of whether that meaning was almost concealed in a large amount of other material (as in logs and diaries), whether it was predigested and delivered up in the form of critical incidents, and whether the measurements were obtained via mechanical instruments, paper-and-pencil questionnaires, or interviewer-checked schedules. Thus, there is continuity from the obvious to the hidden, from the purely logical to the emotional, from the quantitative to the qualitative. Lofland (1971) argues that the bedrock of knowing something—persons or situations—is qualitative, rather than quantitative, and that statistical portrayals must always be grounded in the context of direct, face-to-face knowing. Lofland's qualitative knowing can be illustrated by the difference between having personal experience with clients or reading about some other nurse's experience. Lofland asks researchers to combine the humanistic reportage of what the world is qualitatively like for persons who are subjects of research with statistical portrayals that provide an appropriate degree of economy and clarity. Campbell, well known as a quantitative experimentalist, also strongly recommends (1978) a combined qualitative and quantitative approach to "social knowing."

A combined qualitative and quantitative approach should appeal to nurses who may have considerable personal knowledge of events they want to study and have recognized the dilemma of serving at the juncture of scientific and humanistic experiences discussed at the beginning of Chapter 1.

Nursing research literature, in common with the sociological literature Lofland describes, seems somewhat lacking in qualitative study. For example, where are the case studies of what the hospital experience is like around the clock for patients? The question Lofland would have us ask is, "What are the characteristics of acts, activities, meanings, participation, relationships, settings, and the forms they assume and variations they display in this sector of social life I am now observing?"

On-site observations made by the researcher are a logical extension of interview technique. Selltiz et al. (1976) pose four broad questions concerning use of observation: (1) What should be observed? (2) How should observations be recorded? (3) What procedures should be used to assure the accuracy of the observations? (4) What relationships should exist between the observer and the observed? These four questions are not completely different from those which must be asked about any method, but the answers differ, reemphasizing our point that method should be selected after the purpose and problem are very clear. Thus, the first question is apropos only if it applies to specifics after the general strategy of observation has been judged to be appropriate to the problem as either the primary or supplementary data-collection method. The answer to the second question depends on how unobtrusive the process of recording must be, whether it is more feasible to code data in the field or back at the desk, whether behavior should be photographed for further study, and so on. Any of these decisions may require piloting.

The question of assuring accuracy of observation has been problematic for nurses who do research. It is, of course, the problem of reliability, and the difficulty of establishing reliability in studies involving observation is large. The well-known nursing example is evaluation of quality of nursing care (see Hageman; Ventura in this volume; also Haussman and Hegyvary, 1977; Haussman et al., 1976; Jelinek et al., 1974). In the effort to enhance reliability, attention has been paid to refinement of the observation protocol as well as to simultaneous use of more than one observer. Use of a carefully structured, perhaps standardized, instrument and two or more observers are both conditions that lead to the necessity to train observers. Training observers is a tricky business that is beyond the scope of this book; we mention it to call attention to its fundamental importance to reliability, and therefore to validity.

The fourth question, concerning the relationship of the observer and observed, leads to the literature about participant observation. Are the observers in a setting to participate fully in the regular activities as well as observing for the research? Will they be observers only? Or is there some other combination of these two orientations? Any logical, systematic arrangement is possible so long as it is also ethical. The participant observer whose observer identity is kept secret may be called a researcher in some circles, but a stooge or spy in others. Use of such epithets makes different viewpoints clear and underscores the importance of obtaining clearance from the appropriate institutional review boards (IRBs) or committees. One need not look far to find classic studies that would not be permitted under present guidelines for research on human subjects.

Questionnaires

Strictly speaking, questionnaires are interrogation protocols that call for either oral or written responses. In this broad sense, we will discuss both paper-and-pencil protocols and spoken questions, and then add remarks concerning special aspects of each.

"The world is full of well-meaning people who believe that anyone who can write plain English and has a modicum of common sense can produce a good questionnaire" (Oppenheim, 1966, preface). Oppenheim thought this might be so, providing they were willing to go through a sufficient number of piloted revisions—perhaps as many as eight—to establish validity. Other experts, too (Selltiz et al., 1976; Shaw and Wright, 1967), have deplored the fact that questionnaires have too often been used without evidence of validity. It is certain that too many nursing questionnaires have been constructed only to lie idle after one hasty use. It has become evident that with regard to evaluation of nursing care quality, there must be further validation of instruments before additional progress can be made. Thus, it is preferable to search out and use an existing instrument, if an appropriate one can be found. Regardless of the source of the instrument, the researcher should describe its limitations and probably report split-half reliability. In the words of Likert (1932):

> The ease and simplicity with which attitude scales can be checked for split-half reliability and internal consistency would seem to make it desirable to determine the

reliability and examine the internal consistency of each attitude scale for each group upon which it is used. It is certainly reasonable to suppose that just as an intelligence test which has been standardized upon one cultural group is not applicable to another so an attitude scale which has been constructed for one cultural group will hardly be applicable in its existing form to other cultural groups.

(Perhaps it should be pointed out that this is much easier to do today than when Likert first proposed it, since we now have computers to do the required calculations.)

When the split-half method is used, the single test administered to the group is split into two by obtaining one score on all odd-numbered items and another score on all even-numbered items. The correlation between these two sets of scores estimates the reliability of the entire test (Green, 1970). According to Thorndike and Hagen (1969), any measure of reliability based on a single testing is really a measure of internal consistency.

To date the best resource for research instruments for nursing is the two-volume work titled *Instruments for Measuring Nursing Practice and Other Health Care Variables*, developed by the Western Council on Higher Education for Nursing (WCHEN) of the Western Interstate Commission for Higher Educa-tion and published by DHEW. The compilation contains reproductions and critiques of 135 psychosocial instruments and 19 physiological protocols plus annotations, references, appendixes, and indexes. Figure 6-1 shows the model used for the classification of psychosocial instruments. Other sources for instru-ments on some health topics include Buros (1974) and Shaw and Wright (1967).

Investigators should also feel free to write to authors of either copyrighted or uncopyrighted instruments to ask for permission to use an instrument either in toto or as a basis for a revised version. Many, probably most, researchers will respond favorably. To correspond on any matter of research interest is consis-tent with the aim of a vigorous research community in nursing. If permission is refused, it is apparent that the copyright must be observed as assiduously with regard to certain instruments as it is with regard to ideas in the literature review or copied materials in the library or classroom. Multiple copies of copyrighted material may not be made for any purpose without explicit permission from the copyright holder (Smith, 1976). Some materials must remain uncopyrighted and in the public domain because their development was supported by public fund-ing. Individuals can claim a copyright even when it is not registered, although such a claim must be dealt with by legal authorities.

If no suitable instrument can be found, then developing one should be regarded as a project in itself. Table 6-2 illustrates a specialized instrument developed to measure environmental fear of public health nurses. Presumably such a group would be highly motivated to cooperate in instrument development or to respond to it after its development. It therefore seems likely that the instrument has a high degree of internal validity. We have also included (Table 6-3) the editor's critique of the instrument to illustrate the expert help these volumes provide.

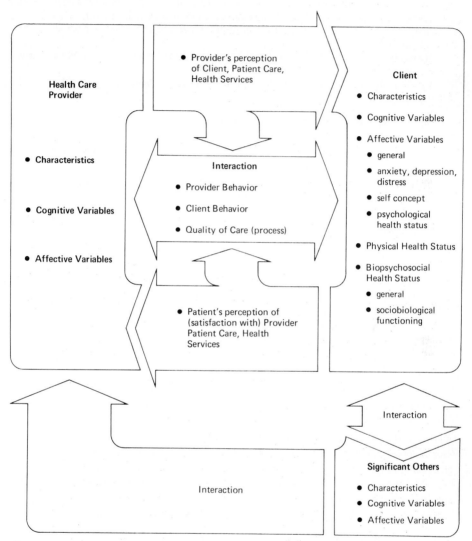

Figure 6-1   Bloch model for the classification of psychosocial instruments.

Although we have had a good deal to say about the care with which research instruments should be constructed under ideal circumstances, nurses should not use lack of a validated instrument as an excuse to avoid data collection on pressing problems. Falkner and Robinson (1976) devised an interview schedule

Table 6-2   Environmental Fear Scale

There have been a good many stories in the newspapers and on television recently about "crime in the streets." The stories are frequently about a woman being attacked, having her purse snatched, being threatened by a large group of young people, etc. Many women have stated that they are afraid to be on the streets alone.

It would be understandable if public health nurses, women who are frequently on the streets alone, share this fear.

Are you afraid? (Please check the blank which best describes how you feel for each statement.)

Never	Infrequently	Sometimes	Often	Always	
_____	_____	_____	_____	_____	Driving along the street
_____	_____	_____	_____	_____	Walking along the street.
_____	_____	_____	_____	_____	Waiting on the street (for a bus, a light change)
_____	_____	_____	_____	_____	Getting into and out of your car
_____	_____	_____	_____	_____	Going into the home
_____	_____	_____	_____	_____	During the home visits
_____	_____	_____	_____	_____	In the halls of a building
_____	_____	_____	_____	_____	On the stairs in a building
_____	_____	_____	_____	_____	In the elevator
_____	_____	_____	_____	_____	Other (please specify)

Source: Mary R. Castles and Patricia M. Keith, in Western Council on Higher Education for Nursing, *Instruments for measuring nursing practice and other health care variables*. Washington, D.C.: DHEW.

Table 6-3   Information and Critique for the Environmental Fear Scale

Variable: Public health nurses' fear of the environment. It is operationally defined as "the perception of threat and the frequency of threat associated with a given spatial area."

Description:
Nature and content: This is a one-page, self-report rating scale. The first item asks, "Are you ever afraid during your working day?" The next eight items specify environmental areas where fear might be experienced. Space is provided for the respondent to specify other areas where she may have experienced fear. Five response alternatives are provided: never, infrequently, sometimes, often, always.

There is a brief introductory paragraph at the top of the form preceding the directions. Administration and scoring: The instrument is self-administered, and no particular arrangements or settings are required. It can be completed in approximately 5 minutes. Subject scores are obtained by summing across the 10 items; total possible scores range from 1 to 50.

Development:
Rationale: The authors stated that the instrument was not based on any specific theory.

Source of items: The items were derived from unstructured interviews with graduate students who had recent public health experience.
Procedure for development: From the interviews mentioned above, items were developed, submitted to another sample of public health nurses, and revised based upon input from that sample.
Reliability and validity: Cronbach's alpha produced a reliability coefficient of .91; the Cornell Technique of Scalogram Analysis produced a reliability coefficient of .93. In addition to face validity, there is evidence of construct validity as shown by the fact that respondents whose

Table 6-3 Information and Critique for the Environmental Fear Scale (*Continued*)

families and colleagues expressed concern about their safety scored higher than others. The instrument was utilized in a sample of 159 public health nurses, students, and staff employed by or assigned to official and nonofficial agencies who were working in neighborhoods with various social, economic, and racial characteristics.

Use in research: A description of the instrument and its use is contained in the articles referenced below.
Comments: This instrument appears to have potential for development into a useful tool for measuring environmental fear. A more refined scoring system would increase the instrument's reliability, i.e., assigning numerical frequencies to the answer choices as opposed to the present choices. In addition, in order to be assigned a score of 50, a respondent would have to have completed the tenth item, "Other"; no specific information was provided relative to that item.

Some evidence of validity is shown in the difference in scores for nurses whose families and colleagues expressed concern for their safety, as compared with other nurses. As the items are now written (e.g., going into the home, during the home visits), its applicability is limited to public health nurses or others who make home visits. However, it would be easy to adapt the instrument as a tool for measuring environmental fear for a more general population. This might be useful, for example, in the study of health-seeking behavior (e.g., going to clinics, etc.). The instrument might also be adapted to development of an environmental fear scale for hospital patients.

References:

Castles, Mary R., and Patricia M. Keith: Correlates of environmental fear in the role of the public health nurse. *Nursing Research*, 1971, *20*, 245–249.
Keith, Patricia M., and Mary R. Castles: Fear and rejection of patients by health practitioners. *Social Science and Medicine*, 1975, *9*, 500–505.

Source: Mary Reardon Castles, college of nursing, Wayne State University, Detroit, Michigan 48202. In Western Council on Higher Education for Nursing, *Instruments for measuring nursing practice and other health care variables*. Washington, D.C.: DHEW.

that enabled them to identify 50 different decubitus ulcer treatments that were in use in the institutions they studied. The treatments were accompanied by extreme inconsistency in responsibility for planning, delivery, and evaluation of the care. Other researchers, too (Francis, 1977; Hightower et al., 1977), studied "abused tasks" and were able to use the results to achieve substantial change in their nursing service.

Watkin (1974) mentioned questionnaire construction along with sampling as points where expert consultation may be helpful. Even so, he covers the most essential points: that questionnaires should employ neutral words that do not suggest to a respondent that one answer is better than another; that written protocols should be pleasing to look at and simple for the respondent to complete; and that feedback should be offered or provided when feasible. As professional practitioners with some knowledge of research, we should probably refuse to have anything to do with questionnaires that fail to meet these basic criteria. Ware's Health Perceptions Questionnaire (Table 6-4) appears to meet them admirably. Aspinall (1975) reported a questionnaire that provided more accurate and systematic patient admission information than was obtained by nurses in face-to-face interviews.

Table 6-4   Health Perceptions Questionnaire (HPQ)

Please read each of the following statements, and then circle one of the numbers on each line to indicate whether the statement is true or false *for you*.

There are no right or wrong answers.
If a statement is definitely true for you, circle 5.
If it is mostly true for you, circle 4.
If you don't know whether it is true or false, circle 3.
If it is mostly false for you, circle 2.
If is definitely false for you, circle 1.
Some of the statements may look or seem like others,
but each statement is different and should be rated
by itself.

	Definitely true	Mostly true	Don't know	Mostly false	Definitely false
According to the doctors I've seen, my health is now excellent	5	4	3	2	1
I try to avoid letting illness interfere with my life	5	4	3	2	1
I seem to get sick a little easier than other people	5	4	3	2	1
I feel better now than I ever have before	5	4	3	2	1
I will probably be sick a lot in the future	5	4	3	2	1
I never worry about my health	5	4	3	2	1
Most people get sick a little easier than I do	5	4	3	2	1
I don't like to go to the doctor	5	4	3	2	1
I am somewhat ill	5	4	3	2	1
In the future, I expect to have better health than other people I know	5	4	3	2	1
I was so sick once I thought I might die	5	4	3	2	1
I'm not as healthy now as I used to be	5	4	3	2	1
I worry about my health more than other people worry about their health	5	4	3	2	1
When I'm sick, I try to keep going as usual	5	4	3	2	1
My body seems to resist illness very well	5	4	3	2	1
Getting sick once in a while is a part of my life	5	4	3	2	1
I am as healthy as anybody I know	5	4	3	2	1
I think my health will be worse in the future than it is now	5	4	3	2	1
I've never had an illness that lasted a long period of time	5	4	3	2	1
Others seem more concerned about their health than I am about mine	5	4	3	2	1

Table 6-4 Health Perceptions Questionnaire (HPQ) (*Continued*)

When I'm sick, I try to keep it to myself	5	4	3	2	1
My health is excellent	5	4	3	2	1
I expect to have a very healthy life	5	4	3	2	1
My health is a concern in my life	5	4	3	2	1
I accept that sometimes I'm just going to be sick	5	4	3	2	1
I have been feeling bad lately	5	4	3	2	1
It doesn't bother me to go to a doctor	5	4	3	2	1
I have never been seriously ill	5	4	3	2	1
When there is something going around, I usually catch it	5	4	3	2	1
Doctors say that I am now in poor health	5	4	3	2	1
When I think I am getting sick, I fight it	5	4	3	2	1
I feel about as good now as I ever have	5	4	3	2	1

Source: John E. Ware, Jr., in Western Council on Higher Education for Nursing, *Instruments for measuring nursing practice and other health care variables*. Washington, D.C.: DHEW.

Paper-and-pencil questionnaires may be preceded, followed by, or combined with interviews. Question construction is similar (see Interviews, above).

The mailed questionnaire presents a special set of difficulties which have become an area of research in themselves. Marshall and Gee (1976) collected a bibliography of some 110 items and abstracted 19 of them. Some of the conclusions were as follows:

Anderson and Berdie   Effectiveness of different follow-up techniques varied according to the group of respondents involved.

Berdie   The response rate of professors was not affected by length of questionnaire (up to four pages).

Carpenter   Reducing personalization of questionnaires reduced response rate, although not greatly.

Champion and Sear   Response rates were greater for "egoistic" rather than "altruistic" types of cover letters.

Cox, Anderson, and Fulcher   Response rate to personalized questionnaires was better than to nonpersonalized, but there was no difference in response rate between the group that received follow-up letters and the group that did not.

Dillman and Frey   A phone call reminder caused earlier return of questionnaires, but did not affect response rate.

Etzel and Walker   Sending a duplicate questionnaire and return envelope with the follow-up did not cause a higher response rate than follow-up without duplicate.

Fuller   There was no difference in response rates between Navy enlisted men who remained anonymous and those who did not; officers who put their service numbers on questionnaires recorded more pro-Navy statements than officers who remained anonymous.

Hackler and Bourgette   Monetary reward ($1) increased response rate at any stage (with questionnaire, after a mailed reminder, and/or after a phone call).

Hensley   Response rates were higher when types of postage on inner and outer envelope were different (metered postage and a commemorative stamp were the best combination).

Hinrichs   Response rate was better when respondents felt singled out as part of a sample than when an entire population was studied.

Huck and Gleason   Responses were as good when an "intent postcard" for the respondent to return was included with the questionnaire as when a reminder postcard was sent later.

Linsky   Personalization of the cover letter affected response rate more than stressing the social utility of the research, explaining the place and importance of the respondent in the study, or appealing for help. Linsky reviewed all the research done on mail questionnaires since 1935 and concluded that there is strong evidence for the positive effect of five variables, including (1) the use of one or more follow-up reminders, (2) contact with respondents before sending the questionnaire, (3) type of postage on outgoing and return mail, (4) cash rewards included with the questionnaire, and (5) the sponsoring organization and title of the person signing the cover letter.

Mason, Dressel, and Bain   No significant differences in response rate were found between those receiving long or short questionnaires or between those having their name and address or a code number on the form.

Sheth and Roscoe   Some follow-up methods work better in certain geographic areas than in others.

Stevens   The difference in response rates for precoded and uncoded questionnaires was not significant.

Wiseman   A monetary reward of 10 cents and a postcard reminder each increased response rate by 8 percent.

Checklists, Inventories, and Grids

Checklists, inventories, and grids are close relatives in that they all deal with dichotomous, yes-or-no answers. A check stands for a "yes," and we have all seen health histories and physical examination forms, for example, that are set up as checklists. The validity of these forms varies widely, depending on the care with which they have been piloted. For example, the reader may have seen rather amateurish forms developed to collect information for a physical examination for summer camp and be able to contrast this with one or more of the extremely sophisticated forms developed for the client's self-report of health history. Some are designed for computer use, others to make "yes" answers almost impossible for the primary health care provider to overlook. If there proved to be an advantage to it, this information could easily be put on a grid that separated illnesses according to the decades of a person's life. We have provided as Table 6-5 a grid example that may prove to be a helpful worksheet for students who are reading research papers. It also serves to illustrate the way three variables—in this case method, setting, and statistics—can be put on a table. For most health conditions, a grid would provide little additional information and be unnecessarily confusing. One notable exception, however, is the duration of the habit of cigarette smoking. Here, too, a grid is impractical because every year is important, and a grid might have to show spaces to check 70 years or so of cigarette smoking. The answer to this problem provides the classic example of an index. An index is not an instrument in itself, but a method of scoring. Thus the numbers of years the person has smoked, multiplied by the number of packs smoked per day, provides an index to smoking behavior that is called *pack years*.

In theory, there is no limit to the number of items that can be included in an index score. Oppenheim (1966) pointed out a method for resolving doubt concerning whether to include an item in an index score. He advised calculating the index without the item, then correlating the item with the index as a whole, and deciding on the basis of the correlation whether it should be included.

Indexes should be used more often in nursing research. If they are constructed carefully, they act as "data crunchers," helping to provide the clear and parsimonious picture that is the aim of data analysts.

Logs and Diaries

When respondents or communicators have not provided the consciously stripped-down data of critical incidents, sometimes logs, diaries, process recordings, letters, written histories, minutes of meetings, recollections, or other general materials can be content-analyzed to obtain needed data.

Content analysis is not a single technique with clearly defined right or wrong, but a whole catalog of techniques that are used by various professional communicators to identify recurring themes. Although it is beyond the scope of this book to present the numerous techniques and copious materials pertinent to content analysis, interested researchers can consult with a communications expert for help in designing a procedure for the current need. Berelson (1971), Holsti (1969), or Carney (1972) will introduce you to the literature of content analysis. Meanwhile, feel confident that a clearly defined, consistently applied, piloted procedure is defensible.

The Fox et al. (1965) study of stressful situations encountered by student nurses is a classic nursing study that used content analysis.

Although the research diary is expensive and difficult to design and analyze, it may be the best solution for problems having to do with food intake, insomnia, dreams, bed-wetting, or other behavior that is difficult or impossible to recall accurately after the passage of time. Typically, diaries deal with behavior rather than attitudes, interests, or emotions (Oppenheim, 1966), although a diary of emotions is conceivable. As the name implies, diaries deal with a specified span of time that must be decided on the basis of the problem. As is well recognized, a diary of food intake for only 1 day may be extremely atypical, but over a 1- or 2-week period may be much more accurate, assuming that the reporter is honest and dutiful.

In order to maintain the respondent's motivation, the researcher may want to visit or phone during the diary period. She should give careful thought to composing a clear form that looks interesting and important and has adequate space for recording. Although the researcher instructs the respondent in person, it is still a good idea to include written instructions that emphasize the need for

Table 6-5 Student's Grid for Classifying Research Studies

Method for data collection	Observation	Interview	Questionnaire/Self-reports (diaries, etc.)	Institutional records	Combinations
Real-life settings Statistics					
%					
C.T.					
Var.					
Cor.					
Surveys					
%					
C.T.					
Var.					
Cor.					
Laboratory experiment					
%					
C.T.					
Var.					
Cor.					

Key: % = percent or proportion; C.T. = central tendency (means); Var. = variances, ranges, deviations; Cor. = correlations.

accuracy and frankness, the danger of allowing the diary to influence one's behavior, and the importance of filling it out at regular intervals rather than at the end of the reporting period.

The Delphi Technique

The original Project Delphi was an Air Force–sponsored study by Rand Corporation. Its objective was to "obtain the most reliable consensus . . . of a large group of experts . . . by a series of intensive questionnaires interspersed with controlled opinion feedback" (Linstone and Turoff, 1975). The original problem asked experts to give opinion from the point of view of a Soviet strategic planner, and the method was almost forced into being by the cold war conditions of the 1950s. Because "hard" data—facts and figures—could not be obtained at the time, subjective expert opinion seemed to be the best available source of information. The justifications for the first study are still valid for many applications of Delphi today, notably those in health care evaluation.

After 25 years of evolution, there are almost as many variations of Delphi as there are investigators who have employed it, but the conventional Delphi uses iterative polling with feedback to elicit a forecast from experts by means of a more or less forced consensus. The most essential elements are three: iteration (repetition) of the rounds of questioning, polling, or asking "experts" for opinions on something; providing feedback of information respondents need to take into consideration before their next response; consensus (general agreement) to approach the policy-making function that Delphi often serves. That is, if the experts think a certain thing will happen, we can and probably should prepare for it.

This explication of Delphi is vastly oversimplified. We have mentioned Delphi mostly to forewarn the innocent. Sackman (1975) provided a critique of Delphi which ended with 16 evaluative conclusions. He showed that Delphis often fall short of recognized professional social science standards for establishing conceptual frameworks, for questionnaire and item design, pilot testing, sampling, and for measuring reliability and validity. In addition, Sackman cited studies concerning the doubtful value of "expert" opinion (which, some studies reported, roughly corresponded to that of randomly selected housewives). He noted further that Delphi inhibits healthy adversary processes such as playing devil's advocate, and so forth. Others, too, have noted that directors of Delphi studies sometimes push too hard for consensus, thus cutting off expressions of individuality and too often avoiding group and face-to-face discussions, even when such discussions might have been economically or geographically feasible.

In summary, investigators who plan to use Delphi are obligated to investigate the literature on opinion polling and questionnaire construction and to put to use what is already known about avoiding bias. Delphi, if used as a heuristic (exploratory) device, should not then be interpreted as a scientific prediction. In short, it should not be used to provide an unwarranted illusion of precision.

Q: List the seven categories of measurement methods discussed in this chapter and attach the names of some nursing research variables to each category, using as a basis your conviction that the variable could be specified by a measurement variate operationalized by the method of the category. Can you think of a nursing research variable which cannot be specified by variates based on any of the methods discussed in this chapter?

REFERENCES

Argyle, Michael: An appraisal of the new approach to the study of social behavior. In Michael Brenner, Peter Marsh, and Marilyn Brenner (Eds.), *The social contexts of method*. London: Croom Helm, 1978.

Aspinall, Mary Jo: Development of a patient-centered admission questionnaire and its comparison with the nursing interview. *Nursing Research*, 1975, *24*(5).

Berelson, Bernard: *Content analysis in communications research*. New York: Hafner, 1971 (facsimile of 1952 ed.).

Bermosk, Loretta Sue, and Raymond J. Corsini: *Critical incidents in nursing*. Philadelphia: Saunders, 1973.

Brenner, Michael: Interviewing: The social phenomenology of a research instrument. In Michael Brenner, Peter Marsh, and Marilyn Brenner (Eds.), *The social contexts of method*. London: Croom Helm, 1978.

Buros, Oscar K.: *Tests in print*. Highland Park, N.J.: Gryphon, 1974.

Campbell, Donald T.: Qualitative knowing in action research. In M. Brenner, P. Marsh, and M. Brenner (Eds.), *The social contexts of method*. London: Croom Helm, 1978.

Cannell, Charles F., and Robert L. Kahn: Interviewing. In Gardner Lindzey, and Elliot Aronson, *The handbook of social psychology*. Reading, Mass.: Addison-Wesley, 1954, 1968.

Carney, Thomas F.: *Content analysis*. Winnipeg: University of Manitoba, 1972.

Falkner, Karen, and Mary Ellen Atwood Robinson: Development of criteria and protocol for client decubitus ulcers evaluation. Unpublished master's thesis, SUNY at Buffalo, 1976.

Flanagan, John C.: The critical incident technique. *Psychological Bulletin*, 1954, *51*, 327–358.

Fox, David J., Lorraine K. Diamond, and associates: *Satisfying and stressful situations in basic programs in nursing education*. New York: Columbia University Teachers College, Bureau of Publications, 1965.

Francis, Gloria: Nursing personnel functions study: Who is doing what in the hospital? *Supervisor Nurse*, 1977 (April).

Friedrichs, Jürgen, and Hartmut Lüdtke: *Participant observation*. Lexington, Mass.: Lexington Books, 1975.

Green, John A.: *Measurement and evaluation*. New York: Dodd, Mead, 1970.

Hagen, Elizabeth, and Luverne Wolff: *Nursing leadership behavior in general hospitals*. New York: Columbia University Teachers College, 1961.

Hardin, C. A.: "Critical incident": What does it mean to research? *Nursing Research*, 1955, *3*(3).

Haussman, R. K., Dieter, and Sue T. Hegyvary: Monitoring quality of nursing care, part III. Hyattsville, Md.: U.S. DHEW, Division of Nursing, 1977. (DHEW Publication no. HRA 77-70)

———, ———, and John F. Newman: Monitoring quality of nursing care, part II. Bethesda, Md.: U.S. DHEW, Division of Nursing, 1976. (DHEW Publication no. HRA 76-7)

Hightower, Lina, Rebecca Patterson, and Linda Pearson: Putting nursing research to work. *Supervisor Nurse*, 1977 (April).

Holsti, Ole R.: *Content analysis for the social sciences and humanities*. Reading, Mass.: Addison-Wesley, 1969.

Hyman, Herbert H.: *Interviewing in social research*. Chicago: University of Chicago, 1954.

Jelinek, Richard C., R. K. Dieter Haussman, Sue T. Hegyvary, and John F. Newman: A methodology for monitoring quality of nursing care, part I. Bethesda, Md.: U.S. DHEW, Division of Nursing, 1974. (Stock no. 017-044-00095-9)

Johnson, John M.: *Doing field research*. New York: Free Press, 1975.

Kramer, Marlene: *Reality shock*. St. Louis: Mosby, 1974.

Likert, Rensis: The method of constructing an attitude scale, 1932. In Gary M. Maranell, *Scaling*. Chicago: Aldine, 1974.

Linstone, Harold A., and Murray Turoff: *The Delphi method*. Reading, Mass.: Addison-Wesley, 1975.

Lofland, John: *Analyzing social settings*. Belmont, Calif.: Wadsworth, 1971.

Marshall, Brian G., and Carol Ann Gee: Mail questionnaire research. Council of Planning Librarians, Exchange Bibliography, 1976 (March).

Maslow, A. H.: Problem-centering vs. means-centering in science. *Philosophy of Science*, 1946, *13*, 326–331.

Nixon, John E.: The mechanics of questionnaire construction. *Journal of Educational Research*, 1954, *57*(7).

Oppenheim, A. N.: *Questionnaire design and attitude measurement*. New York: Basic Books, 1966.

Sackman, Harold: *Delphi critique*. Lexington, Mass.: Heath, 1975.

Selltiz, Claire et al.: *Research methods in social relations*. New York: Holt, 1959, 1965, 1976.

Shaw, Marvin E., and Jack M. Wright: *Scales for the measurement of attitudes*. New York: McGraw-Hill, 1967.

Smith, Eldred R.: Memorandum. University Library, SUNYAB, Buffalo, New York, November 17, 1976.

Thorndike, Robert L., and Elizabeth Hagen: *Measurement and evaluation in psychology and education*. New York: Wiley, 1969.

Watkin, Brian: Attitude surveys. *Nursing Mirror*, 1974, *138*(13), 55.

Webb, Eugene J., Donald T. Campbell, Richard D. Schwartz, and Lee Sechrest: *Unobtrusive measures*. Chicago: Rand McNally, 1966.

Weick, Karl E.: Systematic observational methods. In Gardner Lindzey, and Elliot Aronson, *The handbook of social psychology*. Reading, Mass.: Addison-Wesley, 1968.

Chapter 7

What Settings and Persons Are Researched?

Previous chapters have explored the purposes for which research in nursing is done and the measurement methods which are employed. Samples of subjects have been referred to in the vaguest way as the source of *N* sets of scores. But nursing research has to be conducted somewhere, sometime, on someone, and the planning decisions about setting and sample are just as crucial as the choices of problem and measurement methods. This chapter explains why and how setting and sample are selected.

THE PROBLEM OF GENERALIZABILITY

Research is not done simply to satisfy curiosity about the events which are studied. Those events have become historical as soon as they are recorded, and although history is interesting to some of us, it does not command public resources for that reason. Public resources (research support) are made available because of the public's need to foresee and control what is going to happen. The presentiment that historical events may to some extent be repeated is the basis of support for research. However, if we are to be clear about generalizability we must perceive exactly wherein the repeatability of history resides. Obviously an event is unique in its happening in one time and place. Another event, in another time and place, may resemble the first event in some or many respects, but it is another event. *It is the pattern of events that may appear to be repetitive.* Thus when an event of type B always seems to follow an event of type

A, we say that A causes B. We are really observing a pattern of relationships between events which are similar enough to be typed or classified as A events and B events. In nursing research we do not expect to find such simple cause-effect patterns, but rather elaborate correlational networks among events which are more or less repetitive. This can be illustrated in research which classifies type A and B personality tendencies as precursors of heart attacks (Friedman and Rosenman, 1974). Persons with type A personalities are not automatically condemned to become victims of heart disease. If they have a heart attack, their personality cannot be designated as the sole cause. The point is that personality type correlates to some extent with the incidence of fatal or serious heart attacks. It has been fairly well established that this pattern repeats itself. Thus, people are advised to reduce their stress-producing type A activities in the effort to prevent heart attacks. In research terminology this represents an effort to predict and control future events by recognizing and manipulating patterns. Unfortunately, the desired control can be illusory. Wishful thinking can project a pattern where none exists or can distort a perceived pattern fantastically. When good research has been done it is, after all, just good history that has been written. The problem remains to decide wisely to what new settings the discovered patterns apply. This is the problem of generalizability.

Semmelweis finally perceived a pattern in events in the Vienna Lying-In Hospital which generalized to events in childbearing settings everywhere. We honor him as one of the greatest health care researchers because he found a pattern in some parochial events which had universal applicability. Yet professional judgment is required in each obstetrical setting to see how the pattern applies at that time and place under those unique circumstances. Thus, at the present time in the United States the problem of postpartum infection is not the overriding cause of most maternal mortality as it was in Semmelweis's day, but is confounded with a variety of illness-wellness factors including, for example, the mother's total drug diet—a construct that includes everything ingested, injected, and smoked. Seldom does health research uncover patterns of such universality as that discovered by Semmelweis, and deciding the limits of generalizability of most research findings is a continual, unavoidable problem for professional judgment. In this chapter we plan to suggest some guidelines for decisions about the limits of generalizability, but first we need to study the scientific principles on which claims of generalizability are based.

RULES FOR GENERALIZING

If it were possible to reduce professional judgment to the act of following a definite set of rules, both the rewards and the risks of professional stature would disappear. Have no fear that we are going to demystify the judgments nurses must make about the applicability of general knowledge to specific nursing situations. We can delineate some principles which properly guide judgment up to a point where a veil descends and only time can tell who is wise and who is foolish. Respect for these principles can probably increase the probability of wisdom. The three principles of research design which promote generalizability for research findings are (1) random assignment, (2) random selection, and (3) replication. This trinity of sanctified research behaviors is taken up in the three subsections which follow.

Internal Validity

In the section titled Validity in Chapter 5, the validity of a measurement procedure was said to be an interpretation of what it measures. Validity is a crucial characteristic of research measurements. It is essential to have a good idea of what each scale measures, or we will not know what we are talking about when we discuss statistics computed from the measurements. Just as the validity of a particular measurement device can be questioned, the validity of an entire research design can be questioned. The validity of a research design is an interpretation of the design in terms of the type and limits of generalization it permits. The issue of the type of generalization permissible from a design is called the *internal validity* issue, whereas the limits of generalizability issue is called the *external validity* issue. The two types of internal validity a design may provide are (1) descriptive validity and (2) causative validity. Both of these are concerned with the statements that may be made about the data collected in the research as a result of the ways those data were collected and analyzed.

Internal validity is concerned solely with the kinds of statements that are possible about the data in hand. It is not concerned with issues regarding what might be said about other possible data sets as a result of what is learned from the data set under consideration.

Descriptive validity refers to the completeness, accuracy, and insightfulness of the description of the phenomena under study afforded by the data analyses. We emphasize the analyses rather than the data because only analyses are reported. The analyses cannot be better than the data. The completeness and accuracy of the data contain the potential for these characteristics of the analyses. However, the analyses can be worse than the data, and frequently are. It is sad that some researchers collect excellent data and do miserable analyses, while other researchers collect bad data and massage them with sophisticated analytic techniques. Both of these eventualities are wasteful. We emphasize the desirability of teamwork in research because the people who can collect excellent data are seldom the people who can perform excellent analyses.

Completeness of the picture of events captured in data sets is a vital issue. Too often researchers measure only two, three, or four aspects of a situation which is far more complex in its dimensions. In the recent past the arithmetic difficulties of analyzing extensively multivariate research data sets were insuperable. The computer has revolutionized the field of social research data analysis and it is no longer excusable to oversimplify descriptions of social phenomena. Thus, a modern plan for studying attrition of students from nursing schools would have to include characteristics of the structure and organization of the schools, their processes of instruction, the recruitment and support of students, students' reasons for entering and leaving, as well as (perhaps) the personality traits of students that were commonly studied in the 1960s. The plan for a research study has to visualize all the relevant dimensions of the phenomena to be investigated and specify measurement procedures for all of them. The research plan which is adequate today is not only a multivariate plan, it is an adequately multivariate plan. In planning, when you think you have listed all the relevant facets of the problem situation, think again. After the research has been done there is no recovery from a supportable charge that the measurements were incomplete. Jargon for the list of dimensions brought under measurement in a research study (i.e., the list of research variates) is the *specification*. The charge of a *specification error* in the criticism of a study is the assertion that some crucial aspect(s) of the phenomena examined was not measured. A correct charge of this error is a knockout blow. It must be guarded against in the planning stage.

Frequently the relevance of a facet of the situation is clearly recognized, but a measurement procedure for assessing that facet either does not exist, or is too expensive, or is otherwise impossible to apply. This is when we realize that research is no rose garden. Ideals are as seldom fully achieved in research as in any other human enterprise. On the other hand, just doing the best one can is not always enough, and sometimes it makes sense to abandon a research plan because of the measurement difficulties that arise.

When plenty of money is available to pay for a study, a shotgun approach to specification sometimes is used. That is, the well-heeled but feckless researchers just go ahead and take every conceivable measurement. We do not endorse this approach because it is wasteful and seldom leads to sharp, insightful analytic outcomes. Subjecting persons to unnecessary data collecting may be ethically questionable, too. We do concede that occasionally the initial exploration of an important new problem may call for a shotgun approach. Still, some federal agencies seem to be too gullible about whether "more" and "bigger" imply "better." What we would like to see in a specification are *all* the variates which experience indicates are relevant, plus one or two additional variates which hunch suggests might turn out to be more relevant than previous results would lead one to expect.

The requirement of accuracy of description breaks down into the needs for (1) reasonable reliability of the measurements taken and (2) enough objects or subjects measured to provide adequate degrees of freedom for intended analyses. Reliability was discussed in Chapter 5. A research report should discuss the probable reliabilities of the measurements obtained and should make a strong case for the presumption of substantial reliability for each measurement device under the conditions of its employment in the research. Sometimes it is a good investment to actually include research on the reliabilities of the variates in the research plan, so that good numerical estimates of reliabilities will be available for the analyses of relationships among the variates. Availability of such reliability coefficients for the variates makes it possible to *disattenuate* the correlations among the variates, which means to adjust them for the effects of measurement errors. (Measurement errors always make correlations smaller in absolute value than they would be if the variates were perfectly measured; thus correlations are said to be attenuated by unreliabilities.) We will not be able to teach you the techniques of disattenuation (and indeed they are seldom used because of their expense and difficulty), but if you are able to recruit a sufficiently skilled analyst to your team you may want to explore in this area.

The degrees of freedom issue, or sample size issue, is an important one which will never be settled to everyone's satisfaction. We once heard a prominent statistician say, "Sample size is the only issue of real interest to a consulting statistician." At least it is true that if you consult a professional statistician about your research design you should expect to hear a great deal of advice about your sample size. Although we are not statisticians, we do need to understand that the adequacy of description is related to the number of objects or subjects measured. One common sense reason is that people are more impressed by a description of a large number of cases than by a description of a small number of cases, and quite properly so. Nursing research is not often going to discover lawful regularities which permit statements of exactly what can be expected in each new case. What we hope to discover are trends in cases which can be extrapolated to permit statements of what can be expected approximately in new cases, over an aggregate of new cases. An approximate regularity in the research cases leads to the expectation of a similar approximate regularity in some new set of cases. It makes sense to hesitate to extrapolate from data unless a reasonable amount of data underlie the generalization. It makes sense that more data should be more impressive than less data, other things being equal. What should be equal is the extent of scatter of the cases around the trend line or average which is the generalization. When there is very little scatter of cases around the statistical generalization, a small sample can be quite impressive, but when there is a great deal of scatter around the generalization, a rather large sample may be unimpressive. In Chapter 9 we provide a measure of the scatter of the cases around a statistical generalization, which provides a sort of "goodness of fit" measure for the generalization. As a rule we will assert that tight-fitting generalizations can be useful even when derived from moderate-sized samples, but loose-fitting generalizations are useful only when derived from rather large samples.

A more technical reason why adequacy of description is related to sample size involves the degrees of freedom requirements of various statistical generalizations. *Degrees of freedom* is a measurement concerned with the extent to which the sample size interacts with a statistic to bias the range of values the statistic is likely to take. You would have to study statistics at length to achieve an understanding of this, so we ask you to take our word for it that the correlational statistics which we emphasize in Chapter 9 are seriously biased in the direction of running too large when sample sizes are too small. Thus there are minimal sample sizes for the analytic procedures we recommend, and it is always nice to have a large rather than moderate sample size, especially when you do not know ahead of time (at the research planning stage) how much the data are likely to scatter around the generalization. It turns out that degrees of freedom requirements are related to the number of research variates and the number of constructs (thus the number of variables) involved, as well as to the goodness of fit of the generalization. We can only give some rule-of-thumb advice, as follows:

    1 Multiply the number of variables by 20 for a moderate-sized sample, and by 40 for a large sample.
    2 Multiply the number of variates by 10 for a moderate-sized sample, and by 20 for a large sample.

Usually these rules will give different answers, and we would suggest playing it safe by applying the more punishing rule. In planning, you sometimes know what the constructs are before you choose the indicating variates for the corresponding variables, and thus the first rule is useful before the second rule can be applied. On the other hand, sometimes the available theory is insufficient to permit a priori closure on the constructs, but you do know what the list of variates to be measured is, making the second rule useful at this stage. To recapitulate, strong generalizations to which the data fit tightly can be extrapolated from moderate-sized samples, but weak generalizations to which the data fit loosely should be extrapolated only from large samples.

    Another issue about the sample is its representativeness, and we are assuming that, large or moderate, the research sample is reasonably representative of the new sample to which extrapolation will be made. Proper statisticians are very concerned about the requirement of randomization in qualifying samples as representative. However, small random samples can be quite unrepresentative by chance. We are not concerned about randomization because we are convinced that the very act of randomizing in nursing research more often than not distorts the reality to which it is necessary to generalize. We do not urge you to randomize, but we do urge you to think out the reasons why what is approximately true of your research cases may also be approximately true of the new cases to which you intend to apply your research findings. Our rule is that you should select your research cases to be reasonably representative. Often this will not be very convincing and it will be necessary to hedge your bets, guard against disastrous failure of generalization, and wait to see what happens. Policy making, even when informed by good research, is risky. Later in this chapter we describe a strategy of replication that is the best procedure we can suggest. Meanwhile, expect any consulting statistician to be outraged when you propose to select a research sample without randomizing, and remember that you have hired the consultant to advise you, but you are in charge.

    The real value of the description research renders of the phenomena studied depends on the extent to which understanding is generated by the research report. Few aspects of human experience are more mysterious, and more difficult to communicate about or to program for, than the experience of understanding. Suppose we had a research report which described in detail some variety of ways to organize teams of hospital nurses and showed some definite relationships between organizational features and outcomes of nursing measured upon patients. This research might describe some arrangements for nursing and/or apparent consequences of organization which you had not previously known about. After reading the report, you would be able to say, "Now I know that . . . ," but would you say, "Now I understand that. . . ."? What are the special characteristics of new knowledge that lead us to claim new understanding? How does an insight differ from a collection of facts? Maybe it is when we feel that we see *into* things, when we see beneath the surface of events to their inner workings, when we begin to sense *why* things happen, and how they happen, that we claim understanding.

A description has to be an abstraction. It extracts from the data set some essential features of the phenomena which have been observed and measured. How do we know what the essential features of a process are? Experience provides the test of understandings, but if we lack appropriate experience, how can we test our insights? We can only call on our critical intelligence to tell us whether new abstractions of important phenomena we read about in research reports seem to generate understanding rather than just information. What we are likely to be impressed by are descriptions which employ strong analytic tools to expose an underlying, simplifying structure of the data, so that we feel we are getting down to the skeleton, to the bare bones, as it were. The basic device for creating insightful descriptions in scientific research is the use of constructs as structural components, and the scaling from many variates of a few variables to represent the constructs at the empirical level. (Please review the presentation on constructs, variables, and variates in the first section of Chapter 5 at this time.)

When descriptive validity is high enough on the insightfulness scale it begins to shade into *causative validity*. The causative type of internal validity belongs to studies which support strong inferences about the probable causes of the events studied. It is almost impossible to be certain or definitive about the causes of complex social outcomes, such as the outcomes of nursing, simply because a host of influences play on such outcomes. Many popular research designs are woefully inadequate to support any speculation about causation, however, and we do need to decide what features in designs best support causal arguments. Nursing research is applied science which has to be justified by the extent to which it contributes to improvements in nursing practice. It is not possible to justify decisions about nursing practice without some knowledge of the causal influences of nursing practices on patient outcomes. The enormous impediments to the acquisition of such causal knowledge do not free nursing researchers from the responsibility of attempting to produce it.

The strongest logical support for causal inference is provided by the classic *randomized experiment*. This design calls for random assignment of individuals from a pool of available subjects to one of two or more treatment groups. A subject has been randomly assigned to a treatment when it is the case that he or she had the same fair chance of being assigned to any group. The idea is that assignment to one of two or more treatments takes place entirely by chance, just as in a fair game of chance. Under random assignment, all the individual differences among subjects that might affect the outcomes of the study should be more or less equally spread out among the treatment groups, giving no treatment an unfair advantage, and logic suggests that any significant differences in outcomes among the groups must have been caused by the treatment differences.

The genius of the randomized experiment is that it seems to eliminate all possible causes of large outcome differences among the treatment groups other than the planned variations in treatment. (Small outcome differences can be explained as "possibly due to chance.") Why isn't this method ideal for nursing research? Many have thought it to be so. In our judgment, randomized experiments often create such artificial nursing environments that we cannot assume that what happens in the experimental situation resembles what would happen in other, everyday situations. There is no random assignment in ordinary nursing contexts, and all the variables which the experimental design makes uncorrelated with treatments and outcomes tend to be correlated with both in everyday life. Thus, the experiment may leave much to be desired in terms of its external validity, even though its internal causative validity may be substantial.

Even the internal validity of a nursing experiment is not likely to be as impressive as the internal validity of experiments on simple physical processes. In most nursing research the treatment construct will be a complex one, really a category for a number of different facets or dimensions along which the two or several treatment programs differ. This complexity of medical and nursing care plans is such that the experiment will not be able to reveal which facets or dimensions of the care make the most difference in the outcomes. Usually there will be more than one outcome dimension to complicate matters further. Consult Cooley and Lohnes (1976, pp. 169–175 and 246–250) for elaboration of this critique.

In all research on social phenomena, including research on nursing, it will probably be necessary to conceptualize at the construct level and to scale at the empirical level a complex of environmental variables which comprise relevant aspects of treatment, so that the independent or causal variables will be multiple. It will be possible to manipulate some of these by health care policies, and it will not be possible to manipulate others. Some will have substantially more influence on the outcomes than others, and often it will be the case that inflexible background variables are stronger causes of outcomes than are professionally controlled dimensions of nursing. That's the way it happens. We hope this leads you to develop instant suspicion of any statement about "the cause" of anything. As though multiple independent and correlated causative variables were not confusing enough, another severe complication is that all the dependent variables will tend to be intercorrelated in ways that suggest they are causally influencing each other. These realities of social research create very serious problems for causal inference, but we are going to show you in Chapter 11 how causal inferences can be supported by analytical models for research data. We believe these devices will make it possible for you to create causative validity for properly specified research studies. We do not say it will be easy.

Q: Select a report of a nursing research from a journal or other source and
     discuss the internal validity of the major generalization produced.

External Validity

Historians usually hope to improve their readers' understandings of a broader
reach of human affairs than just the particular events they write about. A history
of a particular revolution is intended to describe that one revolution comprehen-
sively and accurately, but the author intends that at least some of the insights
promulgated will apply at least loosely to other revolutions. Although they
concede that history never repeats itself exactly, historians believe that some
patterns in human affairs are nearly enough repeated so that discernment of
patterns in the record of the past can be instructive as we face the future. Nursing
research reports are history documents, however scientific the measurements
and analyses they report. The *external validity* of a research design is an estimate
of the extent to which the findings of the study can be generalized to times and
places other than the time-and-place–specialized source of the data. This estimate is named the *limits of generalizability* to emphasize that it is natural to be
excessively optimistic about the extent to which knowledge of the particular
stretches toward universality. Perhaps there is no universal knowledge which
nursing research can generate. The mix of institution (agency), patient, physician, nurse, disease would seem to be almost infinitely variable and therefore to
defy generalization in the laboratory sense.

    We might expect that the best estimates of limits of generalizability for
research findings would be made by the people with the broadest experience in
the field of application and with the best intelligence. There is a mature wisdom
which cannot be fabricated or faked, so that the leadership figures in a profession
either have it or they do not. Fortunately, energetic activity can sometimes be a
substitute for inspired intuition. We describe a program for discovering the limits
of generalizability of research knowledge, called replication strategy, in the
following section.

    Random selection of research subjects from a particular universe of subjects
is the classic way to guarantee generalizability of research knowledge based on
the randomly selected sample to the universe (also called the *population*) which
is sampled. A sample is randomly selected if every member of the population had
a known nonzero probability of being selected. In simple random sampling this
probability of being selected is the same for all members of the population. Fair
lotteries are examples of random-selection schemes. How to insure that every
member of a population has an equal chance of being selected opens up quite a
can of worms, and usually in practice only an approximation to a completely fair
procedure can be operationalized, but the theoretical assumption that a sample
was randomly drawn provides a foundation stone for the edifice of survey
statistics.

    The reason that randomizing is supposed to produce a sample peculiarly
representative of the population from which it is drawn is that any bias in the
sample can only be accidental, i.e, due to chance. No systematic bias of the

researcher is allowed to influence the selection of subjects. Imagine a researcher who likes women more than men. If this investigator draws a sample of patients by a randomizing procedure, personal preference cannot influence the sex ratio for the sample. Thus we may hope that the sex ratio for the sample will mirror (somewhat imperfectly) the sex ratio for the population, and if it does not, the bias will be due to chance alone rather than to researcher prejudice. The hazards of chance are the only hazards statistics admits of. Statistical inference can be described as a collection of procedures for estimating the hazards of chance when randomizing has been the basis for sampling.

Facts about a population of subjects are termed *parameters*. For example, the mean or arithmetic average of the scores on a variate for all the members of a population is a much-sought-after parameter. We might want to know the mean caloric intake of all adults between the ages of 25 and 50 in the United States in June of 1979. Since it is not practical to measure caloric intake of this immense population for a day, much less for a month, we readily concede that we cannot know the desired parameter exactly. It may be practical to test a more or less randomly selected sample, perhaps 6 out of 100,000 in the population, with the hope that the mean score for this sample will approximate the mean score for the population. In this sense, the statistic estimates the population parameter. The indicated research would call for a national survey of adult caloric intakes. Assessed once, in June of 1979, the mean of the sample might estimate the mean of the population rather accurately, but it would not be a very interesting number. Assessed annually, the trend in the statistics over the years would command considerable attention.

In a survey, subjects are randomly selected to be representative of a real population. In an experiment, subjects are randomly assigned to two or more treatments from a pool of available subjects. The sample assigned to a particular treatment is thought to be representative of a hypothetical treatment population, and it is thought that the statistics for the treatment sample may adequately estimate the parameters for the imagined treatment population. We have already suggested that random assignment may yield treatment populations which are entirely mythical and unlike anything that will ever exist in nature outside the experiment. We now want to suggest that extant populations which can be sampled randomly in surveys are seldom the universes to which research knowledge has to be generalized. Like time, a population is a flowing river into which one can never wade twice at the same place. Everything in nature is changing, and human societies seem to be changing incredibly fast. Exact random selection from a population would not alter the fact that the research study was a piece of history, at best reporting accurately on a reality which no longer existed. The future in which we must apply what we learn from nursing research has not been and could not have been sampled. Therefore, the rules of statistical inference, even when applied to exactly randomized samples, cannot dictate the limits of generalizability of knowledge.

True randomization, either of selection or assignment, is almost never achieved in any substantial research project. Randomization is always a plan for selecting or assigning subjects, but it is a plan which is frustrated in actuality by accidents, by malice, by sloth, by indifference, by circumstances uncatalogable. When you want to disconcert a researcher, ask casually what was done about missing data in the data set. Applied social science simply is not done under the conditions statisticians dream of. The moral is that you must depend on your experience and your intelligence, not your statistician, to estimate the limits of generalizability promised by your research design or achieved by your research findings.

Q: How could a sample for a national adult caloric-intake survey be drawn? Try to invent a method which is both practical, cost-effective, and reasonably randomizing. Assume that the adult population between the ages of 25 and 50 comprises approximately 100 million Americans, each of whom should have an equal chance of being in the sample, at least theoretically. Sample $N = 600$.

Q: For the same research report selected in response to the Q in the previous section, discuss the external validity of the major generalization. How would you state the limits of generalizability? Does your statement agree with that in the report?

Replication Strategy

Eventually a generalization about nursing has to be proved in practice. Even if they are based on research, nursing practices which do not yield desirable results will sooner or later be pushed out by new practices that are more successful. The test of practice can be slow and dangerous, however. In medicine, purging and bleeding patients was practiced for centuries without widespread awareness of its unproductiveness. In 1849, J. Dietl did an experiment on 380 pneumonia patients in which he purged some of them with tartar emetics, leeched some of them, and simply put some of them to bed on a light diet. He observed the mortality rates to be 20.7 percent for the purged, 20.4 percent for the bled, and 7.4 percent for the bedded, from which he concluded that bleeding and purging were downright harmful to patients (Wold, 1956). Nevertheless physicians continued to bleed and purge for a long time after Dietl's experiment. Replications of this experiment might have helped persuade physicians to alter their practices.

Replication strategy is the testing of research findings by showing that they can be repeated in new situations. If new studies verify that the generalization from a research study applies in the new situations, in the sense that the same pattern of events is discovered again and again, the external validity of the generalization is established. When new situations are found in which the old pattern of events is not repeated, the limits of the generalization have been passed. Limits of generalizability are not usually sharp boundary lines in time and space, out to which the generalization is valid and beyond which it is invalid. Instead there is likely to be a gradual tapering off of validity as circumstances become less and less like those of the original study. For this reason a replication strategy should attempt to provide a variety of replications of the research under a graduated series of increasingly dissimilar circumstances. Such an ideal (and perhaps prohibitively expensive) strategy permits the mapping of validity contours for a finding.

There are three kinds of replications:

1 *Exact replication*—This method requires drawing a new random sample from the same population sampled for the original research, then executing precisely the same measurement program upon the new sample as was executed upon the original sample. If some variable was manipulated in certain ways in the original research (a treatment variable), it must be manipulated in the same ways in the new study. Following these rules, if they can be followed, will produce a classic replication study. This is often presented in textbooks as the ideal, but in fact it is likely to be either impractical or uninformative. In the light of what we said before about the dynamic movement of real populations, it is obviously not possible to sample the same real population again at a later time. The hypothetical treatment populations visualized by the theory of randomized experiments do have a timelessness about them that permits their being sampled again, but they also have an unworldliness that leaves us uninformed about how well a generalization will apply in the real world, however many times it survives replications of the experiment which originally justified it.

2 *Approximate replication*—This method involves repeating the research study under conditions very similar to those of the original study, especially with respect to the measurement program. The sample of subjects is drawn from a population similar to that of the first study. Differences between the original and the replication study in manipulations (treatments), measurements, settings, and samples are described as thoroughly as possible. If the findings of the old research do not replicate under this method, the conclusion is that the findings were due to *capitalization on chance*, and they ought not to be trusted at all as guides to practice.

3 *Replication under new conditions*—This method requires searching for an old pattern of events with a new research design executed in a new setting on a sample from a new population. The only constants between the original research and the replication research are theoretical constants, namely that both studies involve the same constructs and the new research tests that generalization about relationships among the constructs which was validated by the first research. The measurement devices for operationalizing the constructs in the new research may be different in whole or part from those of the old research. That is, the two sets of measurement procedures must have the same construct validities but not necessarily the same mechanics. In our earlier terminology, the specification must be the same for both studies. If there are manipulations of a treatment variable they need not be exactly the same manipulations as those of the first study. Schedules, doses, instruments, etc. may be different, as long as the treatment construct remains the same. The institutional or societal setting for the study and the sex, age, ethnicity, etc. of the population may be quite different. If the original generalization is found to apply in this type of replication, a presumption of its substantial robustness is warranted. If a series of replications under new conditions could be arranged, each under unique conditions, and the generalization was found to apply reasonably well under all these replications, the courage of some strong conviction should be engendered. Ideally, at least, the most important generalizations in a theory of nursing should have passed such a series of different tests.

A useful aspect of a strategy of replications under new conditions is that it does not obligate the researcher to randomize anything or anyone, ever. Neither is she required to compute or discuss any statistical inference procedures. Randomizing is really a strategy for getting good information cheaply. The costs of getting good information without randomizing are probably bearable in research on nursing, and there are real advantages to paying those costs and abjuring randomization. Naturally, professional statisticians will never give this advice, but it is obligatory that nursing researchers, their sponsors, and their editors think this issue through for themselves and not defer to statisticians.

Q: For the research study selected in response to the Q in the Internal Validity section, what replication strategy would seem to be appropriate? How would such a strategy extend the limits of generalizability, assuming that the finding stood up under the replications?

SETTINGS AND SAMPLES

Settings and samples shade into each other in nursing research because the relevant populations for generalizations about nursing are always aggregates of people who are connected with particular delivery systems for nursing care. Thus when a setting is selected as the place where research will be done, a population comes with it. It may be that one setting serves many distinct groups of clients, so that a choice among populations is possible. Or, if nurses rather than patients are to be sampled, several classes of nurses may be employed or learning in a single setting, enabling a choice among nurse populations. Alternately, a desired population may be selected (e.g., inner-city elderly people paying for health care by medicaid) and it may be necessary to study several settings in which members of that population receive nursing care. There is not a one-to-one correspondence between settings and samples, but they are linked.

It is usually easier to select sample members systematically rather than randomly within a setting. For example, every tenth nurse may be interviewed, starting at a randomly selected position among the first 10 nurses on a roster and then counting down 10 for each successive subject. Patients may also be sampled systematically by taking, for example, every twentieth patient in the admissions file. Either systematically or randomly, subjects should be selected by a scheme that protects the research against the researcher's biases or laziness (some people are much more cooperative and easier to work with than others). This effort to get a representative sample from the setting does not change the fact that the setting and other circumstances surrounding the research have been selected quite arbitrarily and are not representative of any universe of settings and circumstances. We can learn from experience, but we must be on guard against the temptation to try to draw universal truths from parochial data. It is sometimes easier for the reader of a research report to behave intelligently in judging the limits of generalizability of the finding than it is for the proud researcher who would like to believe that she has done the absolutely crucial study of an issue.

REFERENCES

Cooley, William W., and Paul R. Lohnes: *Evaluation research in education*. New York: Irvington/Halsted/Wiley, 1976.

Friedman, M., and R. H. Rosenman: *Type A behavior and your heart*. Greenwich, Conn.: Fawcett, 1974.

Wold, H.: Causal inferences from observational data: A review of ends and means. *Journal of the Royal Statistical Society, Series A*, 1956, *119*, 351–390. Reprinted in M. C. Wittrock, and D. E. Wiley (Eds.): *The evaluation of instruction: Issues and problems*. New York: Holt, 1970.

Chapter 8

Where and Upon Whom Will You Do Your Research?

This chapter encourages you to apply the generalizations about selection of sites and subjects put forward in Chapter 7 to your own ideas about nursing research which needs to be done, and which you might possibly attempt to do.

NEGOTIATING A SITE

The most cogent statement we have found regarding the changing nature of researcher access to clinical settings is Hodgman's (1978):

> Gaining access to clinical agencies for the conduct of research is a much more complicated and time-consuming process now than in the past. Two developments contributing to this situation are the increased concern for the protection of the rights of human subjects, as evidenced in the proliferation of institutional review boards, and the development of agency-based nursing research departments.

We have addressed the human rights issues in the last section of Chapter 5 and will have more to say in the following section of this chapter. Now we want to discuss the stake nursing research departments have in reviewing outside proposals, since the researcher is asking them for their sponsorship and support.

Whatever a researcher does in an institution reflects on the whole and uses up some of the research potential, whether that potential be research subjects or patience and good will of staff. If there is no research department in a given service agency, then a nursing service or other administrator assumes the responsibility. Wherever field research is done, right to access belongs to someone (Fiedler, 1978), and researchers, whether from inside or outside an agency, must obtain permission.

Yet another layer of review exists on the patient care unit where nurses may have the right of approval (or veto) of a project. Although this may seem like too much to the researcher who is eager to begin data collection, we as nurses should easily understand that the professional staff on the unit is more capable than anyone else of judging whether the proposed study is administratively feasible and clinically sound. As patient advocates in the practice role, we would want to have some say about access to the patient, and such decisions are an integral part of the primary nurse role.

The researcher and her advisers should see to it that the research application hangs together before it is presented to personnel at the research site. That is, it should show adequate integration of prior research, thoughtful statement of the problem, careful selection or development of instruments, clear description of procedures, and adequate consideration of human rights guidelines. The service agency's point of view includes other concerns that are well stated in the excellent Beth Israel Hospital criteria in the Appendix in the back of this chapter. At present these criteria may not be typical, but they are the wave of the future.

Experience suggests that the most frequent mistake research students make is that they fail to allow sufficient time to negotiate the necessary arrangements at the research site. Hodgman has remarked on the importance of speaking informally with the director of nursing or research personnel well in advance to find out whether the institution is likely to be able to provide the necessary data. Such early contacts can inform the researcher whether she is following a realistic plan, may save time and effort, and will probably avert frustration.

Now we have warned the researcher against contacting the agency too soon, and also too late. This should provide a clue that arranging for a research site can be a delicate interpersonal matter as well as a research routine. You should proceed carefully on the best local advice you can obtain.

HUMAN SUBJECTS CLEARANCE

The regulation of access to human subjects, the establishment of institutional review boards, and the various activities involved in obtaining permission to conduct studies all hinge on the ethical principle of informed consent. A spokesman for the Federal Drug Administration explicated the principle well in the *Federal Register* (1979):

> The concept of "informed consent" is not a narrow or technical concept, limited in application to this or that particular kind of research on human subjects. Rather, the concept has a broad sweep; and, like the concepts of "due process of law" and "equal protection of the laws," it reflects fundamental social value judgments about how people should be treated. Like those other concepts, too, the concept of "informed consent" changes and grows in light of increasing experience in its application and more precise identification of problems to be addressed in its articulation. (p. 47718)

The same source quotes a hearing record of the New York State Board of Regents, which in turn quotes Barber (source unknown) to the effect that patients have the right to know they are being asked to volunteer and to refuse to participate in a study for any reason, intelligent or otherwise, well informed, or prejudiced. No one has a right to withhold from prospective volunteers any fact which may influence their decision. In short, it is the patient's right to be "emotional" or "irrational."

The rules newly proposed by HED operationalize informed consent this way:

46.112 Informed consent.
(a) Except as provided elsewhere in this section, no subject may be involved in research covered by these regulations without the legally effective informed consent of the subject or the subject's legally authorized representative. This consent shall be sought under circumstances that provide the subject (or the subject's legally authorized representative) sufficient opportunity to consider whether or not to participate and that minimize the possibility of coercion or undue influence. The information that is given to the subject or the subject's legally authorized representative must be in a language understandable to the subject or the legally authorized representative. No informed consent, whether oral or written, may include any exculpatory language through which the subject or the subject's legally authorized representative is made to waive, or to appear to waive, the subject's legal rights, including any release of the institution or its agents from liability for negligence.

(1) *Basic elements of informed consent*. In seeking informed consent, the following information shall be provided:

(A) A statement that the activity involves research, and that the Institutional Review Board has approved the solicitation of subjects to participate in the research;

(B) An explanation of the scope, aims, and purposes of the research, and the procedures to be followed (including identification of any treatments or procedures which are experimental), and the expected duration of the subject's participation;

(C) A description of any reasonably foreseeable risks or discomforts to the subject (including likely results if an experimental treatment should prove ineffective);

(D) A description of any benefits to the subject or to others which may reasonably be expected from the research;

(E) A disclosure of appropriate alternative procedures or courses of treatment, if any, that might be advantageous to the subject;

(F) A statement that new information developed during the course of the research which may relate to the subject's willingness to continue participation will be provided to the subject;

(G) A statement describing the extent to which confidentiality of records identifying the subject will be maintained;

(H) An offer to answer any questions the subject (or the subject's representative) may have about the research, the subject's rights, or related matters;

(I) For research involving more than minimal risk, an explanation as to whether compensation and medical treatment are available if injury occurs and, if so, what they consist of or where further information may be obtained;

(J) Who should be contacted if harm occurs or there are questions or problems; and

(K) A statement that participation is voluntary, refusal to participate will involve no penalty or loss of benefits to which the subject is otherwise entitled, and the subject may discontinue participation at any time without penalty or loss of benefits to which the subject is otherwise entitled. (p. 47,696)

The above should make it clear that all research involving human subjects—even if those subjects are one's "own" patients or coworkers—must be processed through the appropriate IRBs.

All this discussion of informed consent assumes, of course, that the researcher has access to prospective subjects. Even after the strictly legal requirements have been cleared, researchers, especially nurse researchers, have problems of access to subjects. Like research sites, subjects may be under someone's protection, but this is a gray area so far as definitude of rules goes. In approaching a child, do you need permission of parents, school principal, teacher, or all of these? And what about the child? What age child would you ask for formal consent? Although formal consent from the child is not legally required, would it enhance rapport? Regarding hospitalized persons, can a physician refuse or give access to his patients? Is this a right or a responsibility of the physician? As family members or patients we might expect protection from the doctor, but as researchers we may feel that doctors claim more right than they have. What about patients who have gone home? Although they can give their own permission, should the physician still be notified about the study?

If the researcher is approaching children, prisoners, mental patients, or any other group of individuals not able to fend for themselves, the IRB will take special care in examining the proposal and making recommendations. They may or may not make recommendations about informing physicians or requesting permission from them. Your best guidance on this may come from giving thought to four questions: What does professional courtesy demand? What is the local custom? What do advisers say? If I were the physician, how interested would I be in the study, and at what stage might I want to know about it? Clearly the nature of the study makes a great deal of difference. Most doctors might be mildly interested to know that someone is studying patients who are on general diets to find out how their diets changed upon admission to the hospital; they would certainly be greatly concerned about a study that requires an expenditure of energy from an open-heart surgical patient. What we are really saying is that after the researcher has observed general guidelines and is approaching individual subjects, consideration must be given to the particular situation. Discretion and advice must be used.

Discretion must be exercised with regard to all sponsors, individuals, and institutions. For graduate students especially, this means that no letters or protocols under the name of the university or college should go out until they have been fully approved. We may sometimes envy the freedom of Mendel in his pea patch, but persons who elect to study humans in complex settings must paddle their canoes through numerous currents and countercurrents. (There! We have deliberately contributed a mixed metaphor which the reader can refer to in connection with Chapter 13.)

Sometimes information about research subjects is obtained from inanimate objects such as patient records. Although hospitals are quick to claim ownership of patient charts, attorneys often claim that records really belong to patients. Physicians have sometimes tried to exert more claim on these records than the courts were willing to allow, yet it seems obvious that all these claims are legitimate in some measure. No one party can remove or destroy a record. Thus there seems to be an element of community or government ownership. This should serve to reemphasize the question about local custom. Access to the records of a given institution will be determined by the institution's policy, traditions, and perhaps its legal adviser.

When you have finally gained access, how will you document the informed consent? HEW has never required that all consents be in writing, and does not now propose to do so. The newly proposed rules differ little from the old, and make very clear what the researcher owes to the IRB and to the research subject. We present them here:

46.113 Documentation of informed consent.
(a) Except as provided in paragraph (b), informed consent shall be documented in writing (and a copy provided to the subject or the subject's legally authorized representative) through either of the following methods:
(1) A written consent document embodying the elements of informed consent. This may be read to the subject or to his or her legally authorized representative, but in any event the subject or his or her legally authorized representative must be given adequate opportunity to read it. This document is to be signed by the subject or his or her legally authorized representative, and a copy supplied to the subject or representative. The Board shall retain approved sample copies of the consent form.
(2) A "short form" written consent document indicating that the elements of informed consent have been presented orally to the subject or his or her legally authorized representative. Written summaries of what is to be said to the subject (or representative) are to be approved by the Board. The short form is to be signed by the subject or his or her legally authorized representative and by a witness to the oral presentation and to the subject's signature, or that of the representative. A copy of the approved summary is to be signed by the persons officially obtaining the consent and by the witness. Copies of the form and the summary shall be provided to the subject or representative. The Board shall retain approved sample copies of the consent form and the summaries.
(b) The Board may waive the requirement for the researcher to obtain documentation of consent for some or all subjects if it finds (and documents) either:
(1) That the only record linking the subject and the research would be the consent document, the only significant risk would be potential harm resulting from a breach of confidentiality, each subject will be asked whether he or she wants there to be documentation linking the subject with the research, and the subject's wishes will govern; or
(2) That the research presents no more than minimal risk of harm to subjects and involves no procedures for which written consent is normally required outside of the research context.
In many cases covered by this paragraph it may be appropriate for the Board to require the investigator to provide subjects with a written statement regarding the

research, but not to request their signature, or to require that oral consent be witnessed.

(c) In those cases when new information is provided to the subject during the course of the research, the information shall be reviewed and approved by the Board and a copy retained in its records. (p. 47,697)

PILOT STUDIES

Oppenheim (1966) called attention to various research elements that might be piloted advantageously, such as letters of introduction, ways of reducing non-response, color of questionnaire paper, effect of age and sex of interviewer, the ordinal position of multiple responses, and length of questionnaire or sections of it. Fortunately, some of these items have been studied separately. (We called attention to some studies on mail questionnaires in Chapter 6.) What the researcher is most likely to be interested in pretesting is the collection of background data, measures specifying the independent variables, and criterion measures.

Probably the single most helpful pilot step is for the researcher to ask herself often, "Why do I want this answer? What will I do with it after I get it?" Beyond these questions, the next step is to explore in unstructured interviews with key informants. These informants should be comparable to subjects in the main study, but normally they cannot be used as part of the sample once they have been used in the pilots. The exploratory talks are likely to proceed in tandem with appropriate reading.

After the researcher has a fairly clear mental picture of the data collection, Oppenheim suggests shifting to an assembly-line format in which small subsections are tested and then fitted into larger subassemblies and finally into the total. Finally, the questionnaire as a whole must be piloted.

How will the researcher know when a question is "bad"? A poor question may be misunderstood because it is too colloquial, technical, or abstract. Or it may be too obvious and therefore produce a narrow range of responses. It may be too vague, or ask for information the respondent does not have or cannot remember. It may be a leading question that biases answers, or it may be a reasonable-sounding question which produces answers that cannot be compared. "What brought you to the hospital?" will get responses all the way from the name of an ambulance company to "a fractured femur"!

Unstructured exploratory questions can gradually be turned into closed questions with a choice of precoded answers. This may not be feasible or desirable for every question, and one or two free questions may be worth the extra coding difficulty.

Piloting will not solve all the problems the researcher might want to solve before going on to the main data-collection process. As we indicated, some of the questions are worthy of full-scale research by measurement experts. The researcher will finally be forced to draw an arbitrary line between further piloting and the main study. But it is likely that, looking back, she will feel that the pilot or pilots paid off handsomely.

Q: Under what circumstances could the pilot study data be incorporated in the research sample?

RELIABILITY, VALIDITY, AND GENERALIZABILITY

Reliability and validity are often spoken of together as though they were twins. Reliability, in fact, is more like a mother to validity, since no valid interpretation can be made of variances and covariances from unreliable measurements. Some research writers do not even discuss reliability as a separate issue, preferring to let the achieved validity coefficients of their variables testify to the reliabilities which must have been obtained.

Even if the mechanics of recording observations, coding, and analyzing have been perfect, data still contain bias resulting from methods of data collection. For example, in Chapter 6 we pointed out that an interviewer is a participant who cannot help affecting the milieu. Every method of data collection has its own deficiencies and generates its own unique variance which has nothing to do with the issues under research. Webb et al. (1966) suggest as a remedy the use of the concept of triangulation. Triangulation is not esoteric, but rather an idea we all use in everyday life. When we hear a fresh piece of gossip, we are likely to discount it until we hear it from a different, apparently unrelated source. In the same way, Webb et al. point out, a second method of data collection—even a relatively weak one—will have weaknesses that are different from those of the first method. The two methods used in conjunction can offer strong protection against unreliable information and its devastating effect on apparent validity. That is, a variate may appear to have low validity in the data analysis, when in fact it was simply measured very unreliably. We have defined reliability as reproducibility. It is quite likely that when two or more variates are used as indicators of one variable, their measurement errors will tend to cancel in the process of summing the weighted variate scores into a variable score, so that the reliability of the variable score can be much higher than the average reliability of the variates. Test makers use this theorem all the time to produce highly reliable test scores as the sum of scores on a great many test items of very low average reliability. This tendency of errors of measurement to cancel under summation is so trustworthy that it long ago led to the adage of test makers: Other things being equal, the longer the test, the more reliable its score. Of course, the items or variates which are added together to create a test or variable score must have the same validity, which is to say that they must be indicators of the same variable, for this to work.

Every sample, every setting, every time period differs from every other. What we call unreliability in a data-collecting instrument or method we may have to call uniqueness when we are talking about people, places, times. Whatever we call the differences, they exist. Thus Webb et al. argued for variation in samples, settings, times, as well as data-collection methods. Such variation offers advantages similar to those offered by randomization in selection or assignment of subjects and is very close to the idea of replication that was discussed in Chapter 7.

Now we ask the question: Why do some researchers who are strongly convinced of the value of randomization show such lack of interest in replication? As previously noted, replication provides a similar service to randomization in mapping the contours of validity or limits of generalizability. While no one would want to discourage originality, researchers need to strive for a reasonable balance between highly original research projects and those which replicate successful projects. An old problem studied by a different method, or in a different place, or with a different kind of data analysis, or perhaps merely at a different time, can be a meaningful study and might be more important than some other highly novel study.

Should your research design include one or both types of randomization? We do not know. We have suggested that it is not essential that it do so, which is contrary to some advice you may hear. If you are to be able to answer this question for yourself it is essential that you perceive clearly what randomization can and cannot contribute. If you have a clear grasp of this, you will be ahead of some of the experts.

Clearheadedness on randomization requires that one distinguish between the population which has been (or is to be) studied, which we may call the *research population*, and the population to which it is necessary to generalize the findings, which we may call the *theoretical population*. Two concepts closely related to the notion of the research population are sample and delimitation. The *sample* is the actual collection of subjects or objects which has been studied (or is to be studied). Its members are the units of analysis for statistical modeling of the data. The research population is the aggregate of subjects or objects in the real world which had the opportunity to be in the sample, whether or not they were part of the sample; it is the full set of potential units of analysis available at the site or sites where the data were collected. Sometimes the sample and the research population will be identical because every possible unit of analysis the site provided actually entered into the research data. Usually, however, the design will call for selecting *some* of the available units to stand for all of them. A representative sample of the research population is desired. Now we may say that the research population is the *delimitation* of the obvious validity of the research findings. The boundaries of the research population delimit exactly the direct applicability of the findings.

The validity of the findings within their delimitation can be challenged if it can be argued or shown that the sample is biased, which is to say that it is unrepresentative of the research population. What is at issue is the internal validity of the study.

Random selection from a research population is a way to try to get a representative sample. It does not guarantee a representative sample, partly because chance can lead to an unrepresentative sample quite easily, especially when sample size is small, and partly because loss of sampled units (the specter of missing data) is usually unavoidable and not randomly distributed. There are other ways to try to get a representative sample. Systematic selection of subjects within some strata of the population may work well. Statisticians favor random samples because randomization justifies the use of their statistical inference logic. Since we do not intend to use statistical inference in our decision making, we are not as dependent on randomization. Random assignment of individuals from a pool of subjects to treatment groups can create a set of experimental research populations which are properly represented in the research, thus leading to high internal validity for a successful experiment, but both the pool of subjects and the set of treatments can be trivial to the world at large.

However we delimit the knowledge generated by a research study, we will not be able to keep it within that delimitation. Time passes, the stream of life flows. We have to wade in at new points and apply knowledge which, strictly speaking, does not apply. We have to take calculated risks in extending the claim of knowledge beyond the actual delimitations of available findings. The limits of generalizability problem concerns how far we can go. The theoretical population is the universe of subjects or objects which had no chance to be in the sample but to which we choose to apply the findings. We choose! A subjective assessment of risks and possible gains motivates a courageous (or foolhardy) extrapolation into the unknown. That's life. It's how we must live. Whether you should randomize is an interesting question, but whether or not you randomize, you will have to discuss the applicability of your findings to a theoretical population, the members of which had no opportunity to be studied, but for whom decisions have to be made. At some point, technical ability gives way to wisdom.

Q: Can you think of a nursing norm which represents a risky extrapolation from the research population on which the generalization underlying the norm was based? Is the risk justified? Should the norm be tested in further research? How?

REFERENCES

Federal Register, 1979, *44*(158), Tuesday, August 14.

Fiedler, Judith: *Field research*. San Francisco: Jossey-Bass, 1978.

Hodgman, Eileen Callahan: Student research in service agencies. *Nursing Outlook*, 1978, *26*(9).

Oppenheim, A. N.: *Questionnaire design and attitude measurement*. New York: Basic Books, 1966.

Webb, Eugene J., Donald T. Campbell, Richard D. Schwartz, and Lee Sechrest: *Unobtrusive measures*. Chicago: Rand McNally, 1966.

Appendix: Example of a Nursing Staff's Internal Criteria for Research*

BETH ISRAEL HOSPITAL
Boston, Massachusetts
Nursing Services

Nursing Research Review Committee
RESEARCH PROPOSALS

Project title: _____
_____Investigator: _____
Evaluator: _____
Date: _____

EVALUATION CRITERIA

		Yes	No	Don't know	Not applicable
1	Are the projected dates for data collection reasonable?	___	___	___	___
2	Can Beth Israel Hospital provide the data being sought?	___	___	___	___
3	Will carrying out the study seriously interfere with patient care management or unit routines?	___	___	___	___
4	Can assistance requested by the investigator from members of the nursing services be provided?	___	___	___	___
5	If the study involves the investigator's providing care to patients, is the described care consistent with safe and accepted practice?	___	___	___	___
6	Will the proposed study inferfere with or duplicate current or projected nursing research at Beth Israel Hospital?	___	___	___	___
7	Does any aspect of the study conflict with institutional or departmental philosophy, objectives, or policy?	___	___	___	___
8	Is the purpose of the proposed study clearly stated?	___	___	___	___
9	Is the significance of the proposed study to nursing indicated?	___	___	___	___
10	Are the study's methods (sample, tool, data-collection procedures)				
	Adequately described?	___	___	___	___
	Likely to fulfill the purpose of the study?	___	___	___	___

*The authors are grateful to Eileen Hodgman, RN, MSN, director of nursing research programs, Beth Israel Hospital, 330 Brookline Avenue, Boston, MA 02215 for permission to reproduce this document.

11 Is the procedure for obtaining informed con-
   sent adequately described?   ___ ___ ___ _____
      Appropriate?   ___ ___ ___ _____
      Ethical?   ___ ___ ___ _____
12 Is the consent form clear and accurate with
   regard to the study's aims and procedures?   ___ ___ ___ _____
13 Will the study require approval from the Com-
   mittee on Clinical Investigations?   ___ ___ ___ _____
14 Does the application indicate why it is impor-
   tant that the study be conducted?   ___ ___ ___ _____

DECISION FOR SPONSORSHIP (Clinical directors should seek head nurse input before making final decision)

___Recommend for sponsorship
___Recommend only if the following changes are made or issues addressed:

___Do not recommend for sponsorship (Provide legible reasons that can be communicated to the investigator):

If sponsorship is granted, who else should the investigator contact before beginning the study? Why?

Who would particularly benefit from hearing the results of this study?

Ignaz Phillip Semmelweis

The man who was to be one of the greatest benefactors of modern women because of his research victory over puerperal (childbirth) fever was born in Budapest in 1818, the youngest of five children in a shopkeeping family. After attending the Catholic Gymnasium (high school), he studied philosophy for 2 years at the University of Budapest. Then he went to Vienna to study law. In those years Budapest was a remote city (really two cities, Buda and Pesth) in the provinces of the Austro-Hungarian Empire, whereas Vienna was the glittering capital. Throughout his career Semmelweis was handicapped by his lack of fluency in German and the prejudice of Vienna's Germanic medical leadership against a foreigner. A different person would have overcome these obstacles (Hungarians did have full citizenship, and German could be mastered), but Semmelweis remained stubbornly "different." This attitude may have contributed to his determination to solve a problem the medical elite had turned its back upon, but it also prevented the rapid dissemination of his great discovery after it was made.

Semmelweis was stirred to become a doctor when a friend took him to an autopsy. (Autopsies were to be decisive events at several points in his life, including its end.) He studied medicine at the University of Budapest from 1839 to 1841, then spent 3 years completing his medical degree at the famous school in Vienna. Following his graduation in 1844 he took a graduate course for which he was awarded a master's degree in practical midwifery. He was assigned as assistant in the First Obstetric Clinic of the Vienna General Hospital, then (in

1846) under Johann Klein. This clinic was part of the world's largest lying-in hospital, founded by the liberal Empress Maria Theresa in the mid-eighteenth century. It had been illegal for male doctors to examine women or deliver a child until shortly before the founding of the Vienna General, and when Semmelweis joined it the hospital was organized into two lying-in wards, one in which doctors practiced and the other in which nursing sisters practiced midwifery. These were called "doctors' ward" and "sisters' ward."

Maria Theresa had wanted to ensure good care for all pregnant women, including poor and unwed mothers. Her son, Emperor Franz Joseph II, had appointed Dr. Lucas Boer, educated in England and a stickler for cleanliness, as professor and head of the lying-in wards. During Boer's tenure of 33 years, maternal mortality ran at 0.85 percent (i.e., less than 1 percent). Klein, who had trained with Boer, was then appointed. He had not taken Boer's lessons on cleanliness to heart, and mortality rose immediately in the doctors' ward. One of the principal differences in the practice of Boer and Klein was that Boer used "phantoms," or models, to demonstrate midwifery techniques, steadfastly refusing to use dead infants or mothers or parts of them in the horrifying accepted way. Klein, however, reverted to the use of cadavers for his demonstrations to medical students and midwives. Under Klein, maternal mortality averaged 10 percent, 1 month reaching 30 percent. Ten mothers out of a hundred, and usually their infants along with them, died of childbed fever. Sometimes the babies sickened first, sometimes the mothers—but they sickened with pulses so rapid they often could not be counted, dry tongues, fever—and most of the sick ones died discolored, bloated, putrid, delirious. The mothers were mostly primiparas, young girls in their teens having their first baby.

Semmelweis made a vow to discover the cause of childbed fever or die in the attempt. He was a man who loved women. During his university days he frequently availed himself of the wine, women, and songfests of student life. Later, he fell so deeply in love with Marie, who became Frau Semmelweis, that he was frequently the butt of jokes concerning his inability to cover the depth of his feeling. He loved his patients and did not attempt to prevent his feelings for them from showing. He said, "We would rather know less, and preserve the health of our patients more." Nevertheless, he was also a man of logic. He could number himself among the best-educated physicians in the world, having completed 5 years of training at a school that led the field in the integration of laboratory, bedside, and theoretical knowledge. By way of contrast, most American physicians of the day had 1 year of medical school or were the products of an apprenticeship with a general practitioner. Semmelweis was the right man in the right place, for prepared by his education, his intelligence, and his deep empathy and love for women, he was in a position to witness one of the most dramatic natural experiments of all time.

This experiment was provided by the differences in practice between the doctors' ward, where the physicians and student-physicians were constantly moving from cadavers (autopsies were performed in a room immediately adjacent to the ward) and infected patients to patients not yet infected, and the sisters' ward. The staggering fact was that, year after year, the mortality rate in the doctors' ward was much higher than it was in the sisters' ward. Only Semmelweis saw that this had to be significant. Only he had the devotion and perseverance to examine and discard on the evidence all the available theories of the causes of childbed fever, until only one conclusion was possible. Table I-2 consolidates figures Semmelweis ultimately made available in his great statistical treatise of 1861. The first part of the table reports mortality figures and rates

Table I-2   Mortality in Two Wards of Vienna General Hospital

Year	Doctors' ward			Sisters' ward		
	Births	Deaths	%	Births	Deaths	%
1833–1840*						
1833	3737	197	5.3	353	8	2.3
1834	2657	205	7.7	1744	150	8.6
1835	2573	143	5.6	1682	84	5.0
1836	2677	200	7.5	1670	131	7.8
1837	2765	251	9.1	1784	124	7.0
1838	2987	91	3.0	1779	88	4.9
1839	2787	151	5.4	2010	91	4.5
1840	2889	267	9.2	2073	55	2.7
Average	2883	188	6.6	1637	91	5.6
1841–1846†						
1841	3036	237	7.8	2442	86	3.5
1842	3287	518	15.8	2659	202	7.6
1843	3060	274	9.0	2739	164	6.0
1844	3157	260	8.2	2956	68	2.3
1845	3492	241	6.9	3241	66	2.0
1846	4010	459	11.4	3754	105	2.7
Average	3340	332	9.9	2965	115	3.4
1847–1858‡						
1847	3490	176	5.0			
1848	3556	45	1.3			
1849	3858	103	2.7			
1850	3745	74	2.0			
1851	4194	75	1.8			
1852	4471	181	4.6			
1853	4221	94	2.1			
1854	4393	400	9.1			
1855	3659	198	5.4			
1856	3925	156	4.0			
1857	4220	124	3.0			
1858	4203	86	2.0			
Average	3995	143	3.6			

*From Semmelweis, 1861, p. 378.
†*Ibid.*, p. 379.
‡*Ibid.*, p. 379.

for the years 1833 to 1840, when the hospital was divided into two clinics in both of which physicians were allowed to teach. For those years the mortality rates in the two wards were quite similar. The second part reports on the years 1841 to 1846. After October 1840, only male doctors were trained in clinic I and only female midwives were trained in clinic II. The lesson was there to be learned in the carefully compiled records of the hospital. The doctors' ward was more dangerous than the sisters' ward. Admission to the two wards was rotated day by day, with the changeover coming at midnight, and it is told that before midnight the carriages of women in labor could be heard circling the hospital on the days of admission to the doctors' ward, waiting the changeover and the mercy of admission to the sisters' ward.

The modern researcher, faced with a problem, goes first to the literature. She also discusses the problem with experts in the field. Semmelweis had expert opinions on childbed fever available in abundance in the writings and utterances of physicians. Among the causes from *within* the mother which were put forward were

Illegitimacy—most of the victims in the Vienna General were unmarried

Physiological instability of motherhood—milk fever, suppression of the lochia, fibrinous crasis, crasis of the blood, special vulnerability to some external factor because of "loaded" blood and tissues

Psychic causes—fear of labor, delivery, and death

Peritonitis—inflammation of the peritoneum brought on by pregnancy and labor

Contagion—although Henle showed in 1840 that no sharp distinction could be made between contagia and miasma, contagia were commonly regarded as internal, individual reactions to agencies so specific that each could cause one disease and no other

Causes from *without* the mother that were hypothesized included

Zymosis—disease in disguise, i.e, from fermented products of other diseases

Miasma—untoward influences from the cosmos, atmosphere, or soil that entered through the respiratory tract

The primitive laboratory procedures and notions of how research should be carried out in the mid-nineteenth century made it very difficult to dispose of or prove any idea. Even after he had made his great discovery and proved it clinically to his own satisfaction, Semmelweis had the frustrating experience of having his colleagues reject a rather brilliant series of experiments he did on rabbits, in which he successfully infected the animals with puerperal fever by brushing cadaverous material from infected women upon them. His critics argued speciously that he had used amounts of cadaverous material far in excess of what physicians would be likely to convey to patients via their dirty hands. (This sounds similar to the rejection of animal experiments involving carcinogens by many industry representatives today.)

An interesting theory of the time was that illegitimacy caused the fever. This was a perfect example of how a spurious variable could mislead researchers. A spurious variable is one that correlates sufficiently with a criterion that it can be mistaken as a cause. Most of the mothers who died in Vienna General were unmarried, but so were most of the mothers who survived. Historians say that marriage was nearly impossible for the poorest socioeconomic classes of Vienna in the mid-nineteenth century. They could not afford it. In the suburbs and countryside where marriage was more prevalent, home delivery with its attendant lesser risk of infection was also more prevalent. It was well known in Vienna that women who delivered in the streets were more likely to survive than those who delivered in the hospital. The most popular opinion among the physicians of the day was that childbed fever was an inevitable aspect of hospital-based obstetrics, a product of unknown agents operating in conjunction with elusive atmospheric conditions. In other words, a comfortable if feeble excuse was rampant. Semmelweis's anguish at the plight of his patients was an aspect of his foreignness.

It is important to remember that Semmelweis's search and discovery preceded Pasteur's promulgation of the germ theory by many years, and it was to be 50 years before Pasteur identified the streptococcus as the bacterium responsible for puerperal fever. In 1846, the majority of scientists and physicians believed in the spontaneous generation of living organisms from inanimate matter. There was no vivid notion of infection through the multiplication and transmission of living organisms that were able to maintain their existence in either live or dead human tissue or exudate.

Although not widespread or vivid, some notions of infection did exist, and we can assume that Semmelweis was familiar with them. We know that he was sufficiently impressed with the published positions taken by certain English and Scottish obstetricians that he studied English intensively to prepare for a visit to the Rotunda Hospital in Dublin and other hospitals in the United Kingdom. (He corresponded with these and many other great European hospitals about their mortality records, but never did go to work at Dublin as he had planned.) Few if any scientific breakthroughs actually occur without precursors or signposts. Among the precursors for Semmelweis's discovery were

1546 Girolama Fracastoro put forth a germ theory of infection and recognized the contagiousness of typhus and tuberculosis.

1774 Thomas Kirkland published a treatise on puerperal fever.

1795 Alexander Gordon published a paper on the epidemic of puerperal fever in Aberdeen.

1822 Marie H. B. Gaspard studied pyemia by injecting putrid fluids (pus, vaccine, lymph, blood, bile, urine, saliva, carbonic acid, hydrogen, sulfuretted hydrogen) into dogs, sheep, foxes, pigs.

1835 Agostino Bassi demonstrated that parasites caused a disease of silkworms.

1836   Theodor Schwann concluded that alcoholic fermentation was the work of a live organism.

1838   Pierre F. O. Rayer inoculated a donkey with pus from a patient who had glanders.

1840   Friedrich G. J. Henle showed that no sharp distinction between miasma and contagia was possible because carriers of disease were living materials that colonized the host body.

Semmelweis tortured himself with internal arguments over the logic of the various hypothesized etiologies of the fever. Gradually he persuaded himself that none of them could be correct. Thus he prepared his mind for the flash of insight which came when one of his colleagues died of the fever after slicing himself during an autopsy on a fever victim. Suddenly he was convinced that transfer of cadaverous material on dirty hands of physicians and students was the cause. What cleansing technique would suffice? Luckily, Semmelweis hit upon a wash of chlorinated lime solution, which he doggedly insisted that everyone attending deliveries on his ward use. The result made history. In 1846, the mortality rate in the doctors' ward was 11.4 percent. Semmelweis introduced his chlorine wash late in May of 1847. The rate dropped immediately. In 1848, the mortality rate in the doctors' ward was 1.27 percent. The third part of Table I-2 reports the rates in the doctors' ward for 1847 to 1858. A great victory had been accomplished.

Unfortunately, Semmelweis was not a great communicator. He was a stranger in the Vienna medical community, and his discovery was vigorously resisted. He was perceived as blaming the doctors for the horrendous mortality of their patients, and that was naturally unacceptable to them. His efforts to publicize his discovery in 1847 met with almost total hostility. His profession stonewalled him. He responded by withdrawal, determined to prepare a master-work which would force the acceptance of his achievement. Finally, in 1861, he brought out his great book. In 103 pages and 63 tables he barraged the profession with statistical, laboratory, and logical evidence, all badly organized and poorly described. Instead of acclaim he was met with more controversy. Semmelweis died in 1865, after some years of mental illness, of puerperal fever contracted through a nick he gave himself during an autopsy. It was many years later that his discovery achieved final ascendancy over the prejudices and inertia of physicians. In 1894, a monument was erected in Vienna to honor "woman's greatest friend" (Jones, 1970).

It is noteworthy that Ignaz Phillip Semmelweis was not the first physician to attribute puerperal sepsis to the unsanitariness of birth attendants. Charles White (1778), Robert Collins (1836), and Oliver Wendell Holmes (1843) had already made the attribution, without succeeding in changing the behavior of the medical community. Nor did Semmelweis discover the immediate cause of infection, the germ of the matter, so to speak. Fifty years were to elapse before Pasteur did that. In Semmelweis's time there was no bacteriology, and he described the agent luridly as "cadaveric matter." But where Holmes, Collins, and White vaguely prescribed cleanliness, Semmelweis boldly insisted upon a specific antiseptic procedure he called Chlorwaschungen. He made the physicians, students, and nurses in the wards of his hospital do it, and it worked. He also faced up to the necessity of marshalling compelling statistical evidence for his theory of the proximate cause of childbed fever and the effective prophylaxis. His book presented the statistical case and put across (albeit slowly) the moral where Holmes and others had failed to do so. Semmelweis deserves to be honored as one of humanity's greatest benefactors, but researchers should honor him for having assembled a classic work of social statistics.

REFERENCES

A corner of history. *Preventive Medicine*, 1974, *3*, 574–580.

Bender, G. A.: *Great moments in medicine*. Detroit: Parke-Davis. 1966.

deKruif, P.: *Men against death*. New York: Harcourt, Brace, 1932.

Edgar, J.: Address on Semmelweis: A short sketch of his life and teaching. *Scottish Medical and Surgical Journal*, 1898, *2*, 289–296.

Jones, G. W.: The unbalanced reformer. *Virginia Medical Monthly*, 1970, *97*, 526–527.

McManus, J. F. A.: *The fundamental ideas of medicine*. Springfield, Ill.: Charles C Thomas, 1963.

Oliver Wendell Holmes and the doctrine of Semmelweis. *Lancet*, 1909, *2*, 882.

Reid, R.: *Microbes and men*. New York: Saturday Review Press, 1974.

Robinson, V.: Semmelweis, the obstetrician. *Medical Review of Reviews*, 1912, *18*, 232–246.

———: *Pathfinders in medicine*. New York: Medical Life Press, 1929.

Semmelweis, I. P.: *The etiology, concept and prophylaxis of childbed fever*. Vienna: Hartleben, 1861.

Sigerist, H. E.: *The great doctors*. New York: Doubleday, 1958.

Sinclair, W. J.: *Semmelweis: His life and his doctrine*. Manchester: University Press, 1909.

Thompson, M.: *The cry and the covenant*. London: Heinemann, 1951.

Chapter 9

How Are Data Analyzed to Solve Problems?

DATA FILES AND DATA PROCESSING

The discussion up to this point has been concerned mostly with issues and problems which must be addressed before research data are collected. Consideration has been given to finding a research problem, reviewing the literature on that problem, sketching a theoretical position in terms of the constructs to be used and the probable or possible network of relationships among those constructs, specifying the variables corresponding to the constructs in terms of the observable variates which are to serve as their indicators, and deciding upon the settings and persons to be studied. These are difficult, time-consuming, and therefore expensive preparatory tasks, yet they usually have to be completed before funding for the research project can be sought from a sponsor. The documentation of the outcomes for these tasks comprises the bulk of the research proposal. What remains to be added are a personnel section, a budget, and certain legal appendixes regarding the protection of subjects' rights, an affirmative action posture for the project, and so forth.

Writing an ambitious research proposal today is tantamount to writing a book, but proportionally probably more of the books written get published than proposals written get funded. Authors sometimes have to move their manuscripts around among quite a few publishers before they place them; however, a really good research proposal should be kept circulating until it is funded.

After a proposal is funded there follows a period of frantic activity at the site or sites in which the data are collected. During this period the project staff are required to deploy a staggering mix of management skills, public relations skills, clerical skills, financial control and audit skills, and a variety of domestic skills such as driving, phoning, and housekeeping (otherwise research premises can get rather messy at this stage). It is likely that there will be surprises and emergencies galore. The previous chapter has discussed some of the on-site tasks. It is especially important to anticipate the ways the scenario on site may unfold during the proposal-writing stage, and to provide personnel and budget adequate to cope with what may happen. In the end, of course, the projected scenario will never play perfectly, and some deficiencies in the data collected will have to be remedied during the initial processing of the data, when steps are taken to "clean the data files." Suppose the research has been executed and the data have been collected more or less as planned. What happens next?

First, a data file must be constructed. (In some more complex studies there may be several data files, but we will assume only one is required.) A *data file* is a statement of the data in a form such that a computer can read it. Nonsense, you may think, since you anticipate assembling a data file of modest size and you already own a perfectly good pocket calculator, perhaps one which was sold to you for its statistics capabilities. Sorry, but we do not think you can be permitted to calculate your research statistics on any pocket or desk calculator, however fancy. The reason is that you will inevitably make mistakes in entering the data to such a device. Even if you know that you will not make any entry mistakes, there is absolutely no way for you to guarantee to your public that your handwork will have such uncanny accuracy. Furthermore, we are going to recommend some fairly complicated arithmetic for modeling even modest sets of data, so that the opportunities for copying and entering errors will be greater than you might think. Use your pocket calculator for the many student and domestic chores it is good for, but plan to send your research data to a computer. (Does this mean that all research analyses computed before the computer became available are automatically suspect? Yes!)

Files which the computer can read take several physical forms. The usual form is more suitable. Some machines use cassettes, disks, or floppy disks. Until recently almost all readable files were started by putting the data on punch cards. Tapes would be made by reading cards through the computer and writing their contents out on magnetic tapes. The same procedure was also used for making disks. With the widespread availability of computer terminals it is increasingly popular to type the data directly into the computer memory, then to write it out on whatever long-term storage device is desired (cards, tape, or disk). You may want to make highly organized and very neat handwritten rosters of scores as an aid to entering the data to a readable device—in fact, we urge you to take this step—but we insist that a research data file must be computer-readable.

What happens after the data file has been constructed? First it must be proofread and corrected for entering mistakes. This is usually done by getting a printed listing of the file from the computer, then proofreading by having one person read aloud from the original score roster while another person compares these scores with what appears on the computer printout. If IBM cards are made, there is a method called *verifying*, by which the keypunch operator types all the data a second time while a verifying machine compares the typed data with what was punched on the cards originally. By one method or another it is necessary to make certain that the scores in the data file are the scores which were collected in the research activity.

The next step may surprise you if you have never done a nursing research project. It involves repairing the file for missing and bad data. It is practically impossible to get to this stage of a research project and not discover that there are some subjects who are missing some sources and other subjects who have had scores recorded which could not possibly be true (scores which are *out of range*, meaning that the variate is not supposed to take those values, as when a patient's age in years is recorded as 187). Now this happens after the proofreading stage, so going back to check the original records probably is not going to help (although it never hurts to try, as it may turn out that a proofreading error slipped by). Somehow the research failed to generate a good score on this variate for this subject. Perhaps the subject refused to answer this question, thus producing a missing score, or perhaps a recording error was made, yielding an out-of-range score.

Accounting for missing or incorrect scores is a matter requiring judgment. One absolute rule is that the research report must document exactly what was done about repairing such situations and exactly how many times it was done. The reader who is not informed about the occurrences of "bad" data and what was done about them is not in a position to make an informed judgment of the limits of generalizability of the results. In some cases it is best to discard the subject's scores entirely from the panel of data. But if a great deal has been learned about a subject at considerable expense, it makes no sense to throw away all that information because the subject is missing one piece of descriptive measurement. It does make sense to salvage a crucial criterion (outcome) datum or perhaps even a crucial independent variate which describes the treatment received by a subject (when the research is intended to evaluate different treatments). Some strategies exist for such salvaging operations. Cohen and Cohen (1975) devote an entire chapter to the matter of missing data strategies. Theirs is the most complete and trustworthy text we know of on the subject. For most situations they recommend *plugging the mean*. This strategy involves computing an average score on a variate for all the subjects who have believable scores, and then replacing a missing score or a score out of range with this average. Sometimes it is better to plug with the mode or the median of the available scores, rather than the mean. In each case of a missing datum, one must make a thoughtful decision and an honest disclosure of what was done and why.

The contemporary researcher has a responsibility to archive her data files in a way that permits sharing the data with interested colleagues or critics. Probably the data were collected with the support of public funds or charitable funds which were tax-exempt, and therefore there is a moral and often a legal sense in which they are in the public domain in any case. Nursing research is a public enterprise, however it is funded, and sometimes the greatest contribution a set of data can make to public knowledge arises when it is merged with data collected in a variety of research projects, or when it is cleverly reanalyzed by a borrower. No modern researcher should be possessive of her data. Sharing is so much the norm today that not being willing to share properly raises the suspicion that one is not able to share, perhaps because the claim to have collected the data described in a research report was fraudulent. Good management involves storing the data file in a form which is readily copied and machine-readable, usually on an IBM card deck or a computer magnetic tape. It is, of course, reasonable to require the borrower to pay the costs of copying, packing, and mailing.

Q: Make a report on the missing data in the Project TALENT sample of Appendix B. How seriously is this sample biased by missing data, in your judgment? Why?

SCORE DISTRIBUTIONS

The first step in data analysis is the computation and presentation of descriptive statistics. We do statistics to summarize the experience gained by the execution of the research design. Abstracting, reducing, simplifying, and generalizing are fundamental tools of intelligence. We would drown in a welter of impressions and memories (and a sea of data) if we did not summarize. We do summarize constantly and inevitably in pictures, words, and numbers. The counting and measuring expressed in statistical summaries sometimes carry an aura of scientism that may blind us to the possibility that they are poorly made. Statistics can be misused in comically or tragically misleading ways. Many summaries of experience are just wastefully irrelevant, somehow getting published even though they actually summarize oceans of trivia with elegant and meaningless statistics.

Meaning is the key to good statistics. The two purposes of statistics are to help us understand experience and to help us communicate understandings we have achieved to others who need them. Understanding and communication are promoted by good statistics. We could give many examples of the promotion of misunderstanding and confusion by poor statistics, but we are not going to involve ourselves with such examples. As you develop your insights and skills you will find examples of poor statistics in your professional reading all too readily. We want to emphasize *how statistics can create understanding* and *how statistics can communicate understanding* so that you will be able to evaluate the statistics you find in the research you read and be able to provide good statistics in the reports you write. Since most nurses will not be researchers, we urge all to learn to make intelligent evaluation of statistics they read. A professional person who cannot evaluate statistics is handicapped. It's that simple.

Meaning and summarizing are inextricably entangled. Every way of understanding a collection of events involves some kind of summarizing. Every way of extracting the meaning of a particular event involves some method for relating it to a summary of a collection of events. It is just because summaries are so unavoidable in intellectual work that they are so potentially dangerous. They can be worked too hard and kept intact too long. There are always some events in a collection of events which are not very well described by the summary fitted to the aggregate. When we get down to cases, as nurses must, we have to use summaries cautiously, respecting differences as well as similarities. A case may follow the trend for most cases in its class or it may surprise us. Knowledge of an aggregate of such cases conveyed by some sort of summary can be used intelligently to guide our expectations regarding a new case, but should not make us blind to evidence that a unique case has arisen if indeed it has. Statistics as summaries have the advantage that they encapsulate information about the extent of variation in an aggregate as well as about averages or trends. Alas, times, circumstances, and relationships change and knowledge suffers obsolescence. We have to view all summaries of experience, including statistics, as history. The question of the current relevance of history is an inescapable problem. Human intelligence feeds on problems such as this and would starve without a steady diet of them, but statistics do not solve such value problems. If we do not hide in a welter of statistics, if we think hard about what good statistical summaries of relevant past experience can teach us, we may find illumination in statistics.

Florence Nightingale was a great pioneer in the use of statistics as an information base for social policies. She invented splendid graphic representations of data summaries, such as the pie diagram of which Figure 9-1 is an example. So deep was her devotion to statistical method that her biographer, E. T. Cook, termed her "the passionate statistician." In 1891 she wrote to Galton, urging him to lend his support to her project to create a chair in social statistics at Oxford, statistics not yet being a university subject, to her dismay. She was convinced that social policy could be successful only if it were guided by statistical evidence. "We sweep annually into our elementary schools hundreds of thousands of children, spending millions of money," she said to Galton. "Do we know: (1) what proportion of children forget their whole education after leaving school; whether *all* they have been taught is *waste*? (2) what are the results upon the lives and conduct of children in after life who don't forget all they have been taught?" How marvelous for her to have seen so early that the justification of curriculum decisions in a democracy's schools would have to be largely statistical! Although he was the inventor of the correlation method to which we attach so much importance, Galton did not possess Nightingale's enlightened vision on the relation of statistics to policy, and he did not soldier for her. Thus the chair at Oxford did not materialize. Upon Galton's death and at his bequest, Karl Pearson assumed a new Galton chair of eugenics at the University of London and organized Galton's laboratories there into a new department of applied statistics (this took place in 1911, 1 year after Nightingale died). By that

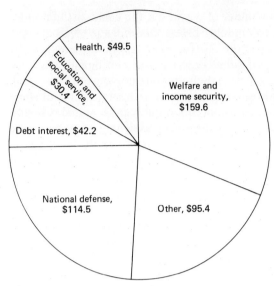

Figure 9-1 Pie diagram of the 1979 U.S. federal budget, in billions. (*Data from Time, December 4, 1978, p. 34.*)

time Pearson had given formal mathematical definition to all the statistical methods we advocate in this text.

Scales and Scores

A measurement scale is a device for assigning numbers to stand for individual differences among objects or subjects as observed by some rule. Throughout this text we will talk about scores assigned to subjects, but in some cases in nursing research the variates will actually be measured on objects (e.g., a room, the temperature of which is measured). The basic requirement for a scale is that there must be at least two different numbers assigned in the distribution of scores for all the research subjects. A score *distribution* is the set of scores assigned to the research subjects on a particular variate. The distribution has the property of *variance* when there are at least two different scores that occur in the distribution. Without some variation in scores, the score distribution would be worthless as a research finding, in that it could not be used to explain the variance in any other variate and would not have any variance which could be explained by anything else. (Of course, if informed people had expected some variance in a particular variate and found none, that would be important to report. Thus, if sex is a variate in a study of nurses but all the nurses in the sample turn out to be females, whereas it was reasonable to expect to find some males, it is important to report that no male nurses were found. However, nothing further can be done with the sex distribution, and sex has to be eliminated from the list of research variates because it has no variance.) Only when there is some variability in scores do we have anything on which to perform statistical analysis.

Scales may be classified in a number of ways, but the basic distinction we will need is between nominal and continuous scales. *Nominal* scales (from Latin *nomen* meaning name, as in nomenclature) are based on taxonomies, and can be operated by counting the number of subjects in each of two or more cells or categories of a taxonomy. Sex is a simple dichotomous nominal variate. Each subject may be counted as a female or a male, at least in theory. (Think of some reasons why it might be difficult to determine sex reliably in an actual research situation.) It is also possible to score sex by arbitrarily assigning a number to the subject depending on the observed (or claimed) sex, as for example 0 = female, 1 = male. Usually we will want to scale nominal variates by this method, called *dummy coding*. When there are three or more cells or categories in the taxonomy, we will create a dichotomous nominal variate for each cell, assigning the score 0 if the subject does not belong to the cell and the score 1 if the subject does belong to the cell. Thus, in a four-cell taxonomy of religious preferences, a subject whose preference was given as Protestant would be scored as follows:

Dummy variate	Score
1 Catholic?	0
2 Protestant?	1
3 Other religion?	0
4 No religion?	0

What scores would you assign on the four dummy variates for a person who reported having no religion? What about a subject claiming to be an agnostic, or an atheist? You are reminded that the second section of Chapter 5 established the need for very precise and exhaustive rules for scoring responses to a variate. The immediate practical value is that we are anticipating the use of computer data processing. In each cell the coding must be absolute (all that is not black is white). The computer will obey doggedly, but, like a dog, it must be told clearly whether to sit or fetch.

A *continuous* scale is one on which a higher numerical score represents the observation that the subject displays "more" of the characteristic under measurement, whereas a lower score represents the subject as displaying "less" of the characteristic. Age and SAT verbal test are two examples of continuous variates in educational research. The important thing about continuous variates is that we are willing to average the scale scores assigned. Strangely, we are also willing to average dichotomous nominal variates which have been dummy-coded. Thus, to say that 100 subjects have an average age of 192 months and an average SAT verbal score of 503 is somehow meaningful. If sex is scored as a dummy variate with 0 = female and 1 = male, the statement that the 100 subjects have a sex average of .65 implies that 65 percent of the subjects are males. Can you see why this is so?

Q: In Appendix B, variate 11 is a dummy code. What proportion of the subjects took an academic curriculum in high school?

Statistics

Statistics capture the behaviors of subjects in the aggregate. Individuals are known in statistical reasoning by their positions within the distribution of scores for all subjects. It is essential that we have some summary of the distribution, and indeed, as a plural noun, statistics are descriptive characteristics of sample distributions. (As a singular noun, statistics is a method, a theory, a body of empirical knowledge, and perhaps some other things.) Sir Ronald Fisher, one of the most inventive and influential of twentieth-century statisticians, said, "A statistic is a value calculated from an observed sample with a view to characterizing the population from which it is drawn" (1950, p. 41). That is a statistician's view of what a statistic is. Unfortunately, we usually have to attempt to generalize our statistics to populations other than the one from which the sample was drawn. In addition, Fisher's definition assumes that we drew the sample randomly, which we cannot always do. The point of view of this book is that some of the descriptive statistics which statisticians have invented and popularized are extremely useful in nursing research, while much of the higher theory of statistics is largely irrelevant at best and dangerously misleading at worst. A comparison of the contents of this chapter with the statistics sections of competitive books on nursing research is likely to show that our point of view makes a difference in the syllabus.

Averages

A natural question to ask about a set of scores is, "Where is the center of the distribution?" If the distribution is symmetric around its most frequent score, as is the fictitious SAT verbal distribution in Figure 9-2, the maximum ordinate (i.e., the most frequent score) is obviously the answer. This most frequent score is called the *mode*. When the distribution is not symmetric, as in the fictitious skewed income distribution of Figure 9-3, the most frequent score is not necessarily the best measure of the center of the distribution (often called the *central tendency*). A very attractive center for skewed distributions is the score which separates the lower 50 percent of the subjects from the upper 50 percent. This is the *median*, and is also known as the 50th percentile. However, the statistician's

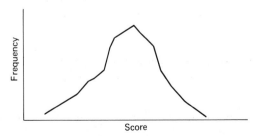

Figure 9-2   Distribution of SAT verbal scores.

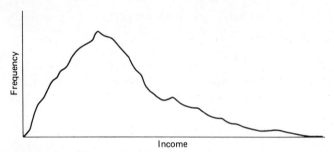

Figure 9-3   Distribution of income.

favorite center, and ours, is neither of these, but is instead the arithmetic average, or *mean*. Expressed algebraically, the mean is

$$m = \frac{X_1 + X_2 + \cdots + X_N}{N} \tag{1}$$

where X_1 is the score of the first subject, etc.; N is the number of subjects in the sample. The usual way to write the cumulative summation of the scores is to use a summation operator, provided by the symbol Σ, and a subscript j on the score X, which is understood to take the values from 1 to N. In this notation the mean is

$$m = \frac{\Sigma X_j}{N} \tag{2}$$

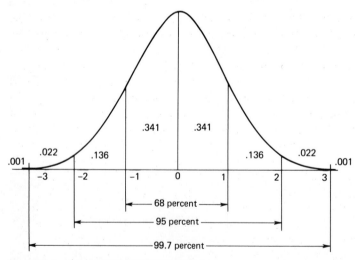

Figure 9-4   Areas of the $N(0,1)$ distribution.

A very convenient facet of symmetric distributions is that the three measures of central tendency (mean, median, mode) coincide. Idealized or theoretical distributions in statistics are often symmetric, as in the case of the normal curve. Actual research distributions are not likely to be exactly symmetric, but there is a good reason, stated by the central limit theorem, why they are often close to it.

Central Limit Theorem

Many of the variates used in nursing research are scaled by adding together into a scale score the responses of a subject to a number of items. An attitude toward pain variate might be scaled by adding together the subject's scores on a set of items which inquire into feelings about different painful situations, where each item is scored so that the higher item scores would indicate the more stoic or less fearful responses to pain. Then the sum of item scores would be a scale score such that subjects with lower scores would seem to be more afraid of pain and subjects with higher scores would seem to be more determined to master pain. Now, if this attitude scale is administered to a research sample, what will the score distribution look like? Common sense says we do not know and cannot anticipate, but there is a remarkable theorem from mathematical statistics which asserts that the score distribution will tend to be symmetric and approximately the shape of a normal curve. Figure 9-4 is an example of a normal curve. Formally, the central limit theorem states that a sum of n independent, random observations from any population distribution whatever will tend toward a normal sampling distribution. The theorem applies in our imaginary attitude toward pain distribution because the separate items added together to make the scale score can be thought of as having been selected independently and randomly from a population of possible items about handling pain. The n of the theorem is the number of items combined in the scale. The larger n is, the more nearly symmetric and normal we can expect the score distribution to be. The central limit theorem describes a phenomenon which is mysterious but trustworthy, and it occurs in so many scalings of variates in nursing research that it is well for us to know some facts about normal curves and appropriate for us to employ statistics which are ideal for normal distributions. The mean, variance, and correlation, which are the three basic statistics we advocate, are ideal for normal distributions.

Frequency Polygons

A frequency polygon is made by counting the number of times each score value occurs in the score distribution (thus getting the *frequency* of each score value), plotting these counts as the ordinates (vertical heights of the curve) over each of the score values on the abscissa (horizontal axis), and finally connecting adjacent points with straight line segments. Figure 9-5 is a polygon for 50 scores. Notice that the lowest score in the distribution is 1, and it occurs once. The highest score is 9, which also occurs once. The score values of 5, 6, and 7 are tied for highest

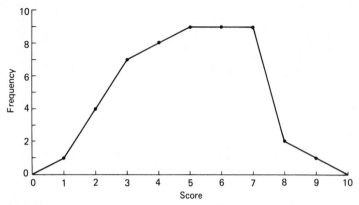

Figure 9-5 Polygon for 50 scores.

frequency, and all occur nine times. It is hard to determine by inspection what the mode and median are for this distribution, but the mean can be computed by multiplying each score value by its frequency, summing these products, and dividing by the sample size, which is 50. Symbolically, this formulation of the mean is

$$m = \frac{\Sigma\ (X_j f_j)}{N} \tag{3}$$

where the range of j is the lowest and highest score values. Arithmetically, this formulation produces

$$
\begin{aligned}
m &= [(1 \times 1) + (2 \times 4) + (3 \times 7) + (4 \times 8) \\
&\quad + (5 \times 9) + (6 \times 9) + (7 \times 9) + (8 \times 2) + (9 \times 1)]\ /\ 50 \\
&= 4.98
\end{aligned}
$$

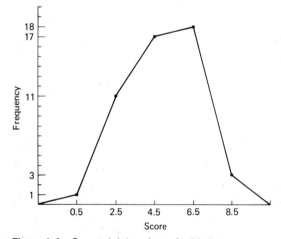

Figure 9-6 Grouped-data polygon for 50 scores.

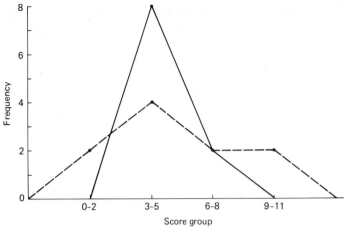

Figure 9-7 Polygons for two groups of 10 subjects each.

Often in research the range of score values that occur is so large in relation to the number of subjects, N, that it is useful to group scores before counting frequencies. For example, the scores in the distribution of Figure 9-5 may be grouped as 0–1, 2–3, 4–5, 6–7, 8–9 to produce the polygon of Figure 9-6. Now the polygon has a modal score category (group 6–7 with a frequency of 18), and it is possible to see that the median falls in the score category 4–5, but the loss of detail makes it impossible to compute the mean precisely. However, multiplying each score category midpoint by the category frequency, summing these products, and dividing by N yields

$$m = [(.5 \times 1) + (2.5 \times 11) + (4.5 \times 17) + (6.5 \times 18) + (8.5 \times 3)] / 50$$
$$= 4.94$$

which is not too far off the mark. Since decisions about how to group the scores and how to scale the vertical and horizontal axes are left up to the researcher, polygons can be made to look smooth or jagged, tall and slim, or squat and long, as the researcher likes. The reader has to wonder whether the researcher has grouped the scores and chosen axis scales appropriately. If so, the frequency polygon often gives a good impression of the score distribution. Polygons are not reported more often simply because they are troublesome to prepare and expensive to print.

Polygons are especially interesting when they are available on the same grid for two or more different groups of subjects (or for one group of subjects observed at two or more different times). Figure 9-7 puts a grouped-data polygon for one group of subjects (solid line) on the same grid with a polygon for a second group of subjects (dashed line) for the following two groups of 10 subjects each:

Group 1: 3 4 4 5 5 5 5 5 7 7 ($m_1 = 5$)
Group 2: 1 2 3 3 4 5 6 6 9 11 ($m_2 = 5$)

(Verify that the mean is 5 for each group.) This figure confirms what inspection of the data reveals, namely, that while the two distributions have the same mean, there is more scatter of scores around the mean in the second group than there is in the first group. If we think of the mean as locating the central tendency of a group, we may say that the members of the first group do not show as much variation around the group location as do the members of the second. Wouldn't it be helpful to have an index of the amount of scatter in a group of scores?

Q: Make a grouped-data frequency polygon for variate 3 in Appendix B. Does it appear that the English test scores are approximately normal in distribution? Would it be reasonable to hypothesize that the English test scores of all nursing aspirants among the nation's female eleventh graders in 1960 were normally distributed? Why?

Variances

A statistic which describes the amount of scatter of the scores in a distribution is defined as

$$s^2 = \frac{\Sigma(X_j - m)^2}{N} \tag{4}$$

This algebra defines the *variance* as the average squared deviation from the mean. Notice that the mean is subtracted from each score, X_j (where j takes integer values from 1 to N), so that the score of the jth subject is expressed as a "deviation from the mean," $X_j - m$; then these are squared and all the squares are summed; and finally the sum of squared deviations is divided by the sample size, N, giving an average squared deviation. This formula is the definition of variance, but an algebraically equivalent formula which is easier to compute is

$$s^2 = \frac{\Sigma X_j^2 - [(\Sigma X_j)^2 / N]}{N} \tag{5}$$

This computing formula for the variance requires ΣX_j^2, the sum of squared scores and $(\Sigma X_j)^2$, the square of the sum of scores.

Variance is a marvelous measure of the extent of variation in a score distribution because we have tools for partitioning a variance into a part which is explained by a relationship we are studying and an unexplained part. These tools are the subjects of the next three major sections of this chapter. One problem with the variance as a descriptive statistic, however, is that it is expressed in the metric of squared scores, and it is often convenient to take the square root of the variance, which is called the *standard deviation*, as an alternative measure of scatter. The standard deviation, for which we use the symbol s, might seem to be much more suitable as a measure of variability because it is in the metric of the scores. Unfortunately, it is not possible to partition s, which is why we will usually concern ourselves with s^2.

Q: What are the variances for each of the two groups of 10 scores given in the last section as the basis of Figure 9-7?

Standard Scores

The standard deviation is a most useful yardstick for measuring a deviation of a subject from a group mean. Defining a standard score as

$$z_j = \frac{X_j - m}{s} \tag{6}$$

we get a score which tells by its sign whether the subject is above or below the mean, and by its magnitude how many standard deviation units the subject is from the mean. With z scores the direction and extent of the subject's deviance in two different score distributions can be compared, as all z score distributions are in the same metric. For example, if a subject is age 10 in an age distribution for the research sample with mean 9 and standard deviation 2, the subject has

$$z_{A_j} = \frac{10 - 9}{2} = .5$$

If the same subject is weight 90 in a weight distribution for the research sample with mean 85 and standard deviation 1.8, the subject has

$$z_{W_j} = \frac{90 - 85}{1.8} = 2.78$$

The comparison of these two z scores permits us to say that this subject is overage and overweight in the sample, but only half a standard deviation above the age mean and almost three standard deviations above the weight mean. Obviously the sample has considerable age variation and not much weight variation. Perhaps it is composed of subjects who were chosen to be of a given height, regardless of age and weight. In this sample the subject is not very deviant with respect to age but is very deviant with respect to weight.

Normal Curves

Normal curves are a family of curves described by a particular formula. All normal curves follow that set formula, but each particular curve is identified by its own mean and variance. All normal curves are symmetrical around their coinciding mean, median, and mode locations, and all have the bell shape to some extent, although those curves for which the mean is large relative to the variance will appear peaked (tall and narrow), and those for which the mean is small relative to the variance will appear squat. Special interest attaches to that normal curve which has 0 as its mean and 1 as its variance. Figure 9-4 reveals some facts about this special normal curve, designated $N(0,1)$. This $N(0,1)$ is the curve which the z scores will follow when any normal distribution whatever is transformed to a z score distribution by subtracting the mean from each score and dividing that difference by the standard deviation. Whenever we have good reason to believe that the central limit theorem is operating upon a research distribution, we can expect the z score version of the distribution to approximate the shape of the normal curve of Figure 9-4.

CORRELATIONS

Correlation is the most important idea in statistics. It means that two variates are observed to vary together to some extent. When we see that the way in which subjects are spread out on one measurement is similar to the way they are spread out on another measurement, we say that the two measurements are correlated. For example, we notice that taller people also tend to be heavier people. The agreement in ranking of subjects on correlated measurements is never perfect, and sometimes it is so slight that we worry that the measurements only seem to be correlated in the sample in hand, when in fact they are almost uncorrelated in the population. However, it is as unlikely that two measurements are perfectly uncorrelated in a population as it is that they are perfectly correlated. Statistics uses an index of correlation which varies between 0—meaning no correlation— and 1—meaning perfect correlation. The correlation index, or correlation coefficient, usually denoted r, never quite reaches either limit, so that

$$0 < r < 1$$

for all pairs of observed variates. If one variate tends to decrease as the other increases, the range of r is

$$0 > r > -1$$

but in such a case it is possible to multiply all scores on one of the variates by -1 (called reflecting the variate), after which transformation it will be the case that

$$0 < r < 1$$

A *scatter diagram* is a good device for eyeballing the correlation of two variates, X and Y. This is made by laying out cartesian axes on graph paper for X and Y, then plotting a point for each subject where a vertical line through the subject's X score intercepts a horizontal line through the corresponding Y score. Figure 9-8 is a scatter plot for the data of Table 9-1. When the points stretch out in a recognizable direction we are seeing evidence of correlation. *The more the points stretch out, the greater the correlation*.

An obvious thing about the scatter plot in which correlation is present to a marked degree is that it suggests how to predict one variate from the other, say to predict Y from X. If we eyeball a "line of stretch" or "line of best fit" through the

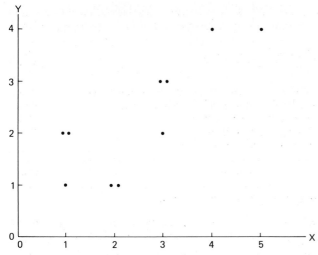

Figure 9-8 Scatter plot for 10 subjects.

points, as we have done in Figure 9-9, we can predict Y_i by erecting a vertical line over X_i, then erecting a horizontal line through the point where the vertical line crosses the stretch line. Where this horizontal line crosses the Y axis is the predicted Y_i, which we will denote $\hat{Y}_i$. Figure 9-10 shows this scheme for $X_i = 2$ giving $\hat{Y}_i = 2.2$; and $X_i = 4$ giving $\hat{Y}_i = 3.5$.

Notice that in Figure 9-9 a $\bar{Y}$ has been plotted over each possible X score. This $\bar{Y}$ is the mean of all Y scores for that X score, and is called the Y array mean for the X value. These array means are a big help in eyeballing the best-fitting line.

You may have learned in algebra that every straight line can be expressed by an equation of the form

$$\hat{Y}_i = bX_i + a \tag{7}$$

Table 9-1 Data for 10 Subjects

Subject	X	Y
1	1	1
2	1	2
3	1	2
4	2	1
5	2	1
6	3	3
7	3	3
8	3	2
9	4	4
10	5	4

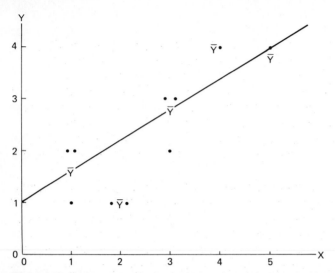

Figure 9-9   Scatter plot with array means and eyeballed regression line.

In Figure 9-11, b is the *slope* of the line (its tilt; given by the tangent of angle Θ, which is length c divided by length d) and a is the *intercept*, that is, the value of Y when $X = 0$, which is where the line of best fit crosses the Y axis. A statistics term for the stretch line or line of best fit to the scatter plot is *regression* line. Equation (7) is called a regression equation, and the act of predicting Y from X on the basis of the correlation of the two variates is called computing the regression of Y on X.

The trouble with eyeballing lines of best fit is that two analysts may disagree

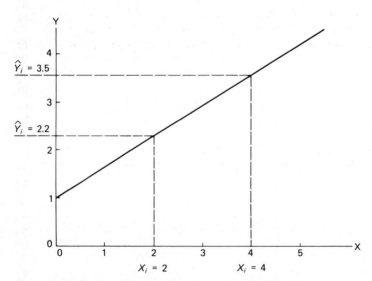

Figure 9-10   Predicted Y scores for two scores on the X variate.

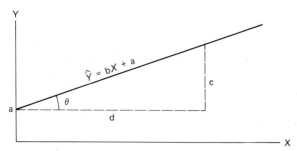

Figure 9-11   Slope and intercept for line of best fit.

on where the line should be put. Statistics favors a rule for placing the line which is called the *least squares* rule, because it results from using calculus to minimize the sum of squared errors of prediction.

$$\sum_{i}^{N} (\hat{Y}_i - Y_i)^2 \text{ (minimized)} \tag{8}$$

The rule for b to satisfy Equation (8) is

$$b = \frac{\Sigma XY - [(\Sigma X)(\Sigma Y)/N]}{\Sigma X^2 - [(\Sigma X)^2/N]} \tag{9}$$

and the intercept is made from this slope coefficient b and the means of X and Y.

$$a = m_Y - bm_X \tag{10}$$

The use of differential calculus to derive b and a assures us that no other slope and intercept can be chosen to locate a prediction line for which the sum of squared errors of prediction across the entire sample will be smaller than the least squares for this line.

Technical note: Closely related to the numerator of b in Equation (9) is a useful quantity called the *covariance*. If we let s_{XY} be the symbol for the covariance of X and Y, then

$$s_{XY} = \frac{1}{N}\left[\Sigma XY - \frac{(\Sigma X)(\Sigma Y)}{N}\right]$$

The bivariate statistic s_{XY} is the natural mate or counterpart for the univariate statistics s_X^2 and s_Y^2. It has the same advantage as the variance, which is that theorems exist for its partition in research analyses. We do not need s_{XY} in our present discussion of correlation and regression, but in Chapter 11 we will teach you a dramatic and powerful method for partitioning the variances and covariances of a set of research variates. A memorable and informative formula for the covariance in relation to the correlation is

$$s_{XY} = r_{XY} s_X s_Y$$

from which you can see that when $s_X = s_Y = 1.000$, as is the case for standardized variates, the covariance is the correlation. We strongly recommend standardization of research variates in nursing research precisely to take advantage of this equality.

Sir Francis Galton first proposed the use of linear regression in social sciences toward the end of the nineteenth century, and his student Karl Pearson developed the algebra for fitting the least squares regression at just about the turn of the century. It is an interesting fact that Florence Nightingale was in correspondence with both of these men about her vision of a chair in social statistics at one of the leading British universities. In due time Pearson came to be the first occupant of such a chair, at the University of London and named for Galton. We do not know of a chair in any university named for that "passionate statistician" Florence Nightingale, but there should be one.

Closely associated with the slope coefficient is the *correlation* coefficient, which is defined as

$$r = \frac{N\Sigma XY - (\Sigma X)(\Sigma Y)}{\sqrt{[N\Sigma X^2 - (\Sigma X)^2][N\Sigma Y^2 - (\Sigma Y)^2]}} \tag{11}$$

This is often called the Pearson product-moment correlation coefficient, because Pearson first gave its algebra and the form of the algebra is recognized as a product-moment by statisticians. You may also hear it called zero-order correlation or bivariate correlation. Whatever it is called, r is the most ubiquitous of statistics.

The statistics of the regression line and the correlation coefficient may be computed for the data of Table 9-1 by placing the accumulations (sums of scores, sums of squares, and sum of cross products) for the scores given in the table into place in the equations.

$$b = \frac{\Sigma XY - \Sigma X(\Sigma Y)/N}{\Sigma X^2 - (\Sigma X)^2/N} = \frac{69 - 25(23)/10}{79 - (25)^2/10}$$

$$= \frac{11.5}{16.5} = .697$$

$$a = m_Y - bm_X = 2.3 - .697(2.5) = 2.3 - 1.743 = .557$$

$$r = \frac{N\Sigma XY - \Sigma X(\Sigma Y)}{\sqrt{[N\Sigma X^2 - (\Sigma X)^2][N\Sigma Y^2 - (\Sigma Y)^2]}} = \frac{10(69) - 25(23)}{\sqrt{[10(79) - (25)^2][10(65) - (23)^2]}}$$

$$= \frac{690 - 575}{\sqrt{(790 - 625)(650 - 529)}} = \frac{115}{\sqrt{19,965}} = \frac{115}{141.3} = .814$$

How well does the regression of Y on X account for the distribution of Y? Recall that the measure of the scatter of scores on Y is the variance of Y, denoted $s_Y{}^2$. Pearsonian regression partitions the unconditional variance of Y into independent, additive variances, the first of which is the predictable variance of Y given its regression on X, and the second of which is the variance of errors from regression, which is minimized.

$$s_Y{}^2 = s_{\hat{Y}}{}^2 + s_e{}^2 \tag{12}$$

Another way of talking about Equation (12) is to say that the variance of the data has been partitioned into the variance due to the regression fit plus the variance of residuals from the fit. Two important facts are

$$s_{\hat{Y}}{}^2 = r^2 s_Y{}^2 \tag{13}$$
$$s_e{}^2 = (1 - r^2)s_Y{}^2 \tag{14}$$

Thus r^2 is the proportion of the variance of Y that is accounted for by the regression of Y on X, and $1 - r^2$ is the proportion of variance of Y *not* accounted for, or the residual variance. This ability of r^2 to express the proportion of the variance in the dependent variable accounted for by the regression fit makes r^2 the most useful index to the strength of regression.

For the data of Table 9-1 the regression equation turned out

$$\hat{Y}_i = .697 X_i + .557$$

The predicted Y score for a person having $X = 1$ is therefore 1.25, but in the sample, two of the people for whom $X = 1$ had $Y = 2$ and the third had $Y = 1$. It will always be the case that the actual Y scores in a given array will scatter around the predicted score. Assuming that this scatter of actual scores around the predicted score is the same in all the arrays, an estimate of its standard deviation is provided by

$$s_e = \left(\sqrt{1 - r^2}\right) s_Y \tag{15}$$

and if we further assume that the scatter around predicted values in the arrays is normally distributed, a 95 percent confidence interval for $\hat{Y}_i$ is given by

$$(\hat{Y}_i - 2s_e) <\text{- - - -}> (\hat{Y}_i + 2s_e)$$

It is customary to assume that 95 times out of 100 this interval will contain the actual value of Y_i. Usually correlations and regressions are computed to help us to understand the relation between X and Y, without any view to making actual predictions, but when the regression equation is put to work to produce predicted scores it is vital that those predictions be interpreted in the light of s_e (called the standard error of estimate in this context). Unless r is close to 1, predictions can be very fallible.

Q: Find a research report which contains correlation coefficients. Discuss the interpretations of the correlations. Can you add anything to the interpretations put forward in the report? (Hint: Did the authors interpret r^2 as explained variance?)

MULTIPLE CORRELATIONS

Practical research on nursing can never be done with a bivariate data set. There always are more than two variates that must be measured and analyzed, even if interest centers on the relationship of one key independent variate to one key dependent variate. In the SUNYAB thermometer study, interest was centered on the relationship between the sheath variate (whether or not the thermometer was sheathed) and the temperature reading. However, the length of time the thermometer was in the mouth was another variate, and yet another variate was the site where the data were collected (school or hospital). There are always circumstances or conditions that have to be taken into consideration. Since data sets are multivariate rather than bivariate, we have to employ multivariate analysis procedures to answer research questions or to test theoretical propositions. The multivariate methods we recommend are built up from the full set of all bivariate correlations among the multiple variates. If there are p variates in a study, there are $p(p - 1)/2$ different bivariate correlations. The first step in research analysis is to compute these correlations and to think about them. First interest attaches to the correlations of the predictors with the criterion (or criteria). (This simple predictor value is often termed the *simple validity* of a predictor for the criterion. It is given as r_{jp} for the jth independent variate, assuming the pth variate is the criterion.) The comparison of simple validities is not the entire story, because the intercorrelations among the predictors must be taken into account. Looking at the correlations among the predictors, one views them as indicators of redundancy. (Redundancy is overlapping variance. Since the information about subjects is contained in the scatter of scores, overlap in variance of two variates is also overlap in information.) The most redundant predictor is probably the most expendable, or the one we could best get along without.

   A technical measure of the information a particular predictor contributes to a set of predictors is its *uniqueness* (U_j) in the set. This U_j is the part of the predictability of the criterion from the set of predictors which is lost if the jth predictor is withdrawn from the set. If we let U stand for the part of the criterion variance which is predictable from the full set of predictors (where U can be thought of as the *usefulness* of the set), and let U_{*j} stand for the part of the criterion variance which is predictable from all the independent variates except the jth one, then

$$U_j = U - U_{*j} \tag{16}$$

If the independent variates were mutually uncorrelated, then it would follow that

$$U = U_1 + U_2 + \cdots + U_q \tag{17}$$

if there were q independent variates in all. However, independent variates never are mutually uncorrelated, so a leftover piece c (for *commonality*) occurs.

$$U = U_1 + U_2 + \cdots + U_q + c \tag{18}$$
Or
$$c = U - (U_1 + U_2 + \cdots + U_q) \tag{19}$$

This commonality is the result of the joint action, or confounded action, of the independent variates on the criterion. The existence of c is implied by the correlations among the independent variates, which makes it an unavoidable nuisance. If only c were zero, we would have the lovely situation where

$$U_j = r_{jp}^2 \tag{20}$$

That is, the square of the simple validity of the jth predictor would be the uniqueness of that predictor. Another version of Equation (17) for uncorrelated predictors would be

$$U = r_{1p}^2 + r_{2p}^2 + \cdots + r_{qp}^2 \tag{21}$$

It may seem cruel to emphasize in Equations (17), (20), and (21) a lovely situation pertaining to uncorrelated predictors at the same time that we emphasize that such a situation never arises naturally in measurements. Soon, however, we are going to unveil a simple scheme by which correlated predictor variates can be transformed into uncorrelated predictor variables, with the lovely simplifying result of abolishing c and making Equations (17), (20), and (21) applicable. *Voilà*, the coach from the pumpkin.

For the moment, Equations (16), (18), and (19) describe the situation for multivariate correlations. What they do not tell us is how to compute U and U_{*j}. We recommend computing these statistics by a method we shall term *sweeping out*. This is a method which sweeps one variate out of the correlation table entirely, then sweeps out a second variate, and so forth, until all the independent variates have been swept out. Each time one of the independent variates is swept out of the table of correlations, it takes some of the variance of each of the other variates along with it, on the basis of its correlations with the other variates. This includes some criterion variance as well. When all the independent variates have been swept out, the remaining (or residual) criterion variance is reported as d^2. Then

$$U = 1 - d^2 \tag{22}$$

When the first $q - 1$ predictors have been swept out, the residual criterion variance may be designated $d_{*q}{}^2$, and then

$$U_{*q} = 1 - d_{*q}{}^2 \tag{23}$$

and

$$U_q = U - U_{*q} \tag{24}$$

as an application of Equation (16). The way to compute U_{*j} is to put the jth independent variate in last position (i.e., position q) among the predictors and recompute the sweep-out of $q - 1$ variates. This may seem awkward, but a computer can be instructed to cycle these sweep-out operations readily. In MODEL we provide a computer program capable of managing this analysis. The only arithmetic involved in sweeping out is addition, subtraction, multiplication, division, and taking square roots. Because of the last, the method has been called *square root factor analysis* in some books. The arithmetic is simple but repetitive, since it has to be applied to the whole table of correlations. The algebra of the sweep-out method is given in Cooley and Lohnes (1971, pp. 137–144). Appendix A lists the computer program MODEL, which incorporates the matrix algebra of the sweep-out method. You should have no trouble getting this program mounted in any computer center you have access to. Chapter 10 teaches you how to use this program to analyze your data.

Table 9-2 analyzes intercorrelations among five variates borrowed from a splendid research project done in Australia by John Keeves (1972). The correlations can be found in Table 11-1. In Chapter 11 we analyze these correlations in a way which tests a hypothesized causal model for the 1969 science achievement

Table 9-2 Partition of Variance for 1969 Science Achievement

Symbol	Definition	Value
U_1	Uniqueness for 1968 science achievement	.508
U_2	Uniqueness for 1968 science attitude	.010
U_3	Uniqueness for science class processes	.006
U_4	Uniqueness for peer science and mathematics activities	.004
c	Commonality, or confounded contribution, of the four predictors	.068
U	Usefulness of the four predictors	.596
e	Unexplained variance in the criterion	.464
s^2	Total variance for 1969 science achievement	1.000

criterion, but here we analyze them by the multivariate correlation method of this section. The questions we want to answer are: (1) What is the usefulness U of the four predictor variates working together to explain the variance in the 1969 science achievement criterion? (2) What is the uniqueness U_j of each of the four predictors, and what is the commonality c which estimates their confounded, inseparable contribution to the explanation of criterion variance? Our method is to run the MODEL computer program four times, each time specifying that four factors are to be extracted and that each one of the four predictors is to specify a different one of the four factors. All this is managed by simple setup procedures for a MODEL run, as explained in the next chapter. The trick for the present analysis is to rearrange the correlation matrix for runs 2, 3, and 4 so that for run 2 the 1968 science achievement predictor is factored last (i.e., as the fourth factor); for run 3 the 1968 science attitude predictor is factored last; and for run 4 the science class processes predictor is factored last. When these four runs are completed, the last line of a table of CONTRIBUTIONS OF DOMAINS TO KEY CRITERION VARIANCE, which is found in the output, reports the value of U as the cumulative proportion of criterion variance explained by the four predictors (this will be the same number for all four runs), and the third line of that table reports the cumulative proportion of criterion variance explained by the first three predictors working together *but without the fourth predictor*. This is U_{*j} of Equation (16), and when we have four values of U_{*j} we can compute each of the U_j. This sounds complicated because you have not studied the MODEL program yet, but it is actually easy with MODEL doing most of the work. In Chapter 10 we will encourage you to compute this analysis yourself. The results of this work are displayed in Table 9-2, where we see that the four predictors working together can explain .596 of the 1969 mathematics variance (or 59.6 percent of it), and the 1968 science achievement predictor makes the largest unique contribution of .508, while the peer science and mathematics activities predictor makes the smallest unique contribution of .004. Can you figure out why the uniqueness of the pretest of science achievement is so disproportionately large in comparison with the other three uniquenesses? The commonality is .068, which indicates the piece of the explained variance that cannot be attributed to any one predictor but must be viewed as the joint contributions of the four predictors.

Q: Write a paragraph interpreting the research results reported in Table 9-2.

REFERENCES

Cohen, Jacob, and Patricia Cohen: *Applied multiple regression/correlation analysis for the behavioral sciences*. New York: Wiley, 1975.
Cooley, William W., and Paul R. Lohnes: *Multivariate data analysis*. New York: Wiley, 1971.
Fisher, Sir Ronald A.: *The design of experiments* (6th ed.). New York: Hafner, 1950.
Keeves, John P.: *Educational environment and student achievement*. Melbourne: Australian Council for Educational Research, 1972.

How Will You Analyze Your Data?

This chapter shows you how to analyze data by the methods recommended in Chapter 9. You are taught the use of the computer program called MODEL, the code for which is presented in Appendix A. A consultant in any research computer center will have no difficulty getting this program stored in the center's program library and showing you how to access it. Your consultant will also show you how to create and save a data file (perhaps starting by punching IBM cards for your data, or by typing the data directly into the computer memory from a terminal). As a student researcher, you will enjoy learning to use the computer. If you ever become a funded researcher or a member of a research team, you may want to contract for your computing tasks with a paid consultant (these are easy to find around computer centers), but you will still want to understand the use of the MODEL program so that you can direct your consultant properly. The instruction in this chapter is provided by worked examples of data analyses that were made by means of the MODEL program.

RUNNING MODEL

Younger readers of this text have probably had experiences with computers in high school and college, but some of us were not so fortunate, and fear of computing is still prevalent among us. We guarantee that this fear can be overcome in half a day if you will just take your book with you to the campus computing center, ask for the help of a staff member there, present the program listing in Appendix A, and explain that you want to learn how to enter this program into the computer, attach some data to it, and run it. You will be shown how to:

1 Open a computing account and identify yourself as a legal user to the computer
2 Type the program into a storage location assigned to you
3 Call the FORTRAN system to compile your program (which means finding your typing errors for you and, after you correct them, making the program executable)
4 Type in your data and attach the data to an execution request
5 Locate your printout

Half a day's work, we promise. Once you have made this effort, your MODEL program will be in residence at your computing center and you will be able to use it again simply by supplying new data to it. Your friends can use it, too. If your instructor has already installed the MODEL program at your computing center, ask how this was accomplished, so that you can visualize how you could do the same at some new location you might move to. A nice thing about the MODEL program is that many of the small, inexpensive computers which are now being sold so widely can mount it. If you have access to a small computer, ask whether it can compile FORTRAN. If it can, it can probably handle MODEL. Remember that measurement and statistical research designs mandate computerized data analyses. If you are interested in doing such research, it is a good investment to jump in and learn how to use a computer. If you simply cannot overcome your fear of or distaste for computers, it is also the case that the world is full of people who love to run computers and who will work for you for peanuts, by comparison with the other costs of research.

The instructions for running MODEL, as found at the beginning of the program listing, are as follows (in CAPS). Interspersed (in ordinary text) are interpretations of the instructions.

```
    INPUT
1)  SETUP VALUES
        COLS   4–5   M = NUMBER OF VARIATES (LITTLE P IN TEXT)
        COLS   6–10  N = NUMBER OF SUBJECTS
        COLS   14–15 NAF = NUMBER OF FACTORS (LITTLE N IN TEXT)
        COLUMN 20    K1 = 0   TO COMPUTE FROM SCORES
                        = 1   TO READ IN UPPER-TRIANGULAR R MATRIX
        COLUMN 25    K2 = 0   IF NO REMAKE OF R IS REQUIRED
                        = 1   TO REMAKE R MATRIX (I.E., TO EDIT R)
        COLUMN 30    M1 = NUMBER OF VARIATES IN REMAKE R
                         (M1 = 0 IF K2 = 0)
        COLUMN 35    K3 = 0   TO READ DATA FROM DATAPE FILE
                        = 1   TO READ DATA FROM INPUT FILE
```

All this describes the first line of the input file for running MODEL. You are required to enter in spaces 4–5 of the line (COLS, or columns on an IBM card, are spaces in a line typed in at a terminal) an integer representing the total count of variates in your study. In the last section of Chapter 9 this count was symbolized as p, but MODEL calls it M. (When you are given several spaces to enter a number, always crowd your number all the way to the right if you do not need all the assigned spaces. Thus if M = 23, the digits 2 and 3 would be entered in spaces 4 and 5, but if M = 9, the digit 9 must be entered in space 5 of the setup line.)

It may seem irksome that MODEL should ask you to enter in spaces 6–10 a value for N, which is the total number of subjects in your study. Why shouldn't the computer count the subjects for you? Well, many data analysis programs do count N. MODEL does not because it is a program for people who know their data file intimately, and who thus already know the value of N. The reason for the requirement is that MODEL assumes that the file contains a proper score for every subject on every variate (i.e., N × M good scores). Corrections for missing data or scores out of range have to be made before MODEL is run on a data file. In the processing of the file before sending it to MODEL you might as well verify the count of subjects as well as the completeness and correctness of the scores.

The mysterious setup value NAF required next refers to the number of explanatory factors to be hypothesized. This procedure is fully explained in Chapter 11 and several examples of its use are given in Chapter 12. We do want you to learn to create a set of explanatory factors—indeed, it is the most important skill you can acquire from this text—but we wish to save this subject for Chapters 11 and 12. For the moment just put a 1 in space 15 and a single factor will be created out of all your independent variates.

The value of K1 in space 20 depends on whether you are computing from scores (in which case put a zero in space 20) or want to read in correlations previously computed (in which case put a 1 in space 20). For now, we will omit explanations of K2 and K1 and simply ask you to put a zero in space 25 and another zero in space 30. These options for reordering the variates in the correlation matrix are explained in Chapter 11. Your computer consultant can help you decide upon the value of K3 which completes the setup line. This depends on whether you enter your data (scores or correlations) in the same file with which you access the MODEL program (called the INPUT file, in which case use a 1 in space 35), or whether you have filed the data separately in a file which your access instructions will label DATAPE (in which case put a zero in space 35 to cause the reading of data from DATAPE). It is important to note that the required setup lines are expected in the INPUT file whether the data are to be found there or in DATAPE.

   2)   FORMAT WITHIN BRACKETS (FOR SCORES IF K1 = 0,
        FOR R MATRIX IF K1 = 1)

A format for the data (or for the correlations, if they are being read) must be provided by the second setup line. A format is an instruction to the computer on how to read your data file. Your consultant will write a format for you in a minute if you explain which spaces in a line of the data file contain which variates. The format (5X,5F3.0), for example, would tell the computer to skip the first five spaces of each data line and read five scores from three spaces each. Formats are simple technical devices it is best to request from a technician unless you are going to do a lot of computing, in which case you can learn the format rules from a FORTRAN manual very quickly. (FORTRAN is the language MODEL is coded in, and every computer center has FORTRAN manuals.) One thing you must be sure of in making your data file is that the same format rule applies to every subject's record. That is, every subject must be recorded exactly the same way (the same variates in the same places) as every other subject.

3) DATA FILE (SCORES OR R MATRIX), UNLESS ON DATAPE

4) ORIGINAL POSITION NUMBERS, IN THE FORMAT, OF VARIATES TO BE INCLUDED IN THE REMAKE R, IN THEIR NEW ORDER AND IN TWO-COLUMN FIELDS (OMIT IF K2 = 0)

5) NUMBER OF VARIATES WHICH ARE KEY INDICATORS OF EACH FACTOR, IN FIVE-COLUMN FIELDS.

For now, we do not have to use the line which specifies the new order of the variates in a remake of the correlation matrix, since we have agreed to use K2 = 0. For now, put the count of your independent variates (this will be at least one less than M) in columns 4–5 (if a two-digit count) or in column 5 (if a one-digit count) of the last setup line.

If you have done all this correctly, your job will be computed and you will receive back from the computer what we call an *output*. We will now give an example for which we will show you the complete input and output.

A MAINSTREAMING STUDY

In 1977 Doreen Reed brought these research data to our attention. Reed is an educator of exceptional children who had recently taught a class of 26 children, 8 of whom were identified as mentally handicapped and experimentally "mainstreamed" (i.e., taught in the same classroom) with 18 ordinary children for the school year. Her research hypothesis was that the experience of being mainstreamed would encourage the special children to perform on a cognitive test more like the ordinary children performed, so that mainstreaming might be said to reduce the gap in mental acuity between the exceptional children and the ordinary children. She had administered a suitable cognitive ability test to the children twice, at the start of the school year and again at the end of the school year. Thus her data consisted of three scores for each subject: X_1 = label (0 = special, 1 = ordinary), X_2 = pretest, X_3 = posttest. Here is our input file for sending her data to MODEL.

```
USER, PRL.
MODEL
/EOR
  3  26  1  0  0  0  1
(3F3.0)
  0 23 30
  0 34 38
  0 23 38
  0 24 29
  0 23 28
  0 24 36
  0 16 24
  0 17 27
  1 39 40
  1 42 49
  1 30 36
  1 41 47
  1 44 43
  1 49 47
  1 46 49
  1 23 24
  1 44 49
  1 34 44
  1 38 44
  1 39 46
  1 29 39
  1 33 31
  1 38 39
  1 34 41
  1 34 41
  1 28 35
  2
/EOR
```

We proofread this data entry carefully, and the repetition of scores for subjects 24 and 25 is a faithful copy from Reed's report to us. The output from the MODEL run looked like this:

```
MODEL CORRELATIONAL DATA, PROGRAMMED BY P. R. LOHNES
    3 VARIATES,     26 SUBJECTS,     1 VARIABLES
    VARIATE      MEAN    S. D.
       1          .69     .46
       2        32.65    8.97
       3        38.23    7.68
CORRELATION MATRIX
   ROW 1    1.000
   ROW 2     .718    1.000
   ROW 3     .606     .890    1.000
```

HYPOTHESIS VECTOR   1
        .606   .890   .000
FINAL UNEXPLAINED VARIANCE IN CRITERION = .3050

TEST	COMMONALITY	DISTURBANCE	FACTOR STRUCTURE
1	.801	.446	.895
2	.908	.304	.953
3	.695	.552	.834

CONTRIBUTIONS OF DOMAINS TO KEY CRITERION VARIANCE
FACTOR   1   PROP. VAR.   .695   CUM. PROP.   .695

(There was more to the output, but the additional output lines pertained to the characteristics of the explanatory factor model fitted to the data, and would not be useful to you until you had studied Chapter 11.)

The mean of .69 on the dummy variate for label attached to the child indicates that 69 percent of the sample bore the label 1 = ordinary child. You can verify for yourself that $^{18}/_{26}$ = .69. The comparison of the total sample mean for pretest and for posttest indicates that, on the average, the total sample gain in cognitive ability on this test was 5.58 score points over the school year. In addition, the total sample standard deviation shrank from 9.0 on the pretest to 7.7 on the posttest, indicating that there was less variability in cognitive performances at the end of the school year than at the start of the school year for the 26 children. Averaging these two standard deviations gives 8.4, and if we divide the average gain by this average standard deviation, we observe that the average gain was about two-thirds of a standard deviation, which is quite a bit.

Did the special children constitute a different group than the ordinary children in pretest performance? There are several ways to tackle this question. One can compute a mean for each group on the pretest. Please do so. You should find this comparison:

Ordinary children pretest, m = 36.9
Special children pretest, m = 23.0
Mean difference   = 13.9

Dividing this mean difference by the pretest standard deviation indicates that the two groups differed, on the average, by 1.5 standard deviations on the pretest, which is a very substantial difference. Another way to tackle the question is to plot all 26 children on a measurement line, using one symbol for a special child and a different symbol for a normal child. Figure 10-1 provides such a plot. Although it shows the special children pretty much to the left of (below) the ordinary children, it also reveals that six ordinary children scored lower than the best-scoring special child on the pretest (and four ordinary children scored below the best-scoring pair of special children on the posttest, according to Figure 10-1). A third way to tackle this comparison is by means of the point-biserial correlation between the group membership dummy variate and the pretest variate. This is our favorite way to compare two groups on a measurement

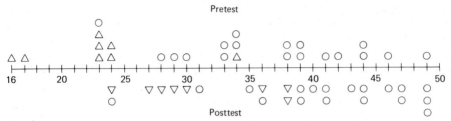

Figure 10-1 Pre- and posttest distributions of special (Δ) and ordinary (o) children. Pretest distributions are shown above the measurement line, and posttest distributions below.

variate, because this statistic can later be assembled with other correlations for a model-building exercise. The MODEL output shows that the correlation of group with pretest was .72. This is a fairly strong correlation, yet its square of .52 indicates that only about half of the variance in pretest is explained by the variance in group membership (or vice versa, if you prefer).

Did the special children constitute a different group than the ordinary children in posttest performance? What does Figure 10-1 seem to show about this issue? If you calculate a posttest mean for each group (please do), you should get this comparison:

Ordinary children posttest, $m = 41.3$
Special children posttest, $m = \underline{31.3}$
Mean difference $ = 10.0$

Dividing this mean difference by the posttest standard deviation indicates that the two groups differed, on the average, by 1.3 standard deviations. The point-biserial correlation of group with posttest was reported by MODEL as .61, indicating that only about 37 percent of the variance in posttest is explained by the variance in group membership (or vice versa).

Are the data consistent with Reed's hypothesis that the mainstreaming of the special children would encourage them to behave more like ordinary children in cognitive performances? The facts that the correlation with group shrank from .72 for pretest to .61 for posttest, and that the standardized mean difference shrank from $z = 1.5$ for pretest to $z = 1.3$ for posttest, suggest an affirmative reply to this question. This was an explanatory observational study conducted in a natural setting. The data cannot prove anything, but they are consistent with the ambition of the mainstreaming intervention. Can you think of a reasonable alternative explanation for the trends in the data? There are some. Put differently, these data lend some support to the program, but do not provide an unequivocal evaluation.

Q: (1) Attach Reed's scores to the MODEL program and execute. Compare your output with ours. (2) Attach the correlation matrix for her data to the MODEL program and execute. Does it make any difference whether MODEL is executed on scores as input or correlations as input?

A THERMOMETER STUDY

In 1977, Graves and Markarian conducted an interesting experiment as a joint master's project. Their primary concern was to determine whether using a plastic sheath on the thermometer while taking an oral temperature biased the temperature readings significantly. They designed their study so that it would also test whether the use of four different times of insertion (3-, 5-, 8-, and 12-minute insertion periods) made for significant differences in temperature readings under either the sheathed or the unsheathed condition. Finally, since they were able to obtain subjects from two different nursing school student bodies (48 volunteers from a hospital school and 43 volunteers from a university school), they were able to look for a significant difference in average temperature between the two groups of subjects.

The research subjects volunteered to read quietly for an hour, refraining from talking, eating, drinking, and smoking, during which time their temperatures were taken eight times. The same thermometer was used for all eight readings on a subject (but 20 thermometers were used in the study), and all the combinations of sheath condition and time condition were administered once to each subject, in a randomized order. This order of conditions was randomized anew for each subject. All readings were taken to the closest even tenth of a degree, making them accurate to one-tenth of a degree. That is, readings of $xx.0$, $xx.2, xx.4, xx.6$, and $xx.8$ were allowed, but readings of $xx.1, xx.3, xx.5, xx.7$, and $xx.9$ were not allowed (where xx stands, usually, for 98).

Graves and Markarian reported their findings (in part) as follows:

1 Site factor

All temperatures from university, $m = 98.67°$F
All temperatures from hospital, $m \quad = 98.53°$F
Mean difference $\qquad = \quad .14°$F

2 Time factor

All temperatures for 3 minutes, $m \qquad = 98.54$
All temperatures for 5 minutes, $m \qquad = 98.58$
All temperatures for 8 minutes, $m \qquad = 98.62$
All temperatures for 12 minutes, $m \qquad = 98.64$
Mean difference, 12 minutes $-$ 3 minutes $= \quad .10$

3 Sheath factor

All temperatures from unsheathed, $m = 98.62$
All temperatures from sheathed, $m \quad = 98.58$
Mean difference $\qquad = \quad .04$

They pointed out that "temperature readings that differ by less than 0.2°F have no practical significance" (p. 29), so none of the factors can be judged to have resulted in a temperature bias of practical concern.

We entered the Graves and Markarian data table to the MODEL program after careful proofreading of what we were sending to the computer. That we did enter their data carefully is confirmed by our having computed with MODEL exactly the same two site means given in their thesis. However, our approach to analysis of their data involved correlation of the factors with each other and with the temperature readings, rather than comparisons of means. We created six variates for correlational analysis, as follows:

Variate	Scoring rule
X_1	0 = hospital subject; 1 = university subject
X_2	Total of all 5-minute temperatures − total of all 3-minute temperatures for each subject
X_3	Total of all 8-minute temperatures − (total 3 minutes + total 5 minutes/2) for each subject
X_4	Total of all 12-minute temperatures − (total 3 minutes + total 5 minutes + total 8 minutes/3) for each subject
X_5	Total of all unsheathed temperatures − total of all sheathed temperatures for each subject
X_6	Average of all eight temperatures for each subject

Computing over a total of 91 subjects, MODEL reported as follows:

Variate	Correlations						Mean	s.d.
X_1	1.00	−.02	−.08	−.10	−.07	.15	.47	.50
X_2	−.02	1.00	−.13	−.27	.25	−.11	.05	.12
X_3	−.08	−.13	1.00	.16	.12	−.07	.06	.10
X_4	−.10	−.27	.16	1.00	−.24	−.17	.05	.11
X_5	−.07	.25	.12	−.24	1.00	.06	.04	.11
X_6	.15	−.11	−.07	−.17	.06	1.00	98.60	.44

From the last row of the correlation table we see that the subject's average temperature correlated trivially with each of the explanatory variates, leading us to the conclusion that none of the explanatory factors (site, time condition, sheath condition) biased the subject's temperature reading to a practically important extent. However, the possible advantages of our correlational approach can only be appreciated when one is able to assess the three-factor model for the data reported by the MODEL program. That mathematical model takes into account the correlations among the variates measuring the explanatory conditions, and fits three uncorrelated explanatory factors. This model, reported here for convenience, will not be meaningful to you now, but after you study Chapter 11 you should refer back to it and interpret it. The communality for variate 6 of .07 can be interpreted as showing that only 7 percent of the variance in average temperatures of the 91 student nurses can be explained by the model for the data. This seems to be a trivial amount of explanation. Where does the other 93 percent of average temperature variation come from?

	Factor structure			
Variate	Site factor	Time factor	Sheath factor	Communality
X_1	1.00	.00	.00	1.00
X_2	−.02	.32	.26	.17
X_3	−.08	.38	.12	.17
X_4	−.10	.77	−.22	.64
X_5	−.07	−.03	.997	1.00
X_6	.15	−.22	.06	.07

A STUDY OF PRIMARY CARE NURSING

In 1977, Hageman compared nursing in two units of a rural hospital for his master's project. One unit was run on a team nursing basis (30 beds in 17 rooms, 23 to 30 patients during the 2-week study period, 9 nurses and 9 assistants), while the other unit was run on a primary care nursing basis (30 beds in 17 rooms, 27 to 33 patients during the period, 9 nurses and 10 assistants). Hageman wanted to know whether the nursing in the primary care unit was better than that in the team unit. The primary care method was newly installed in the unit using it at that time, and thus could have shown some benefits of an initial staff enthusiasm for it. (This phenomenon of temporary benefits from an "experimental" arrangement is called the Hawthorne effect.) Hageman randomly selected records of 10 patients from each unit as the basis for the part of his observations we will consider here. He made ratings of the selected patient records according to the rules of two scaling procedures, the Phaneuf Nursing Audit (PNA) and the Quality of Patient Care Scale (QPACS). He employed comparisons of means as his method of analysis, with these results:

1 Quality of Patient Care total score at posttest time

   Primary care unit, $m = 2.52$
   Team nursing unit, $m = \underline{2.41}$
   Mean difference $= .11$

2 Phaneuf Nursing Audit posttest

   Primary care unit, $m = 165.17$
   Team nursing unit, $m = \underline{134.16}$
   Mean difference $= \overline{31.01}$

Hageman decided that the comparison on the QPACS was not significant, but that the comparison on the PNA was significant. The standard deviations on the PNA averaged 23, so the advantage of the primary care unit over the team nursing unit was, on the average, $z = {}^{31}/_{23} = 1.35$, or 1⅓ standard deviations, which is a very substantial advantage indeed.

Another relevant comparison is provided by Phaneuf Nursing Audit scores computed on sets of 10 randomly selected patient records from each unit from before one of the units changed over to primary care.

3 Phaneuf Nursing Audit pretest

Primary care unit, $m = 126.08$
Team nursing unit, $m = \underline{134.15}$
Mean difference $= -8.07$

With an average standard deviation of 34, this gives $z = -.24$, which suggests that Hageman was right to decide this was an insignificant comparison. Nevertheless, on the basis of data obtained before the changeover, this comparison favored the team nursing unit, and this seeming handicap for the unit which made the changeover makes the PNA posttest comparison even more impressive.

We entered Hageman's scores to the MODEL program and obtained the following correlations. Note that we cannot report correlations of the PNA pretest with the two posttests because different sets of patients were involved in the pre- and posttesting.

Variate	1	2	3	4
Treatment (0 = team; 1 = primary care)	1.00			
Phaneuf nursing pretest	−.11	1.00		
Phaneuf nursing posttest	.56	n.a.	1.00	
Quality of patient care	.19	n.a.	.20	1.00

The correlations make it clear that the only strong contrast exists on the PNA posttest, where nursing method explains 31 percent of the PNA variance, and the comparison favors the primary care unit. What do you suppose might explain the low correlation of .20 between the two posttest measures?

A STUDY OF NURSING CAREER PREDICTORS[1]

In 1960 Project TALENT collected extensive test and questionnaire data from 444,000 American adolescents comprising a national probability sample of high school youth. The original intent was to follow these young people through at least 20 years of career development in order to see how their abilities and interests as measured in high school foreshadowed events in their careers. Unfortunately, it has not been possible to maintain contact with the majority of the subjects. Some have been uncooperative and others have simply moved without leaving forwarding addresses. In 1971 a very intensive, very expensive effort was made to reestablish contact with about 3000 individuals who would be

[1]This section was coauthored by Dr. Lu Pai.

representative of the members of the original eleventh grade sample. This study uses the data for the women in that "11-year follow-up of eleventh graders" sample. The men are not used because so few of them became nurses (6 out of about 1500 men).

The first questions of interest regarding the 1479 women in the file are:

   1 How many of them became registered nurses?

   2 How many of them planned to become nurses when they were in the eleventh grade in 1960?

   3 How many of those who planned to be nurses in 1960 actually had become registered nurses by 1971?

The answers are:

   1 46 out of 1479 women were registered nurses in 1971, leading to the estimate that .031 of this sex-age cohort were registered nurses.

   2 147 out of 1479 women were planning to be nurses when they were in eleventh grade in 1960, leading to the estimate that .106 of this sex-age cohort were planning to be nurses when they were adolescents.

   3 29 of those 147 women who had planned to become nurses in 1960 actually were registered nurses in 1971, leading to the estimate that the odds were .197 that an eleventh grade female student in 1960 whose occupational choice was nurse would be a registered nurse 11 years later. It is also of interest that 17 of those 1332 women who had planned to become something other than a nurse in 1960, or who had no occupational choice at that time, actually were registered nurses in 1971, leading to the estimate that the odds were .013 that an eleventh grade female student who did *not* plan to become a nurse in 1960 would be a registered nurse in 1971. It should be noted that there were some women in other categories of nurse than registered nurse in 1971.

The generalization which is suggested is that there is about one chance in five that a female high school student planning to become a registered nurse will actually do so, and only about one chance in a hundred that a female high school student not planning to become a registered nurse will actually become one. Do you think it would be safe to apply this generalization to other age cohorts? Do you think the estimate that .031 of this age cohort of women became registered nurses can be generalized to other age cohorts? Incidentally, only 25 of the 46 registered nurses were actually employed in nursing in 1971, for which the odds are .543. Why should so many nurses be out of nursing 10 years after graduation from high school?

These data can be summarized as follows:

		RN in 1971?		
		Yes	No	Total
Plan nurse	Yes	29	118	147
in 1960?	No	17	1319	1332
Total		46	1433	1479

Table 10-1   Comparison of Women Planning Careers in Nursing as High School Juniors in 1960 with Other Women in Their Cohort, for Selected 1960 and 1971 Variates

1960 variates	Mean for nursing planners (N = 147)	Mean for other women (N = 1332)	s for total sample	Point-biserial r
1 Mother working?	.921	.913	.872	.003
2 Planning nursing?	1.00	.000	.308	1.00
3 Certainty of choice	2.86	3.23	1.40	−.079
4 Information test	208.	199.	49.9	.057
5 English test	87.0	96.3	13.2	.016
6 Reading test	33.8	31.9	9.83	.056
7 Visualization test	8.73	8.20	3.08	.052
8 Abstract reasoning test	9.37	9.01	2.95	.036
9 Mathematics test	22.7	21.6	9.29	.036
10 Interest in biology and medicine	26.1	15.4	10.3	.313
11 Interest in social service	26.4	24.0	7.52	.098
12 Socioeconomic index	99.8	98.6	9.73	.035
13 High school curriculum (1 = academic, 0 = other)	.590	.351	.484	.148
14 High school grades	26.9	26.2	9.49	.023
1971 variates				
15 Job code nurse?	.122	.006	.131	.265
16 Pay (in thousands)	7.30	6.78	3.82	.041
17 Job satisfaction	4.28	4.15	1.00	.040
18 Importance of job status	1.47	1.38	1.18	.022
19 Importance of job power	.793	.831	1.04	−.011
20 Employed since high school?	2.23	2.21	.513	.009
21 Registered nurse?	.197	.013	.174	.318
22 Highest degree	.857	1.08	.596	−.123
23 Race	1.134	1.130	.720	.002

We have selected 14 variates from the 1960 information and 9 variates from the 1971 information, so that our analyses span 23 variates observed on each of 1479 women. Table 10-1 reports the comparisons of the 147 students who planned to be nurses with the other 1332 students on the selected variates. In terms of the high school variates, the strongest contrast is on interest in biological science and medicine ($r = .31$), which suggests that many women who planned to be nurses did so on the basis of appropriate interests. In this vein, note that the contrast on interest in social service, while weaker ($r = .10$), supports this interpretation. The students planning to be nurses were more likely to be in academic curricula than the other women ($r = .15$), were less certain of their occupational choice ($r = -.08$), were better informed ($r = .06$), better readers ($r = .06$), and better at visualization tasks ($r = .05$). In terms of the 11-year follow-up variates, the women who had planned to be nurses were more likely to have become RNs than the nonplanners ($r = .32$), more likely to be employed as nurses ($r = .27$), better paid ($r = .04$), more satisfied with their jobs ($r = .04$), but less likely to hold advanced degrees ($r = -.12$).

These contrasts assume more meaning when they are compared with the contrasts reported in Table 10-2, which are between the 46 registered nurses and the 1433 other women. On the high school variates, the RNs were more likely to have planned to be nurses ($r = .35$), less certain of their occupational choice ($r = -.08$), more interested in biological science and medicine ($r = .19$), more interested in social service ($r = .07$), better informed ($r = .12$), better readers ($r = .12$), better visualizers ($r = .07$), better abstract reasoners ($r = .11$), better at mathematics ($r = .08$), more likely to be in academic curricula ($r = .13$), and had better grades in high school ($r = .09$). Perhaps the most interesting comparisons between the contrasts in Table 10-1 and those in Table 10-2 concern the set of ability tests taken in high school (variates 4 through 9). In Table 10-1, all six of these contrasts favor the women who chose nursing as a future occupation, and

Table 10-2   Comparison of Women Who Were RNs in 1971 with Other Women in Their Cohort

1960 variates	Mean for RNs ($N = 46$)	Mean for non-RNs ($N = 1433$)	s for total sample	Point-biserial r
1 Mother working?	.854	.916	.872	−.012
2 Planning nursing?	.725	.088	.308	.346
3 Certainty of choice	2.59	3.21	1.40	−.075
4 Information test	233.	198.	49.9	.119
5 English test	90.4	86.2	13.2	.054
6 Reading test	38.6	31.9	9.83	.118
7 Visualization test	9.38	8.21	3.08	.066
8 Abstract reasoning test	10.8	8.99	2.95	.109
9 Mathematics test	25.8	21.6	9.29	.079
10 Interest in biology and medicine	27.7	16.1	10.3	.193
11 Interest in social service	27.0	24.1	7.52	.065
12 Socioeconomic index	101.	98.7	9.73	.047
13 High school curriculum	.732	.364	.484	.129
14 High school grades	31.3	26.1	9.49	.094
1971 variates				
15 Job code nurse?	.543	.001	.131	.717
16 Pay (in thousands)	7.96	6.79	3.82	.061
17 Job satisfaction	4.14	4.16	1.00	−.003
18 Importance of job status	1.47	1.39	1.18	.013
19 Importance of job power	.559	.838	1.04	−.052
20 Employed since high school?	2.44	2.21	.513	.081
21 Registered nurse?	1.00	.000	.174	1.00
22 Highest degree	.786	1.07	.596	−.093
23 Race	1.42	1.12	.720	.073

again in Table 10-2 all six contrasts favor the actual RNs over the other women. However, the contrasts are systematically stronger for the six test variates in Table 10-2 than they are in Table 10-1. Can you interpret this trend?

The most salient finding is that among eleventh graders in 1960 the pool of potential nurses was composed almost entirely of women who had already chosen nursing as a vocational goal. Thus it is particularly interesting to segregate the 147 women who had nursing as a goal in the 1960 high school testing, and ask what discriminates those 29 who became RNs by 1971 from those 118 who did not become RNs. Table 10-3 addresses this discrimination problem. It shows again that the set of six intellectual abilities (variates 4 through 9) strongly discriminates, with the women who became nurses displaying better average abilities than those who did not persist in their career goal. It is reassuring that the RNs had higher average earnings than the non-RNs in 1971, although one could wish that the average earnings of the RNs were higher than $8680. Note from variate 15 that only 59 percent of the RNs were employed as nurses in 1971.

What actually causes some women who want to become nurses to persist to the achievement of RN status, and others who want to become nurses to drop out

Table 10-3   Comparisons of RNs with Non-RNs among Women Who Planned Nursing in 1960

1960 variates	Mean for 1971 RNs (N = 29)	Mean for non-RNs (N = 118)	s for total sample	Point-biserial r
1 Mother working?	.893	.928	.882	−.016
2 Planning nursing?	1.00	1.00	.000	
3 Certainty of choice	2.36	3.00	1.28	−.204
4 Information test	243.	199.	49.3	.351
5 English test	90.5	86.1	15.1	.118
6 Reading test	39.5	32.3	9.71	.296
7 Visualization test	9.59	8.51	3.07	.141
8 Abstract reasoning test	11.1	8.93	2.93	.299
9 Mathematics test	26.2	21.9	9.67	.181
10 Interest in biology and medicine	30.8	25.1	8.97	.252
11 Interest in social service	26.9	26.3	6.27	.035
12 Socioeconomic index	103.	99.0	9.14	.176
13 High school curriculum	.821	.532	.492	.236
14 High school grades	31.3	25.8	9.75	.227
1971 variates				
15 Job code nurse?	.586	.008	.328	.701
16 Pay (in thousands)	8.68	6.82	2.93	.279
17 Job satisfaction	4.39	4.24	1.03	.064
18 Importance of job status	1.36	1.51	1.08	−.058
19 Importance of job power	.591	.862	1.01	−.117
20 Employed since high school?	2.35	2.20	.496	.117
21 Registered nurse?	1.00	.000	.398	1.00
22 Highest degree	.818	.871	.467	−.050

Table 10-4 Correlations among Selected Variates for 147 Women Who Planned Nursing Careers in 1960

Variates grouped into variables	Variates													
	2	3	4	5	6	7	8	9	10	11	12	13	14	15
I Verbal ability														
1 Information	.53	.83	.48	.55	.66	.41	.21	−.07	.43	.48	.44	−.18	.24	.34
2 English test		.50	.31	.38	.63	.19	.18	−.09	.33	.22	.20	−.05	.06	.12
3 Reading test			.40	.56	.61	.26	.19	−.06	.36	.41	.41	−.16	.25	.29
II Reasoning ability														
4 Visualization test				.56	.54	.18	.09	−.10	.24	.26	.28	−.23	.17	.14
5 Abstract reasoning test					.56	.17	.13	−.11	.31	.25	.26	−.14	.23	.30
6 Mathematics test						.20	.23	−.04	.26	.32	.34	−.17	.17	.18
III Interest														
7 Interest in biology and medicine							.32	−.34	.26	.31	.25	.03	.19	.24
8 Interest in social service								−.14	.17	.17	.15	−.05	.04	.03
IV Status														
9 Certainty of occupational choice									−.06	−.13	−.23	−.11	−.14	−.19
10 Socioeconomic index										.36	.02	−.06	.12	.18
11 High school curriculum (1 = academic; 0 = other)											.19	−.02	.13	.23
12 High school grades												−.05	.25	.23
13 Mother working													.01	−.02
1971 criteria														
14 Job code nurse?														.70
15 Registered nurse?														

of the pool of potential RNs? In Chapter 12 we will build a model from these data that demonstrates a multivariate analysis which can support a causal argument, or test a hypothesis about causality. For now, we point to Table 10-4, which reports the intercorrelations among 15 selected variates for the 174 nursing aspirants, as the raw material out of which the causal model of Chapter 12 was fashioned. What can you see in these correlations?

These correlations were computed by the MODEL program. Notice that the variates were grouped into five clusters, the first four of which specified predictor variables, namely

  I   Verbal ability (from variates 1 through 3)
  II Reasoning ability (from variates 4 through 6)
 III Interest (from variates 7, 8)
 IV Status (from variates 9 through 13)

while the fifth cluster was simply termed criteria (from variates 14, 15). The first 13 variates were observed in 1960, the last two in 1971. Short of fitting a hypothesized causal model to these correlations by a method as yet unstudied, what multivariate analysis can we make of them? Well, we can do the "usefulness" and "uniqueness" analysis recommended by Equation (16) of Chapter 9. The usefulness (U) of the set of 13 predictors is the proportion of a criterion variate's variance which is predictable from the set. Focusing on variate 15, registered

```
  15     147    13     1     0     0     1
(15F5.2)
 1.00   .53   .83   .48   .55   .66   .41   .21  -.07   .43   .48   .44  -.18   .24  .3
 1.00   .50   .31   .38   .63   .19   .18  -.09   .33   .22   .20  -.05   .06  .12
 1.00   .40   .56   .61   .26   .19  -.06   .36   .41   .41  -.16   .25  .29
 1.00   .56   .54   .18   .09  -.10   .24   .26   .28  -.23   .17  .14
 1.00   .56   .17   .13  -.11   .31   .25   .26  -.14   .23  .30
 1.00   .20   .23  -.04   .26   .32   .34  -.17   .17  .18
 1.00   .32  -.34   .26   .31   .25   .03   .19  .24
 1.00  -.14   .17   .17   .15  -.05   .04  .03
 1.00  -.06  -.13  -.23  -.11  -.14  -.19
 1.00   .36   .02  -.06   .12  .18
 1.00   .19  -.02   .13  .23
 1.00  -.05   .25  .23
 1.00   .01  -.02
 1.00   .70
 1.00
   1     1     1     1     1     1     1     1     1     1     1     1     1
/EOR
```

Figure 10-2 First MODEL setup.

nurse? as the criterion of interest to us, we can compute U by means of MODEL. A run is initiated for which NAF = 13 and INPUT 5 contains 13 entries of the digit 1 in the right-hand position of 13 five-column fields, specifying one variate for each of 13 factors. Figure 10-2 is a computer readout of the input for the desired MODEL run, and Figure 10-3 is a computer readout of part of the resulting output. In Figure 10-3 the desired numerical value of U is the thirteenth and final CUM. PROP. of the table CONTRIBUTIONS OF DOMAINS TO KEY CRITERION VARIANCE, and thus

$$U = .196$$

```
MODEL CORRELATIONAL DATA, PROGRAMMED BY P.R. LOHNES
    15 VARIATES,    147 SUBJECTS,    13 VARIABLES

CONTRIBUTIONS OF DOMAINS TO KEY CRITERION VARIANCE
FACTOR   1 PROP. VAR. .116 CUM. PROP. .116
FACTOR   2 PROP. VAR. .005 CUM. PROP. .121
FACTOR   3 PROP. VAR. .001 CUM. PROP. .121
FACTOR   4 PROP. VAR. .000 CUM. PROP. .122
FACTOR   5 PROP. VAR. .028 CUM. PROP. .149
FACTOR   6 PROP. VAR. .003 CUM. PROP. .153
FACTOR   7 PROP. VAR. .013 CUM. PROP. .166
FACTOR   8 PROP. VAR. .005 CUM. PROP. .170
FACTOR   9 PROP. VAR. .017 CUM. PROP. .188
FACTOR 10 PROP. VAR. .001 CUM. PROP. .188
FACTOR 11 PROP. VAR. .003 CUM. PROP. .191
FACTOR 12 PROP. VAR. .005 CUM. PROP. .196
FACTOR 13 PROP. VAR. .000 CUM. PROP. .196
```

Figure 10-3 First MODEL output.

```
 15   147   13    1    1    15    1
(15F5.2)
 1.00   .53   .83   .48   .55   .66   .41   .21  -.07   .43   .48   .44  -.18   .24   .3
 1.00   .50   .31   .38   .63   .19   .18  -.09   .33   .22   .20  -.05   .06   .12
 1.00   .40   .56   .61   .26   .19  -.06   .36   .41   .41  -.16   .25   .29
 1.00   .56   .54   .18   .09  -.10   .24   .26   .28  -.23   .17   .14
 1.00   .56   .17   .13  -.11   .31   .25   .26  -.14   .23   .30
 1.00   .20   .23  -.04   .26   .32   .34  -.17   .17   .18
 1.00   .32  -.34   .26   .31   .25   .03   .19   .24
 1.00  -.14   .17   .17   .15  -.05   .04   .03
 1.00  -.06  -.13  -.23  -.11  -.14  -.19
 1.00   .36   .02  -.06   .12   .18
 1.00   .19  -.02   .13   .23
 1.00  -.05   .25   .23
 1.00   .01  -.02
 1.00   .70
 1.00
 2  3  4  5  6  7  8  910111213  11415
    1  1  1  1  1  1  1    1   1   1      1   1
/EOR
```

Figure 10-4 Second MODEL setup.

The uniqueness of the thirteenth predictor (U_{13}) is the part of U which would be lost if the thirteenth predictor were not available, and is the difference between U and U_{*13}, where U_{*13} is the proportion of the criterion variance which is predictable from the other 12 predictors. In Figure 10-3 the desired numerical value of U_{*13} is the twelfth CUM. PROP. of the CONTRIBUTIONS table, and thus

$$U_{*13} = .196$$

Substituting in the equation,

$$U_{13} = U - U_{*13} = .196 - .196 = .000$$

Therefore, the unique contribution of variate 13 (mother working?) to the multivariate prediction of variate 15 (registered nurse?) is .00, or 0 percent of the criterion variance.

If you wanted to compute the uniqueness for any other predictor, you could do so by using the REMAKE feature of the MODEL program to transfer the desired predictor into position 13 among the variates (putting it in row 13 and column 13 of the correlation matrix), and then repeating the run described above. Figure 10-4 is a computer readout of the input for a run which uses REMAKE to put variate 1, information total, into row and column 13 (pushing variates 2 through 13 up and to the left one position), and Figure 10-5 is a computer readout of the relevant part of the output from the resulting run. In this output, the former variate 1 has become variate 13, and computing

$$U_{13} = U - U_{*13} = .196 - .183 = .013$$

```
MODEL CORRELATIONAL DATA, PROGRAMMED BY P.R. LOHNES
   15 VARIATES,        147 SUBJECTS,        13 VARIABLES

CONTRIBUTIONS OF DOMAINS TO KEY CRITERION VARIANCE
FACTOR   1 PROP. VAR. .014 CUM. PROP. .014
FACTOR   2 PROP. VAR. .071 CUM. PROP. .085
FACTOR   3 PROP. VAR. .001 CUM. PROP. .086
FACTOR   4 PROP. VAR. .031 CUM. PROP. .117
FACTOR   5 PROP. VAR. .000 CUM. PROP. .117
FACTOR   6 PROP. VAR. .030 CUM. PROP. .147
FACTOR   7 PROP. VAR. .006 CUM. PROP. .153
FACTOR   8 PROP. VAR. .013 CUM. PROP. .166
FACTOR   9 PROP. VAR. .003 CUM. PROP. .169
FACTOR 10 PROP. VAR. .006 CUM. PROP. .175
FACTOR 11 PROP. VAR. .008 CUM. PROP. .183
FACTOR 12 PROP. VAR. .000 CUM. PROP. .183
FACTOR 13 PROP. VAR. .013 CUM. PROP. .196
```

Figure 10-5   Second MODEL output.

leads us to claim that the unique contribution of variate 1 (information total) to the multivariate prediction of variate 15 (registered nurse?) is .013. Similarly, we have computed the U_j for each of the 13 predictors, and these are presented in Table 10-5. Using Equation (19) of Chapter 9 we were able to compute the commonality (c), representing the joint or confounded action of the predictors as a set, as .112.

Q: Set up and run a MODEL analysis for which there are two explanatory variables with two variates grouped under each, and one criterion, as follows:

Table 10-5   Uniquenesses for 13 Independent Variates when Variate 15 (Registered Nurse?) Is the Criterion ($N = 147$)

Variate	U_j
1 Information test	.013
2 English test	.003
3 Reading test	.000
4 Visualization test	.008
5 Abstract reasoning test	.028
6 Mathematics test	.001
7 Interest in biology and medicine	.004
8 Interest in social service	.006
9 Certainty of choice	.012
10 Socioeconomic index	.001
11 High school curriculum	.003
12 High school grades	.005
13 Mother working?	.000
Commonality	.112
Total explained variance	.196

Variable 1: Aptitude
  Variate 1. Information test
  Variate 2. Reading test
Variable 2: Nursing-related interests
  Variate 3. Interest in biological science and medicine
  Variate 4. Interest in social service
Criterion:
  Variate 5. Registered nurse in 1971?
The format statement for this run is
  (5X, 2F4.0, 12X, 2F3.0, 12X, F1.0)

How are you going to get the Project TALENT data entered into the computer? What are you going to do about the missing data? Write a report on your results.

REFERENCES

Cooley, William W., and Paul R. Lohnes: *Predicting development of young adults*. Palo Alto, Calif.: American Institutes for Research, 1968.

Graves, Ruby, and Martha Markarian: The accuracy of oral plastic sheathed thermometers in the recording of body temperature. Unpublished masters' project, SUNY at Buffalo, 1977.

Hageman, Paul: Evaluation of primary nursing: A comparison of two nursing modalities. Unpublished master's project, SUNY at Buffalo, 1977.

Wise, L. L., D. H. McLaughlin, and L. Steel: *The Project TALENT data handbook*. Palo Alto, Calif.: American Institutes for Research, 1977.

Chapter 11

How Does Analysis Build Theory?

Research on nursing is not an end in itself, but rather an instrument for the improvement of nursing theory. Such theory exists as a set of interconnected propositions. Each theoretical proposition states a relationship between two constructs or among several constructs. Weak theory may state only that two constructs covary, or that a set of constructs covary, in a certain way. Such a theory is essentially descriptive, positing only that a regularity or a pattern will be found in nature. Strong theory asserts propositions about causation. A strong theory posits that changes in a construct or among some constructs cause changes in another construct or constructs. A very strong theory posits the amount of change in the dependent construct(s) that results from a given amount of change in the independent construct(s). The strongest theory explains all the changes that can occur in the dependent construct(s), so that the propositions do not have to be qualified with "other things being equal" clauses. Obviously a theory of nursing should be a strong theory, because the claim of professional competence is based upon it, and because lives may depend upon it. This chapter shows how the correlations which describe a network of observed relationships among research variates can be transformed by analysis into propositions about relationships among variables standing for constructs, such that research support for causal inferences is organized.

In this chapter we present just one scheme for data analysis in support of causal argument, and this one scheme has been selected from among a plethora of mathematical and statistical methods for causal analysis. The dictionary tells us that a plethora is an overabundance, and from the point of view of nursing researchers who do not have the time to become mathematicians or statisticians in order to sort out this cornucopia, an overabundance is what exists. This is a deceptively simple chapter on causal analysis because the authors have exercised an informed judgment in selecting this procrustean bed for your research data. To promote a successful one-semester study effort, or alternatively an economical first pass at self-study of causal analysis, we have chosen a single method to teach. You will not have any trouble locating experts to tell you that we have made the wrong choice. It is unlikely your experts will agree on what the right choice would have been. We have made this choice prudently, and we are confident we have provided a method which is powerful yet learnable, promoting intellectual creativity while disciplining imagination in the way that science requires, namely according to the dictates of the data. No one wants her intelligence confined to a procrustean bed for very long. The method we teach here can introduce you to the logic of causal analysis and prepare you to adventure onward in studies of this vast and difficult subject. Naturally, that is what we hope for you, but realistically we know that many of you will not make that choice, in which case we think you will find this method surprisingly serviceable in a wide variety of research endeavors. If you do team up with an analysis expert who favors a different approach, your perspective on this method should help the two of you to communicate. We remind you that any statistician you choose to work with may be overbearing, but there are some reasons why you might want to resist the analysis of your data by methods that are based on strong assumptions about population distributions and are derived by means of differential calculus. This chapter reviews and extends our arguments against deployment of the logic of statistical inference and the power of calculus in nursing research.

HYPOTHESIZING CAUSALITY

Justifying nursing decisions is the central problem for nursing theory. Since nursing decisions seriously affect the lives of patients, those who make them are morally bound to acknowledge their causal beliefs. The mores of the times require as scientific a basis as possible for the beliefs about causation which justify nursing policies. We have argued that the required research base supporting causal arguments about *why* some patients suffer less and heal faster than others is most likely to be provided by data collected in natural nursing settings. Cooley (1978) has termed this class of research designs *explanatory observational studies* (EOS). While it is true that data from EOS cannot completely prove causation, it also seems to be true that because of the many problems impeding meaningful experiments in nursing, ecological correlations often provide the only evidence regarding probable causation. Wold (1956) described various cases of successful strong inference from correlational data in the physical sciences. This paper should be read by everyone who is tempted to stand firmly on the principle that "correlation cannot prove causation."

Four phases of research on causes of troublesome phenomena are

1 Hypothesizing causality in research planning
2 Testing causal hypotheses against research data
3 Detailing the apparent contributions of causes from the data
4 Predicting future events

In the discussion ahead it is assumed that the researcher knows what the criteria, or dependent variates, are. These are the "troublesome phenomena" which give rise to the theoretical problem. In the thermometer study, the criterion was temperature assigned to the patient, and what was troublesome was the suspicion that a significant part of the variance in temperature assigned might be due to situational factors (sheath, mouth time, site) rather than to intrapatient factors.

Every plan for research implies one or more causal propositions. This implication is contained in the list of independent and control variates the plan presents. The rationale for the inclusion of an independent variate is that it is an indicator for at least one variable standing for a construct which influences the criteria. All this "logic of science" matter may not be spelled out explicitly in the research proposal, but what other reason could explain the inclusion of an independent variate? A control variate may be included because it is thought to be an influence on one or some of the independent variates, regardless of whether it influences the criteria directly, but again a causal argument is implied, regardless of whether it is stated. In urging that hypothesizing causality be accepted as a crucial aspect of research planning, we are merely requiring that causal argument be made explicit, sharp, and logical, rather than left implicit. We are demanding that causal thinking be brought out of the closet, as it were. The danger in implicit argument is that it may be fuzzy, illogical, or contrary to experience, and these defects may go unnoticed. What one intends to do surely tends to reveal what one thinks, but it is better to make explicit statements of what one thinks about probable causes as the justification of what one plans to measure.

If research on nursing is cumulative, as it should be, with the passing of time more will be known about problems than can possibly be learned from a single new research act. Therefore, a priori causal hypotheses will become stronger and better, and new research will become more confirmatory than exploratory. "Our general knowledge of the world may well be worth much more than the data" (Mosteller and Tukey, 1977, p. 323). This should increasingly be the case. However, it is essential to distinguish between the act of making hypotheses about causality during research planning on the basis of the best available knowledge and the act of assessing the degree of a priori confidence one can have in those hypotheses at that time. Both these acts must be performed. When our a priori causal hypotheses are firmly grounded, we may expect new research to confirm them and will be quite surprised if that fails to happen. If our a priori causal hypotheses are only weakly grounded, we may treat them as very tentative and await the results of the research with a nearly open mind. In either case, orderly research planning requires these acts.

Why don't researchers make explicit causal hypotheses in the planning stage? The main reason is that they know from experience that all the relevant variates they propose to measure are going to be intercorrelated. (Unless, that is, they make some of them artificially uncorrelated by the design of a randomized experiment, which we do not recommend.) In EOS data there are no zero correlations at all. This awareness that everything in nature is correlated with everything else holds out the possibility of very complicated webs of influence indeed, and the principle that discretion is the better part of valor may suggest that the safest thing to do is to refrain from a priori hypothesizing. We sympathize (in fact, we used to behave this way), and we realize that the duty we now burden the researcher with may be an onerous one, but we are convinced it is a necessary one. In addition, once you get over the shock of having a priori causal hypotheses demanded in the research plan, the opportunity to put what you know about the problem to work in the creative act of framing hypotheses can be enjoyed, and it is always permissible to assert that the a priori confidence in the hypotheses is slight if the state of knowledge is woeful.

How can relatively simple causal hypotheses be made for a network of correlations among what may be a great many variates? The first principle of causal analysis of nursing problems is that the actual causes of the troublesome phenomena are almost never directly observable. The data collected in research describe the observable differences among subjects in terms of the variances and correlations among variates, but it is unlikely that any variate is itself a direct cause of anything. Rather, the independent variates are indicators of latent causes. Please review the first section of Chapter 5 on the relationships of variates to variables and of variables to constructs. The key idea is that variables, which stand in empirical research for the constructs that are the building blocks of pure thought (i.e., theory), have to be created by mathematical analysis out of the variates which are their indicators. Usually some of the information collected by two or more variates will be combined in a linear equation to create a variable. Algebraically, the variable F might be created from parts of the variates X_1 and X_2 by the formula

$$F = c_1 X_1 + c_2 X_2 \tag{1}$$

Determining the actual weights for the two variates, c_1 and c_2, is part of the task of detailing a model for the data, which we address later in this chapter. Technically, what such a formula does is assign parts of the variances of X_1 and X_2 to the variable F. It is important to appreciate that the information collected by a variate is represented by its variance. How the subjects scatter on a variate is the information the measurement act collects, and the variance is an index to that scatter.

Besides the fact that most variates imperfectly represent the underlying, or latent, causes they are selected to indicate, another hard reality is that most variates also represent to some extent other causes or extraneous variables which they were not selected to indicate. Thus, if X_1 and X_2 are measurement variates selected to indicate variable F_1, and X_3 and X_4 are variates selected to indicate F_2, the fact that all ten correlations among the four variates are nonzero implies that the actual linear functions of the variates which define the variables could each use some information from all four variates.

$$F_1 = c_{11}X_1 + c_{12}X_2 + c_{13}X_3 + c_{14}X_4$$
$$F_2 = c_{21}X_1 + c_{22}X_2 + c_{23}X_3 + c_{24}X_4 \tag{2}$$

The hope would be that c_{11} and c_{12} would be large compared to c_{13} and c_{14}, and that c_{23} and c_{24} would be large compared to c_{21} and c_{22} (comparisons of weights are always made in absolute values, since weights are allowed to be negative). It can happen, however, that a variate selected as an indicator of one variable will make a surprisingly large contribution to the linear function creating another variable.

A different perspective on the relation between variates and variables from this "indicator" perspective is provided by the concept that the latent variables cause the variances of the observable variates. This notion that the hidden variances of the variables are the source of at least parts of the observed variances of the variates gives rise to equations expressing the variates as functions of the variables. Such equations are called *structural equations*. They have this form:

$$X_1 = a_{11}F_1 + a_{12}F_2 + d_1W_1$$
$$X_2 = a_{21}F_1 + a_{22}F_2 + d_2W_2$$
$$X_3 = a_{31}F_1 + a_{32}F_2 + d_3W_3$$
$$X_4 = a_{41}F_1 + a_{42}F_2 + d_4W_4 \tag{3}$$

The coefficients a_{jk} in the structural equations for the variates are called *loadings* of the j variates on the k causal factors ($j = 1, 2, \ldots, p; k = 1, 2, \ldots, n$). The d_jW_j are called *disturbances*, and are the portions of the X_j that are not explained by the causal factors. (Throughout this chapter it is assumed that the variates X_j have been transformed to standard score metrics, so that all variates have zero means and unit standard deviations.) Again, if in the research plan measures X_1 and X_2 were specified as the key indicators of variable F_1, it is to be hoped that a_{11} and a_{21} turn out to be larger than a_{12} and a_{22} (in absolute values), and if X_3 and X_4 were specified as the key indicators of variable F_2, it is to be hoped that a_{32} and a_{42} turn out to be larger than a_{31} and a_{41}. Surprises are possible, and a key indicator of variable F_1 can turn out to have a larger loading on F_2 than on F_1. This might lead to a new understanding of the variate, but it might still have been a good idea to include the variate for what it can contribute to the creation of F_1 on the grounds that "purer" indicators of F_1 are not available. The relation of variates to variables can become quite complicated.

Returning to the question of how causal analysis can simplify a complicated appraisal of nature provided by the correlations and variances among the variates, one answer is that it may be possible to replace many independent variates with a small number of causal factors. Usually the count n of latent causes hypothesized can be less than one-half the count $p - c$ of independent variates (where p is the total count of variates in the research, and c is the count of criterion variates). Sometimes it can be that n is less than one-quarter of $p - c$. Thus from a large set of observed variates it is possible to infer a small set of latent causes. This simplification is a step toward the parsimony which Ockham admonished careful thinkers to seek. (William Ockham, 1280–1349, was an English schoolman and one of the founders of the philosophic school of nominalism, embraced by your authors. His famous "razor" principle can be stated as, "Multiplicity ought not to be posited without necessity.")

How should nursing researchers decide what causes to hypothesize? The review of the literature and the researcher's general sense of the problem situation have to be the sources of guidance. In other words, you will need to call upon a combination of probabilities found in the scientific literature, pattern recognition developed in personal experience, and the logical integration of the two. This triad is, of course, the same we quoted earlier as the base for medical diagnosis. A particular concern should be shown for the natural, or ordinary, language terms for ascribing causation in nursing and related health science circles. The ultimate goal of the researcher is to contribute to the reformulation of policy discussions, and the more respect she can show for the ordinary language of discourse in the policy arena, the easier her communication task is going to be. Offering a lot of new jargon in one package may not facilitate communication and persuasion. It should usually be possible to describe most of the probable causes of criterion variance in quite conventional terms, using the license to invent new names for previously ignored causes sparingly. An ideal research project may be one which puts just one novel cause in place among a set of conventional, well-known causes.

Another way to increase the parsimony of a theory is by accepting as a second principle for causal analysis of nursing problems the notion that causal variables must be mutually uncorrelated. If you really think about this you will be troubled by it. The variables are created to stand for the causal constructs of a theory. Do we mean that theory must be constructed out of independent, uncorrelated constructs? No, we don't. The causal constructs of a theory should be clearly separated from each other, and the more nearly they are capable of independent action, the better. Each should provide a separate influence upon the criterion constructs, but these forces may be acting upon each other as well as upon the criteria, so that they cannot be conceptualized as mutually uncorrelated. The variables created from data can correspond to the theoretical constructs only loosely at best. This variable-to-construct correspondence may be enhanced if the variables are allowed to intercorrelate much as the constructs are thought to intercorrelate and can only be damaged if the variables are forced to be mutually uncorrelated. Why, then, should we accept the principle that variables must be uncorrelated?

The answers are: first, to get parsimony, and second, to get discipline. The causal model for the data is simplified enormously if the causes are made uncorrelated. (If the causes were allowed to be intercorrelated we should have to report those correlations, and most unfortunately, we should have to interpret them. The causal factors are created to explain the correlations among the variates. What would be created to explain the correlations among the causes?) The requirement of zero correlation between each pairing of causes permits the data distributions to exert powerful discipline upon the causal analysis. Correlated causes can be created any way the analyst wants them. Uncorrelated causes can only be created in certain ways permitted by the joint distribution of the variates as measured on the sample. The principle of uncorrelatedness of causes forces a compromise between the imagination of the analyst and the realities of nature as captured in the research data. There is such a thing as destructive discipline, which it is masochistic to embrace. Some experts will tell you vehemently that we are recommending a bad discipline. It may be the case that as one becomes expert at causal analysis this discipline is needed less. Most nursing researchers who are studying this book are not experts at causal analysis. The authors are convinced that the discipline provided by the principle of uncorrelatedness of causes is desirable for their students (and themselves), and that it will be constructive rather than destructive in most applications. Incidentally, the contributions of the two greatest data analysis inventors, Sir Ronald Fisher and Harold Hotelling, were built on this principle.

Motivation for acceptance of the principle of uncorrelatedness of causes may be found in a review of the last section of Chapter 9, which highlighted some remarkable simplifications of the analysis of multiple correlations which become available when the predictors are uncorrelated. If U stands for the proportion of the criterion variance that is accounted for by the influence of the full set of hypothesized causes, then the square of the correlation of each causal factor with the criterion is the independent contribution of that cause to the criterion variance, and U is simply the sum of squared correlations of all the causal factors with the criterion. Denoting the criterion as X_c, and letting r_{ck} be the correlation of the kth causal factor with X_c, then

$$U = r_{c1}{}^2 + r_{c2}{}^2 + \cdots + r_{cn}{}^2 \qquad k = 1, 2, \ldots, n \qquad (4)$$

Denoting the uniqueness (i.e., the independent contribution) of F_k to X_c as U_{ck}, it follows that

$$U_{ck} = r_{ck}{}^2 \qquad\qquad\qquad (5)$$

Looking back in this section to the equations for the independent variates in terms of their loadings on the causal factors plus a disturbance (the structural equations), we can now tell you that the loadings a_{jk} are in fact the correlations of the variates with the factors when the factors are mutually uncorrelated. That is, in the equation

$$X_j = a_{j1}F_1 + a_{j2}F_2 + \cdots + a_{jn}F_n + d_jW_j \tag{6}$$

for uncorrelated F_k

$$a_{jk} = r_{jk} \tag{7}$$

Now suppose the method of analysis provided an equation of the same form for the criterion variate as a linear function of the causal factors plus a disturbance:

$$X_c = a_{c1}F_1 + a_{c2}F_2 + \cdots + a_{cn}F_n + d_cW_c \tag{8}$$

The loadings a_{cj} in this structural equation for the criterion would be correlations of the criterion with the causes, and their squares would be proportions of criterion variance contributed by causes. *Voilà!* Our factorial modeling (FaM) method will do it, for any number of criteria.

The correlations among all the variates are going to discipline the definitions of the causal factors that emerge from analysis. Certain correlations are especially salient and ought to receive special attention. These are the correlations between the key indicators for each cause and the key criterion. The key indicators for a cause are the independent variates that were selected during research planning as the specification variates for that cause. The rule in the FaM method is that an independent variate may be a key indicator for only one cause. The idea of a key criterion variate has not been mentioned previously. If there is only one criterion under measurement, it automatically becomes the key criterion. If there are two or more criteria under measurement, the FaM procedure requires the designation of a key criterion. The key criterion should be selected thoughtfully as the criterion variate it is most important to explain (i.e., to get a good causal model for), because the resulting U (proportion of variance explained by the causal model) is likely to be larger for it than for the other criteria. The FaM method pays particular attention to the correlations of key indicators of causes with the key criterion. We think this is a plus for the method.

Next we must discuss the issue of differential calculus. Some of you know that it is possible to minimize the magnitude of the d_j (or maximize the U_j, which is the same thing) by using calculus to determine what the c_{jk} (or a_{jk}, which are in fixed relation to the c_{jk}) weights should be. Fisher, Hotelling, and all the other great inventors of methods for causal analysis used calculus. Our FaM method does not use calculus to determine the rules for calculating the weights or loadings. Consequently, FaM does not minimize the error terms or maximize the proportions of variance explained. Horrors! We have turned our backs on the mathematical genius of the modern era in analysis. Yes, because your methodologist author has contemplated his 20 years of experience with research methods based on calculus and has decided that those methods almost always overfit the data in social science applications. He has persuaded your nurse author of this, she making an informed judgment, not a reluctant one. She thinks his arguments may apply to nursing research better than they do to some other social science fields. Overfitting means detailing the model to conform snugly to all the distribution details of the data in hand. Calculus can vacuum-form a model to the topography of the data. What you and we must remember is that we need good descriptions of situations we have not had the chance to study, not the best possible descriptions of the situations we have studied. Nursing theory has to be informed by historical data, but its usefulness resides in the anticipation of future events. History does not repeat itself exactly. We think that models that fit history loosely may travel to the future most successfully. Nursing is not an engineering problem, and we need not believe that the mathematics of engineering science is the best mathematics for nursing science.

Q: What is the proportion of variance in the jth independent variate explained by the joint action of all n causal factors upon it? How can the value of d_j be expressed in terms of the a_{jk}?

Setting Up a Causal Analysis

This section provides rules for using the FaM procedure. It assumes the MODEL computer program, as listed in Appendix A, will perform the computations on the data. A word is in order about *when* these tasks of preparing for causal analysis should be performed. Researchers often wait until the data are collected and the data file is prepared before they address the issue of setting up for analysis. At this point the painful discovery may be made that the way the data have been collected prevents the desired analysis. Ideally, the tasks described below should be rehearsed in the research planning stage, before any data are collected. This is really one of the biggest points of this text: *Causal hypotheses should guide the selection of variates* in the research planning activity. Before the site and subjects are selected, before a single datum is collected, each variate in the plan should be justified by its place in the causal hypotheses which will be processed when the data analysis stage is finally reached.

The first task is to list the hypothetical causes. In the example, the two hypothesized causes are *aptitude* and *environment*.

The second task is to specify each cause by a list of variates that are the key indicators of each cause. The rule is that a given independent variate can serve as a key indicator of one, and only one, cause. It is not required that all independent variates be used in this specification step. Some variates may be included because they promise to control some source of variation which is known to be relevant but for which the causal loadings cannot be hypothesized. In the example, the specifications are:

> Variable: Aptitude
> Variate 1: 1968 science achievement
> Variate 2: 1968 science attitude
> Variable: Environment
> Variate 3: Science class processes
> Variate 4: Peer science and mathematics activities

There are no extra independent variates in the example.

The third task is to specify the key criterion. There are two dependent variates in the example, and the 1969 science attitude variate is specified as the key criterion.

The fourth task is to order the variables for analysis. The FaM method creates the causal factors serially in an order specified by the analyst. This order of factoring is important because the actual definition of the first cause factored is completely controlled by the a priori specification, but the actual definition of each factor after the first is disciplined by the requirement of uncorrelatedness of the factors, and this constraint imposed by the correlations among the variates is increasingly strong as the method works down the list of factors. We cannot tell you how to order your causes for analysis. Your knowledge of the problem will be the source of your hunches about which cause should be given first draw on the data, which should be given second draw, and so on. The notion of a "draw on the data" is descriptive of what actually happens in FaM. The first cause factored draws some of the variances and covariances among all the variates from the system. The second cause makes its draw only on the variances and covariances remaining after the first cause is factored out. We speak of the *residual* variances and covariances as what is left of the correlation matrix after one or more factors have been factored out. One rule of thumb we can provide is that when there is a program or treatment cause standing for the nursing innovation you wish to evaluate, it should be the last cause factored. Requiring the policy-manipulatable cause to show its explanatory power on a residual set of variances and covariances *after* all the other hypothesized causes have had their draw on the data makes for a fair game. That is, this arrangement makes it most difficult for the policy-manipulatable variable to show any amount of explanatory power, but if it does, the finding is impressive. In the example, the environment factor included variance from the policy-manipulatable science class processes variate, and clearly should have been factored after the aptitude variable, as it was.

In order to run the MODEL program it is necessary to compute the table of correlations among all the variates (which we call a correlation *matrix*). The REMAKE subroutine is then used to place the variates in the correlation matrix in the following order, unless the matrix has been made with the variates already in order:

1 Variates which are key indicators of the first causal variable

   2   Variates which are key indicators of the second causal variable

     ·

     ·

     ·

   n Variates which are key indicators of the nth causal variable
$n + 1$ Independent variates which do not specify any causal variable (if any)
$n + 2$ Extra criterion, or dependent, variates (if any)
$n + 3$ The key criterion variate

Note that it is permissible but undesirable that a single variate specify a causal variable, that sets $n + 1$ and $n + 2$ may perfectly well contain no variates, and that the key criterion is always the last variate, associated with the last row and the last column, of the correlation matrix when it is properly arranged for factoring. Table 11-1 reports the correlation matrix for the example, properly arranged for factoring.

    The first setup card for the MODEL program contains

   1 p, the total number of variates to be correlated
   2 N, the sample size
   3 n, the number of causal variables hypothesized
   4 $k1 = 0$ if means, standard deviations, and correlations are to be computed from scores
          $= 1$ if correlation matrix is to be read as input
   5 $k2 = 0$ if no REMAKE of correlation matrix is required
          $= 1$ if a REMAKE is required
   6 $p1$, the number of variates to be included in REMAKE matrix ($p1 = 0$ if $k2 = 0$)

If $k1 = 0$, the second setup card contains the format for the score cards enclosed in brackets; if $k1 = 1$, the second setup card contains the format for the input correlation matrix cards enclosed in brackets. If $k2 = 1$, the third setup card contains the original position numbers of the variates which are to be included in the REMAKE correlation matrix in the order in which they are to be placed in the new matrix (if $k2 = 0$, this card is not included in the setup deck). The next setup card contains in n fields the number of variates which are key indicators of each of the n causal factors. After these setup cards, the input deck contains

Table 11-1   Correlation Matrix for Six Keeves Variates

Variate	Values					
1968 science achievement	1.000					
1968 science attitude	.128	1.000				
Science class processes	.178	.177	1.000			
Peer science, math activities	.044	−.080	.060	1.000		
1969 science achievement	.758	.202	.228	.091	1.000	
1969 science attitude	.310	.208	.235	.315	.385	1.000

MODEL CORRELATIONAL DATA, PROGRAMMED BY P.R. LOHNES
   6 VARIATES,   235 SUBJECTS,   2 VARIABLES
CORRELATION MATRIX

ROW 1	1.000					
ROW 2	.128	1.000				
ROW 3	.178	.177	1.000			
ROW 4	.044	−.080	.060	1.000		
ROW 5	.758	.202	.228	.091	1.000	
ROW 6	.310	.208	.235	.315	.385	1.000

HYPOTHESIS VECTOR 1
  .310   .208   0.000   0.000   0.000   0.000
RESIDUAL CRITERION VARIANCE AFTER   1 STAGES = .8754
HYPOTHESIS VECTOR 2
  0.000   0.000   .153   .318   0.000   0.000
FINAL UNEXPLAINED VARIANCE IN CRITERION = .7557

TEST	COMMUNALITY	DISTURBANCE	FACTOR	STRUCTURE
1	.728	.521	.853	.036
2	.396	.777	.627	−.053
3	.263	.858	.233	.457
4	.830	.413	−.008	.911
5	.505	.704	.702	.113
6	.244	.869	.353	.346

CONTRIBUTIONS OF DOMAINS TO KEY CRITERION VARIANCE
FACTOR 1 PROP. VAR. .125 CUM. PROP. .125
FACTOR 2 PROP. VAR. .120 CUM. PROP. .244
FINAL RESIDUAL MATRIX

ROW 1	.272					
ROW 2	−.405	.604				
ROW 3	−.037	.055	.737			
ROW 4	.018	−.027	−.354	.170		
ROW 5	.156	−.232	.013	−.006	.495	
ROW 6	−.003	.005	−.005	.003	.098	.756

TOTAL THEORY PARTITION OF R FOR ALL FACTORS

ROW 1	.728					
ROW 2	.533	.396				
ROW 3	.215	.122	.263			
ROW 4	.026	−.053	.414	.830		
ROW 5	.602	.434	.215	.097	.505	
ROW 6	.313	.203	.240	.312	.287	.244

FACTOR-SCORING COEFFICIENTS

ROW 1	.785	−.073
ROW 2	.527	−.049
ROW 3	0.000	.425
ROW 4	0.000	.885
ROW 5	0.000	0.000
ROW 6	0.000	0.000

PREDICTED CHANGES IN CRITERIA (ROWS) FOR UNIT CHANGES
IN A PARTICULAR MANIPULABLE PREDICTOR (COLUMN)

ROW 1	.543	.364	.048	.100
ROW 2	.252	.169	.147	.306

VARIANCE-COVARIANCE MATRIX FOR FACTORS

ROW 1	1.000	.000
ROW 2	.000	1.000

Figure 11-1   MODEL output for Keeves data example.

either the score cards or the input correlation matrix on cards. (Note that the cards referred to may be IBM punch cards or lines in a memory file, depending on how the computer job is being sent to the batch queue. It is assumed that the necessary cards or lines to acquire the MODEL program from a library source and to command an execution of it precede these setup and data cards or lines which will be demanded during the execution.)

For the example, the correlation matrix was available as the data input, and the six variates were in the proper order in it; thus no REMAKE was required. The setup cards looked like this:

Card 1:	6	235	2	1	0	0
Card 2:	(6F5.3)					
Card 3:	1.000	.128	.178	.044	.758	.310
Card 4:	1.000	.177	−.080	.202	.208	
Card 5:	1.000	.060	.228	.235		
Card 6:	1.000	.091	.315			
Card 7:	1.000	.385				
Card 8:	1.000					
Card 9:	2	2				

Figure 11-1 illustrates the printout from the MODEL run on this setup. The computed values describing the causal factors are fitted to the data, telling how well they explain the variance in each variate and what the disturbances are. The interpretations of these computational results are discussed below.

Q: Explain the lines of input to MODEL given in Figures 10-2 and 10-4. What are these submissions doing? How do they differ?

Partitioning the Variances and Covariances

Partitioning is really what data analysis which supports theorizing is all about. The correlation matrix for the data contains the variances of the p variates in its diagonal from the upper left-hand corner to the lower right-hand corner, and the covariances among the variates in its off-diagonal elements, when the variates have been standardized. That is, the 1.000 entries on the diagonal of the correlation matrix (as in Table 11-1 for the example) are variances of standardized variates. The statistic called a *covariance* is defined algebraically as

$$\text{cov}_{jk} = \frac{\Sigma X_j X_k - (\Sigma X_j)(\Sigma X_k)/N}{N} = r_{jk} s_j s_k \tag{9}$$

but when $m_j = m_k = 0$ and $s_j = s_k = 1$ it follows that $\text{cov}_{jk} = r_{jk}$, so that for standardized variates the covariance is also the correlation, which is a very handy fact. If you enjoy algebra, you should be able to prove this by manipulating the formula for variance given in Chapter 9 and the formula for covariance given above. Like the standard deviation, the correlation is an attractive number because of its metric. However, like the variance, the covariance is attractive because partition theorems exist for it. FaM is based on one such theorem.

FaM partitions the matrix of variances and covariances into a number of independent and additive matrices. The first n of these are "theory" matrices, each of which expresses the values the variances and the covariances among the variates would take on the theoretical assumption that the scatter of the subjects on the p variates was caused entirely by one causal factor. The $n + 1$ partition matrix is a residual, or error, matrix which expresses the parts of the observed variances and covariances that are not explained by the sum of the theory matrices. The residuals represent the shortfalls of the hypothesized causes as explanations of the scatter of the subjects reported by the data matrix.

To make this idea of partitions of the data variance-covariance matrix more formal, we will show you the algebra and the numerical results for the six-variate, two-cause example. The loadings of the variates on the first causal factor, a_{j1}, are reported in the first column of the LOADINGS table on the printout. Each element of the first theory matrix is computed as

$$\hat{r}_{1jk} = a_{j1}a_{k1} \tag{10}$$

When $j = k$ the predicted or theoretical element is part of a variance, and when $j \neq k$ it is part of a covariance. Table 11-2(a) reports the first theoretical partition of the data variance-covariance matrix for the example. Verify that the numbers are computable from the loadings of the six variates on the aptitude cause. If we denote the data matrix given by Table 11-1 as R, we may denote the first theory matrix as $\hat{R}_1$. This $\hat{R}_1$ shows what the variances and covariances among the six variates would be if the aptitude cause accounted for all the scatter of the subjects on the six variates, that is, if all a_{j2} and all d_j were equal to zero. Comparing R and $\hat{R}_1$ reveals that aptitude does not completely account for the data.

The second theory matrix has elements

$$\hat{r}_{2jk} = a_{j2}a_{k2} \tag{11}$$

For the example these are arrayed in matrix $\hat{R}_2$ in Table 11-2(b), which shows what the data table R would have to be if environment had been the complete cause of the scatter of scores in the data.

Since $\hat{R}_1$ and $\hat{R}_2$ are independent and additive, they can be added together to get the two-cause theory matrix, which for n causes can be expressed as

$$\hat{R} = \hat{R}_1 + \hat{R}_2 + \cdots + \hat{R}_n \tag{12}$$

In the example n is 2, so

$$\hat{R} = \hat{R}_1 + \hat{R}_2 \tag{13}$$

Table 11-2   Partition Matrices for Six Keeves Variates

(a) Aptitude factor partition, $\hat{R}_1$	(b) Environment factor partition, $\hat{R}_2$

X						X					
(1)	.727					(1)	.001				
(2)	.535	.394				(2)	−.002	.003			
(3)	.199	.146	.054			(3)	.016	−.024	.209		
(4)	−.006	−.005	−.002	.000		(4)	.033	−.049	.416	.830	
(5)	.598	.440	.163	−.005	.492	(5)	.004	−.006	.051	.103	.013
(6)	.301	.221	.082	−.003	.248	.125	(6)	.012	−.018	.158	.315	.039	.120

(c) Two-cause theory matrix, $\hat{R}$

X					
(1)	.728				
(2)	.533	.396			
(3)	.215	.122	.263		
(4)	.026	−.053	.414	.830	
(5)	.602	.434	.215	.097	.505
(6)	.313	.203	.240	.312	.287	.244

(d) Residual variance-covariance matrix, $\tilde{R}$

X					
(1)	.272				
(2)	−.405	.604			
(3)	−.037	.055	.737		
(4)	.011	−.031	−.356	.170	
(5)	.156	−.232	.013	−.006	.495
(6)	−.003	.005	−.005	.003	.098	.755

Matrices are added or subtracted by adding or subtracting corresponding elements; thus

$$\hat{r}_{jk} = \hat{r}_{1jk} + \hat{r}_{2jk} + \cdots + \hat{r}_{njk} \tag{14}$$

Table 11-2(c) reports the two-cause theory matrix for the example. The residual, or error, matrix denoted $\tilde{R}$ can be obtained by subtraction:

$$\tilde{R} = R - \hat{R} \tag{15}$$

For the example, each element of $\tilde{R}$ is given by

$$\tilde{r}_{jk} = r_{jk} - (\hat{r}_{1jk} + \hat{r}_{2jk}) \tag{16}$$

In general, then, FaM makes it possible to partition the data matrix as follows:

$$R = \hat{R}_1 + \hat{R}_2 + \cdots + \hat{R}_n + \tilde{R} \tag{17}$$

For the example, Table 11-2(d) gives $\tilde{R}$. Verify that 11-2(c) plus 11-2(d) equals Table 11-1, and that this is also true for 11-2(a) plus 11-2(b) plus 11-2(d).

The residual matrix $\tilde{R}$ contains the variances and covariances among the parts of the p variates that are not accounted for by the n hypothesized causes. Remembering that the $d_j W_j$ are the unexplained parts of the X_j, we may say that $\tilde{R}$ is the variance-covariance matrix for the $d_j W_j$. It is possible to explore in $\tilde{R}$ for further structural variables which might carry the explanation of the variances and covariances of the X_j beyond the stopping point provided by the extraction of the n hypothesized causes, but such snooping in the residuals from the hypothesized model is an advanced skill, and requires the support of more complicated computer programs. Cooley and Lohnes (1971, chapters 4 and 5) provide instruction and programs for such operations.

TESTING CAUSAL INFERENCES

The previous section showed how a causal model could be specified and computed. Naturally the research scientist awaits her computer printout with great expectations. Think what she has been through to reach this grand day. She has proposed a research plan, obtained funding, arranged for and supervised data-collection operations on site, created a clean data file, thought out her causal hypotheses within the severe constraints imposed by the FaM method, and set up the MODEL program run, and now the moment of fulfillment is at hand. Soon she will be writing up her findings for publication, and then at the end of a long and arduous journey she will coast into that snug harbor where only published researchers may anchor.

If she is far-seeing, she realizes that her findings will have to be tested on other sites and subjects in replication research projects, and that after a refreshing respite she will have to hoist anchor and sail off on new business. Life is a cycle of arrivals and departures, and one can anchor forever only in still waters.

All that is in the future. Right now the MODEL printout has just arrived. What immediate tests can be made of the degree of success of the hypothesized causal model?

Figure 11-1 is the printout for the example data, borrowed for our pedagogical purposes from a much larger set of variates in an excellent study done by John Keeves (1972). The data describe test results for 215 Australian students collected before (variates 1 and 2) and after (variates 5 and 6) their first form school year (first year in secondary school), as well as a major dimension of variation in the science instruction they received in first form (variate 3) and a measurement of variation in science and mathematics activities of each subject's three best friends during the first form year. The subjects were a random sample of youths making the transition from 42 primary schools to 15 secondary schools in the Canberra district in 1968. How successful is the two-cause theory for the Keeves data?

The first test is the proportion of key criterion variance accounted for by each causal factor, and the sum of these proportions, which is the proportion of

key criterion variance accounted for by all the causes working together. For the
Keeves example, the printout shows that factor 1 (aptitude) accounts for .125 of
the key criterion (1969 science attitude) variance. Furthermore, factor 2 (environment) accounts for another .120 of the key criterion variance, so that the
causal model accounts for a total of .244 of the 1969 science attitude variance (the
computer rounding of numbers sometimes produces anomalies in what should be
sums and differences). Thus, the explanation of the key criterion is only modestly successful. Three-quarters of the posttest science attitude variance remains unexplained.

The second test is the proportion of the additional criterion (variate 5, 1969
science achievement) variance explained. The printout reveals that the proportion of posttest science achievement variance explained by the model is .505.
How does this partition into the proportion explained by aptitude and the
proportion explained by environment? The lazy computer programmer has left
this for us to figure out (maybe so we can enjoy some use of our pocket
calculators). Remembering that

$$U_{jk} = a_{jk}{}^2 \tag{18}$$

(the uniqueness of factor k for this variate is the square of the loading of the
variate on factor k), we can square the two loadings for variate 5, which gives

$$
\begin{aligned}
(.702)^2 &= \underline{.493} \\
(.113)^2 &= \underline{.013} \\
h^2 &= .506
\end{aligned}
$$

(In FaM, the part of a variate's variance which is explained by all the variables is
termed the *communality* and given the symbol h^2. Communality is a special case
of the U statistic previously defined.) Thus, aptitude explains .49 of the variance
in the additional criterion while environment explains only a negligible .01 of it.
For practical purposes we may generalize that the model accounts for half of the
variance in posttest science achievement, and all the work is done by the
aptitude cause. Twice as much achievement outcome variance is explained by
comparison with attitude outcome variance. This is not surprising to educational
researchers who know that achievement variance is almost always better accounted for than attitude outcome variance. Probably there is more measurement error variance in attitude measurements than in achievement measurements, and thus less true-score variance is available for modeling.

Overall, then, the initial test of the model is the extents and ways it accounts
for criteria variances. A judgment of success depends on what one reasonably
expected and hoped to accomplish. In the Keeves data one hoped to see the
environment cause account for more of the criteria variances than it does, and
one is therefore disappointed.

It is also interesting to look at the proportions of variances of the independent variates absorbed by the causes, and how these partition among the causes.

The model of the Keeves data absorbs a majority (.728) of the variance in pretest science achievement, and most of this is taken up by the aptitude factor. In addition, a majority of the peers variate variance is absorbed (.830), mostly by the environment factor, which correlates .911 with variate 4. The other two independent variates are not drawn on heavily by the model. Clearly the researcher intended an environment cause which would involve the science class processes variate heavily, but the data did not sanction such an involvement. In particular, the low predictive validities of variate 3 for the two criteria (i.e., the correlations of X_3 with X_5 and X_6), namely .228 and .235, militated against a heavy loading of variate 3, science class processes, on environment. FaM employs the residual covariances of the key indicators of a causal variable with the key criterion as the specification weight in orienting a factor for the variable. The printout informs you that for the environment factor these specification weights were .153 for variate 3 and .318 for variate 4. This inequality in residual covariances really explains why the peers variate rather than the science class variate exerted the controlling influence on the orientation of the environment factor. This is precisely what we meant when we said that in the FaM method the data discipline the imagination of the researcher. In this case the discipline imposed by the data is painful, because support for the hypothesis of causal influence of the curriculum variate on the test outcomes was desired.

Suppose that one knows one has really good data in hand and can see by scrutinizing the correlation matrix that there is considerable structure to the data, but the hypothesized causal model is a flop. Well, rather than stand on the flop, one might want to rethink the causal inference problem and propose a different specification of causes to the MODEL program. This new hypothesized causal model is based on knowledge of the correlations in the data and is *not* an a priori specification. If the reanalysis is successful it is interesting and has some implications for theory and for future research planning, but its success is not nearly as weighty and convincing as the success of the a priori specification would have been, had it been obtained. Your prior knowledge of situations similar to the data situation has failed you, and the description you now create for the data situation is *not* confirmatory of prior theory and is *not* as confidently generalizable to future situations as a successful a priori model would have been. This reiterates a point made in Chapter 2 that data collection is planned to test a previously stated hypothesis. It may lead to further hypotheses, but you should not consider them to have been adequately tested by data that were collected earlier. Serendipity is not as satisfying as confirmation, but it is challenging. Your discovery may replicate and lead to a new development in theory.

DETAILING CAUSAL MODELS

Suppose we decide our causal model is successful. How do we exposit it? Exactly what are its details?

The causal model is a set of structural equations. There is one structural equation for each criterion variate, and these are of primary interest. The equations show how a subject's observed value on a criterion variate (in standard deviation units, since all variates are assumed to be standardized) may be decomposed into n additive pieces, each of which is the product of a loading weight times the subject's standardized value on a cause, plus an unexplained piece, called the *disturbance*. For the key criterion, which is the pth variate, the structural equation has this form:

$$X_p = a_{p1}F_1 + a_{p2}F_2 + \cdots + a_{pn}F_n + d_pW_p \tag{19}$$

The loading a_{pk} is the measure of the contribution of the kth cause to the pth variate, in the sense that a change in the value of the kth cause of one standard deviation magnitude should yield a change in the pth variate of a_{pk} magnitude. (The structural equation is sometimes called a *production function* because the weight a_{jk} shows how much change in the jth variate a unit change in the kth cause produces.) The loading is also called a *structural parameter*.

The set of all loadings is the *parameterization* of a model for the data. FaM produces pn parameters because it parameterizes a structural equation for each of the p variates in the research (the independent as well as the dependent ones) and provides n parameters for each equation. The d_j are not basic parameters, since they can be computed by subtraction once all the a_{jk} are fitted.

These parameters of a model for the data in hand can be thought of as estimates of what the parameters for a model for other data might turn out to be, and therefore the act of parameterizing is sometimes termed *estimation*. Perhaps our description of it as "detailing" the model provides a good perspective.

For the Keeves example, the structural equation for the key criterion, which is variate 6, 1969 science attitude, is parameterized as

$$X_6 = .353 \text{ aptitude} + .346 \text{ environment} + .869W_6$$

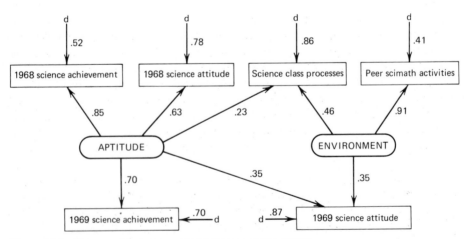

Figure 11-2   Diagram of factorial model for Keeves data example.

Thus the two causes contribute almost equally to the variate, but the large disturbance shows that their joint influence is weak.

The full set of structural equations for the example is detailed as follows:

$$1968 \text{ SciAch} = .853 \text{ aptitude} + .036 \text{ environment} + .521W_1$$
$$1968 \text{ SciAtt} = .627 \text{ aptitude} - .053 \text{ environment} + .777W_2$$
$$\text{SciCProcess} = .233 \text{ aptitude} + .457 \text{ environment} + .858W_3$$
$$\text{PeerActivit} = -.008 \text{ aptitude} + .911 \text{ environment} + .413W_4$$
$$1969 \text{ SciAch} = .702 \text{ aptitude} + .113 \text{ environment} + .704W_5$$
$$1969 \text{ SciAtt} = .353 \text{ aptitude} + .346 \text{ environment} + .869W_6$$

A useful diagraming convention for displaying a causal model is demonstrated by Figure 11-2. Each variate is represented by a rectangle and each cause is represented by a curved-ended box. Arrows representing causal influences are drawn from causes to variates, and the loadings are placed on them. To simplify the view of the model, arrows are omitted for loadings less than .20 in absolute value, as such slight loadings indicate paths of negligible influence. The disturbance for each variate is drawn as d and its value is entered next to it. Such diagrams are very attractive when the complexity of a model is low enough to permit a neat drawing, but sometimes the model is so highly complex that no neat diagram is possible (messiness coming from the necessity of having arrows cross each other). In such a case the parameters and disturbances must be conveyed by a table. Table 11-3 represents one way to arrange a report, in this case for the Keeves example.

This model for the Keeves data is consistent with the theoretical inference that aptitude variation exerts strong causal influence on contemporary science achievement variation and modest causal influence on contemporary science attitude variation among secondary school students, while environment variation exerts no causal influence on current science achievement and modest causal influence on current science attitude. Obviously this model proves nothing about the causation of variance in the Keeves data or anywhere else. However, to the extent that the trends in the Keeves data, as displayed in this model, agree with trends in a number of other studies on adolescents done elsewhere, the theoretical inferences are validated further.

Table 11-3 Factorial Model for Six Keeves Variates

Variate	Loadings for causes, a_{jk}		Disturbance
	Aptitude	Environment	
1968 science achievement	.853	.036	.521
1968 science attitude	.627	−.053	.777
Science class processes	.233	.457	.858
Peer science, math activities	−.008	.911	.413
1969 science achievement	.702	.113	.704
1969 science attitude	.353	.346	.869

A researcher who is combining what she can learn from her data with everything she already knows about the class of problems has to find the courage to make causal interpretations of problem situations. FaM is a technique by which she is challenged to organize her prior knowledge into explicit causal hypotheses and through which she can get a test, based on her data, of those hypotheses. If the model for the data tends to confirm her hypotheses, theory is strengthened. If the model fails to confirm her hypotheses, theory is challenged.

The model for the Keeves data failed to confirm that recent environment variation is an important cause of current science achievement and attitude variation. That is a challenge to science curriculum theory. In fact, however, the hypothesis that environment would be important for explaining the criteria was wishful thinking, in the light of evidence from many other curriculum studies in which similar environment constructs have let down the side. Contemporary curriculum theory seems to incorporate an excess of wishful thinking. Could this be true of nursing theory?

Q: State algebraically the subtraction rule for computing d_j from the known a_{jk}.

PREDICTING FUTURE EVENTS

When research succeeds in validating a theory for a class of problems it is reasonable to ask how the theory can be deployed to predict the results of specific policy decisions. Theory that presumes to explain the causes of variations in the outcomes of nursing care should make it possible to predict the impact of specific manipulations of policy-manipulatable variates. An advantage of a causal model produced by FaM is that the causal variables are independent, and thus the loading for any particular variable shows exactly what the predicted result of a change in that variable is, assuming all other variables remain constant. It will be a variate, however, not a variable, which is directly manipulatable, and since a change in an independent variate can accompany changes of some size in all the variables, the prediction problem is complex. We need to be able to show (1) how much change in each variable is predicted for a given amount of change in a single variate and (2) how much change in a criterion is predicted as the result of that set of changes in the variables.

The MODEL program incorporates the necessary algebra to combine the information about how a manipulated change in a particular predictor variate affects some or all of the causal variables, and how those changes in variables affect each criterion variate. The result is a table that has a column for every predictor variate and a row for each criterion variate. At the intersection of a particular column and row is a number which is the predicted change in that criterion for a unit change (plus one standard deviation) in that predictor. The predicted change is in standard deviation units. Table 11-4 is such a table for the Keeves example. It gives discouraging news about the possible payoffs of improvement in the science curriculum and teaching. It says that, according to the model, an increase of an entire standard deviation in the science class

Table 11-4   Predicted Criterion Changes for Unit Change in an Independent Variate

Criterion	Independent variate			
	1968 science achievement	1968 science attitude	Science class processes	Peer science, math attitudes
1969 science achievement	.543	.364	.048	.100
1969 science attitude	.252	.169	.147	.306

process score of a student is expected to yield only .048 of a standard deviation increase in the student's science achievement score after the instructional year. This suggests that manipulating the science class process variate is not a useful route to improved science achievement test scores. A unit change in science class process score is predicted to yield .147 of a unit change in science attitude score, but even this is a modest yield for a huge improvement in the instructional process variate.

This table of predicted changes in criteria for unit changes in predictors assumes all variates have been rescaled to zero mean and unit standard deviation ($m_X = 0$; $s_X = 1$). Often it will not be reasonable to contemplate a manipulation that would change a predictor score by a full standard deviation unit. Consequences of a change of less than a full unit in a predictor can be calculated by multiplying any number from the table by the decimal fraction representing the contemplated proportion of a unit change in the predictor.

The table of predicted changes does display important consequences of the causal model for the data. However, we must remember that the model is never entirely correct and trustworthy. It only represents the implications of the researcher's preconceived theory of causation for the research data. *Such a model can never prove anything about causation.* Its purpose is to test the reasonableness, and perhaps dramatize the unreasonableness, of a theory about causation. When we believe we have demonstrated a thoroughly convincing and strong theory for the data, the predictions from the model may be quite forceful. When a plausible but weak (or even an implausible) theory has been revealed for what it is, the predictions from the model will have no force. Always, always, always, computed numbers have to be interpreted intelligently. Computing is an aid to intelligence, not a substitute for it.

A DEMONSTRATION RECOVERY OF KNOWN CAUSES

The plight of the researcher is never to know the true causes of the variances and covariances she observes. The most she can do is invent possible causes and test the plausibility of these causal hypotheses against the research data. She can hope to show that her hypothetical causal model is plausible, in that it accounts parsimoniously for a substantial part of the dispersion of criterion scores *and* it is based on sound reasoning, but she cannot hope to prove conclusively that her model is true. It is fun every now and then to create some variates entirely out of known causes, correlate them, and ask one's favorite modeling method to recover the true causes from the correlations if it can. Lu Pai and Paul Lohnes have made this little demonstration for your entertainment and for further elucidation of the FaM method. We began by deciding, let there be two uncorrelated factors which are the true and only sources of the variances and covariances of five variates, such that the true structural equations are

$$X_1 = .92F_1 + .00F_2$$
$$X_2 = .86F_1 + .00F_2$$
$$X_3 = .32F_1 + .71F_2$$
$$X_4 = .42F_1 + .68F_2$$
$$X_5 = .38F_1 + .55F_2$$

Where did we get the loadings? We just made them up to suit ourselves. We agreed to think of F_1 as a causal variable specified by X_1 and X_2. Notice that if F_1 has unit variance, X_1 and X_2 will *not* have unit variance. Actually, $s_1^2 = .8464$ and $s_2^2 = .7376$, because in the present case

$$s_{jk}^2 = a_{j1}^2 + a_{j2}^2$$

The covariance of X_1 with X_2 is $s_{12} = .7912$, because in the present case

$$s_{jk} = a_j a_k$$

We agreed that F_2 should be specified by X_3 and X_4.

Q: What are the variances and the covariance for X_3 and X_4, computed to four decimal places?

X_5 is the designated criterion variate.

Before we compute and model the correlations, it makes an interesting excursion to offer the table of variances and covariances of the five variates to MODEL for analysis, specifying the two causal variables as above. Table 11-5 reports the variance-covariance matrix which was input to MODEL and the structure which MODEL found for it. The dramatic result is that the FaM algorithm manages to recover exactly the true structural coefficients, and the explained variance for each variate is exactly its original variance. In our computer output we also find that the final residual matrix is all zeros, and the total theory partition matrix is exactly the input variance-covariance matrix. This verifies that the two causal variables which have been fitted completely explain all the variances and covariances of the five variates, and in that sense the two variables are the true and complete causes of the five variates.

Table 11-5 FaM Performed on a Fabricated Variance-Covariance Matrix

	Variance-covariance matrix				
X_1	.846	.791	.294	.386	.350
X_2	.791	.740	.275	.361	.327
X_3	.294	.275	.607	.617	.512
X_4	.386	.361	.617	.639	.534
X_5	.350	.327	.512	.534	.447

	Structural model		
	a_{j1}	a_{j2}	$a_{j1}^2 + a_{j2}^2$
X_1	.920	.000	.846
X_2	.860	.000	.740
X_3	.320	.710	.607
X_4	.420	.680	.639
X_5	.380	.550	.447

	Two-factor theory partition, $a_{j1}a_{k1} + a_{j2}a_{k2}$				
X_1	.846	.791	.294	.386	.350
X_2	.791	.740	.275	.361	.327
X_3	.294	.275	.607	.617	.512
X_4	.386	.361	.617	.639	.534
X_5	.350	.327	.512	.534	.447

But this has been an excursion. The MODEL program is supposed to be put to work on a correlation matrix, not a variance-covariance matrix.

Q: What do you expect is the numerical value of the correlation of X_1 with X_2, and why?

Q: What is the correlation matrix for the five variates, to four decimal places, and how did you compute it?

Table 11-6 reports the input correlations and the MODEL output, with the variables specified as discussed above. The communality for each variate is one and the disturbance for each variate is zero, testifying that the two causal variables fitted offer a complete explanation of the five variates; indeed the computer output shows that the total theory partition of the correlation matrix is exactly the correlation matrix itself, and the final residual matrix is all zeros. The only question is whether the two causal variables described by the structure coefficients are the two causes from which the data were generated. Well, the first factor is obviously exactly right, because each of the five variates correlates with it precisely as each correlates with X_1 or X_2, and we know that X_1 and X_2 have to correlate perfectly with F_1 and with each other. The coefficients for the

Table 11-6   FaM Performed on the Correlations of the Fabricated Variates

	Upper triangle of the correlation matrix				
X_1	1.000	1.000	.411	.525	.568
X_2		1.000	.411	.525	.568
X_3			1.000	.992	.984
X_4				1.000	.999
X_5					1.000

Factorial model				
Structure coefficients			h^2	d
X_1	1.000	.000	1.000	.000
X_2	1.000	.000	1.000	.000
X_3	.411	.912	1.000	.000
X_4	.525	.851	1.000	.000
X_5	.568	.823	1.000	.000

	Two-factor theory partition of the correlation matrix				
X_1	1.000	1.000	.411	.525	.568
X_2	1.000	1.000	.411	.525	.568
X_3	.411	.411	1.000	.992	.984
X_4	.525	.525	.992	1.000	.999
X_5	.568	.568	.984	.999	1.000

variates on the second factor eyeball as being roughly proportional to the true generating coefficients, so we suspect that the second fitted factor is right, too.

Why are the structural coefficients returned by MODEL only proportional to the generating coefficients? This follows from the standardization of the variates to unit standard deviation in the process of correlating them. We have to note and remember that FaM provides models for standardized variates, not "raw" variates, when it is used as we have recommended. (A raw variate is one with an arbitrary standard deviation and variance, and is usually the actual observation scale or measurement scale.) If you continue your study of quantitative methods you will find that some methodologists insist that models should always explain the variances of raw variates. Tukey, a very prominent and productive statistician, even claims to have organized a secret society for the abolition of the correlation coefficient, replete with a secret handshake. Clearly, we do not know the handshake. We continue to believe that it is always better in nursing research to cut research variates loose from their arbitrary variances by standardizing them. Our emblem is

$$r_{jk}$$

writ large on everything we touch. To admit that we may be wrong about this causes us a tremendous shudder (and must do the same to you), because it would be a terrible wrong. Shudder we do. We are not godlike in our intellects, and we have had to make hard decisions in delineating a research analysis strategy for ourselves and our students. Fortunately, the student can surpass the teacher. If some day you become convinced that it is better to model raw variances and decide to shift gears accordingly, you still may credit us with having involved you in the great game of mathematical modeling and having moved you some distance into the arena. We hope you will never feel that we thew you unarmed to the lions.

Don't be too impressed by the little game played in this section. FaM coped with this recovery problem perfectly, but when we made up the generating coefficients to suit ourselves we also tailored them to suit FaM nicely. You can invent some generating equations which will give FaM the dickens of a problem if you work at it.

Q: Return to the exercise you did in response to the Q at the end of Chapter 10. Interpret your results on the assumption that you had hypothesized a two-cause model explaining variance in achievement of RN status as a function of aptitude and interest variables. Draw a path diagram for the fitted model. What are the limits of generalizability for your findings?

Q: Invent and specify a three-cause theory for the variance in variates 13 and 14 of the Project TALENT data. Fit the theory to the data by means of the MODEL program. (Someone at the computing center will help you to write a format statement to read the variates you have selected. Be sure to do something reasonable about the missing data.) Report and interpret the results as you would for a journal article.

Q: Locate an interesting correlation matrix in the literature, hypothesize a causal model for it, and run MODEL on it. Report and interpret the results. Would your reanalysis be publishable?

REFERENCES

Cooley, William W.: Explanatory observational studies. *Educational Researcher*, 1978, *7*, 9–15.

————, and Paul R. Lohnes: *Multivariate data analysis*. New York: Wiley, 1971.

Keeves, John P.: *Educational environment and student achievement*. Melbourne: Australian Council for Educational Research, 1972.

Lohnes, Paul R.: Factorial modeling in support of causal inference. *American Educational Research Journal*, 1979, *16*, 323–340.

Mosteller, Frederick, and John W. Tukey: *Data analysis and regression*. Reading, Mass.: Addison-Wesley, 1977.

Wold, H.: Causal inferences from observational data: A review of ends and means. *Journal of the Royal Statistical Society, Series A*, 1956, *119*, 351–390.

Examples of Theoretical Models for Research Data

One way you can develop a "feel" for causal models for research data is to study carefully many examples of such models. This chapter provides 10 examples from a variety of social science fields which we think will reward your study. You might wish that more of the examples represented nursing research, but at the time of this writing it was not possible to find such. Your authors hope that this text will encourage people doing research on nursing to create formal models to marry their theories and their data. We hope you will practice what we preach. Meanwhile, you should be able to imagine parallels in nursing theory for all or most of the issues addressed in these examples. You might discuss among yourselves the possible nursing research designs that would be similar to these. Other questions that can guide your study of these examples include:

1　What constructs were involved in the theory that provoked the research?

2　Were appropriate criterion variates selected?

3　Were appropriate independent variates selected to specify each independent variable? Can you see any grounds on which to charge that a really important specification error invalidates the hypothesized causal model? How would you have improved the specification of the variables?

4　Were the subjects and settings adequate? Were there enough of them? Were they representative of situations and populations to which one might wish to generalize from the data?

5 Were there any surprises in the correlation matrix?

6 How successful was the factorial model in explaining the variances of the criteria?

7 How well did the model confirm the theory which inspired it?

8 Do the intercorrelations suggest to you that a different model should have been tried on the data? (You could use the MODEL program to do this.)

9 How should the research design be changed for replication studies?

You will find that we have not given as much information about some of these studies as you could wish, and you might even want to consult the original sources for some of them. You should also search the nursing research literature available to you for studies which might have profited from analysis by the FaM method. If you find any published correlation matrices you could attempt to reanalyze the data. You might achieve a publishable reanalysis. At any rate, you might inform the authors of this text of your efforts. We would be grateful, and might put your reanalysis in our next edition (the same goes for any original research of yours you share with us).

A MODEL FOR RN ATTAINMENT

The last section of Chapter 10 began the report of an original study of nursing career development which Lohnes and Pai prepared for this book. Please review that section. You will recall that among 1497 young women who were high school juniors in 1960 (and were a representative sample of that national cohort, thanks to Project TALENT's excellent design), only 147 had designated nursing as their career objective. This phase of the study focuses on those 147 women. Table 10-3 compared the 29 of them who actually attained registered nurse (RN) status by 1971 with the 118 who did not become RNs. Please review that table carefully. Most of the comparisons on 14 variates measured in 1960 and on 8 variates measured in 1971 favored the RNs over the non-RNs. Table 10-4 presented the intercorrelations among 15 selected variates for these 147 women, and is the basis for the model to be reported here.

We hypothesized that the criterion of attainment of a nursing career (versus failure to become a nurse) for the women who aspired to nursing in their adolescence would be caused, in part, by variance among them in 1960 on four causal constructs:

I   Verbal ability
II Reasoning ability
III Relevant interests
IV Status in home and school

The hypothesis was that those who had won their way through to nursing would have been superior on all four of these constructs, in adolescence, as a group, to those who did not succeed in becoming nurses.

Specification of research variables to represent the constructs was accomplished by means of subsets of 13 variates measured in 1960, as follows:

I Verbal ability specification
    1 Information test
    2 English test
    3 Reading test
II Reasoning ability specification
    4 Visualization test
    5 Abstract reasoning test
    6 Mathematics test
III Relevant interests specification
    7 Interest in biology and medicine
    8 Interest in social service
IV Status in home and school specification
    9 Certainty of occupational choice
    10 Socioeconomic status
    11 High school curriculum (1 = academic; 0 = other)
    12 High school grades
    13 Mother working?

The criterion domain was constituted by two variates measured in 1971:

    14 Job code nurse? the extra criterion
    15 Registered nurse? the key criterion

The correlation of .70 between these two criterion variates indicates that a number of women who were not RNs were employed as nurses in 1971, and a number of RNs were not so employed at that time.

The portions of key criterion variance accounted for by each factor in turn were:

Causal factor	RN? variance	Cumulative variance
I Verbal ability	.101	.101
II Reasoning ability	.029	.130
III Relevant interests	.024	.154
IV Status in home and school	.022	.176

From this table we see that the theory was not very successful, in that it accounted for barely 18 percent of the key criterion variance. Incidentally, the four factors accounted for only 10 percent of the variance in the other criterion, job code nurse? Our enthusiasm for these hypothesized factors as predictors of RN attainment among women who aspired to become nurses has to be dampened by these results. Even more upsetting to our theorizing is the relatively small contribution to explanation of criterion variance made by factors II, III, and IV. The only reasonably successful factor is I, verbal ability.

We would like to remind you that at the end of Chapter 10 we were able to answer the question, "How much of the key criterion variance is predictable from the combined action of the 13 predictor variates?" in a way which made no reference to a hypothesized causal model for the data. Please review that discussion. You will see that we found that .196 of the key criterion variance could be predicted from the joint action of the 13 independent variates, which is somewhat more than the .176 we now say is explained by the four factors of a causal model. The atheoretical method of analysis by which we did the work at the end of Chapter 10 was introduced in the last section of Chapter 9 under the title Multiple Correlations. If you take a statistics course sometime you will explore the method of multiple correlation at length, and will then learn that the $U = .196$ statistic we arrived at in Chapter 10 for these data is indeed known technically as a *squared multiple correlation coefficient*. This U is a statistic that can be shown by differential calculus to be the proportion of criterion variance accounted for by the best linear function of the predictors which can be obtained. We do *not* favor the use of the multiple correlation method in nursing research for two reasons: (1) we think that the differential calculus method usually overpowers the data available in nursing research, and (2) the multiple correlation method is atheoretical, in that it does not require the researcher to hypothesize any causal model for the phenomenon under study. As shown now by the comparison of the squared multiple correlation coefficient ($U = .196$) and the model communality for the key criterion ($h^2 = .176$), the calculus-based method

Table 12-1　A Model for RN Attainment (N = 147 TALENT Nursing Aspirants)

| Variates | Variables of model | | | | | |
	Verbal ability	Reasoning ability	Interest	Status	d	h^2
1 Information test	.954	−.007	.082	.002	.287	.917
2 English test	.659	−.090	−.058	−.020	.744	.447
3 Reading test	.936	.045	−.072	.006	.340	.884
4 Visualization test	.469	.191	.024	.073	.859	.262
5 Abstract reasoning test	.585	.753	−.028	.016	.299	.911
6 Mathematics test	.706	−.080	−.076	.028	.699	.512
7 Biology and medicine interest	.352	−.024	.902	.039	.245	.940
8 Social service interest	.219	−.034	.000	.152	.963	.072
9 Certainty of choice	−.077	−.085	−.314	−.736	.589	.653
10 Socioeconomic status	.430	.094	.101	.028	.892	.205
11 High school curriculum	.457	−.026	.145	.387	.787	.380
12 High school grades	.433	−.016	.092	.532	.722	.479
13 Mother working?	−.168	−.014	.102	.217	.956	.086
14 Job code nurse?	.239	.111	.123	.133	.948	.102
15 Registered nurse?	.317	.172	.156	.148	.908	.176

will always seem to produce a "better" finding than does the modeling method. We simply claim that while the calculus-based method is more powerful, the modeling method is more reasonable and informative. If you resist our advice, we have shown you in Chapter 10 how to force MODEL to produce a squared multiple correlation coefficient for you.

Table 12-1 reports the factor structure (correlations of variables with variates) and communalities (proportion of each variate's variance accounted for by the four factors). The only variates for which the model explains a majority of the variance are:

Variate	% s^2 explained
1 Information test	91.7
3 Reading test	88.4
5 Abstract reasoning test	91.1
6 Mathematics test	51.2
7 Interest in biology and medicine	94.0
9 Certainty of choice	65.3

These were the six "best" predictor variates, in the sense that they contributed most to the operational definition of the variables. The chief details of the model are depicted in Figure 12-1, which may or may not be more revealing than Table 12-1, depending on your taste for tables versus figures.

It is useful to check the factor structure for the extent to which the variates specifying each variable in the MODEL setup actually contributed to the operational definition of the variable. The three variates for the verbal factor all relate

Table 12-2   Percentage Changes in Criterion Scores Predicted for Unit Increase in Each Independent Variate Standard Score

1960 independent variates	Criteria	
	RN in 1971?	Employed as nurse in 1971?
1 Information test	7.4	5.5
2 English test	2.6	1.9
3 Reading test	6.4	4.7
4 Visualization test	−1.6	−1.0
5 Abstract reasoning test	21.7	13.8
6 Mathematics test	−8.3	−5.3
7 Interest in biology and medicine	11.6	8.4
8 Interest in social service	−2.9	−2.1
9 Certainty of choice	−10.1	−9.1
10 Socioeconomic status	1.2	1.1
11 High school curriculum	6.6	6.0
12 High school grades	8.0	7.2
13 Mother working	2.0	1.8

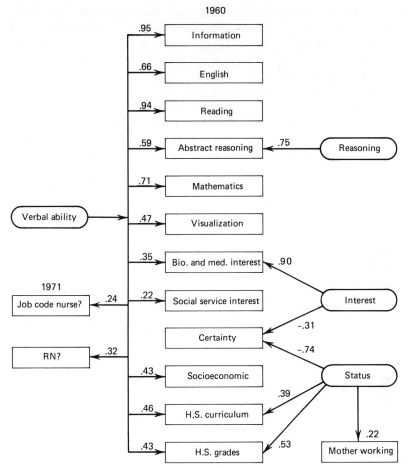

Figure 12-1 Diagram of model for the RN attainment study.

to the factor reasonably well. Two of the three variates for the reasoning factor, visualization and mathematics, do not relate to the factor they were supposed to specify. Mathematics even has a negative correlation with the factor. Clearly something was wrong with the thinking that led to this specification. The same is true with respect to the interest factor. It is very odd that the social service variate correlates exactly .000 with the factor. This should really shock the analysts out of any complacency they might feel about their capacity to hypothesize a suitable causal model for these data. (We were tempted to tinker with our hypotheses after seeing these results, to find a "better" picture to show you, but we resisted the temptation to cheat you of the opportunity to tinker with this problem yourself. You have the correlations and the MODEL program. See what you can do to find a better FaM solution.)

Table 12-2 shows the proportion of a standard deviation change in each criterion score which the model would predict for a full standard deviation increase in each independent variate score. It is clear that the model predicts the best payoff for manipulation of variate 5, abstract reasoning test. The second and third best variates for manipulation are indicated to be variate 7, interest in biology and medicine, and variate 9, certainty of choice. Ironically, the model asserts that activities which would decrease an adolescent girl's certainty that she wanted to be a nurse would probably increase her chances of becoming a nurse. If you see no sense in this, we remind you that correlational models only describe how things happened somewhere historically, and a large grain of common sense is required in the interpretation of their "predictions." It might be safer to interpret this model as telling us to choose a girl who is a good abstract reasoner, who is strongly interested in biology and medicine, and who, while aspiring to be a nurse, is not too certain of this aspiration, if we want to be somewhat confident that we have selected a girl who will become a nurse when she grows up. What do you think of this interpretation?

We note that you have every right to be puzzled and perturbed by the negative signs on variates 4, 6, 8, and 9 in Table 12-2, as these are contrary to reason in the light of the positive point-biserial correlations for these variates in Table 10-3. In the same light, why doesn't variate 13 have negative signs in Table 12-2? These strange results are examples of what statisticians call *suppression*, which is the tendency of predictors to combine in strange ways in poorly specified models. This analysis has tested our theoretical ideas and has found them wanting. That is an important contribution data analysis can make to a scientific enterprise.

CONTRIBUTING FACTORS IN MATHEMATICS LEARNING[1]

In 1960, Project TALENT administered an elaborate battery of mental tests to a national probability sample of hundreds of thousands of American high school students. Lohnes and Cooley (1968) published a small selection of test data for 505 students randomly selected from over 100,000 students who were tested by TALENT as seniors. Langley specified three factors, each indicated by two tests, which he thought might be "the specific factors underlying math ability," and computed factorial models separately for the 271 girls and 234 boys of the Lohnes and Cooley data set. The six independent variates employed by Langley, grouped according to the factors they provided indicators for, were:

g indicators

Information part I: a composite score based on 22 diverse information scales, including such subjects as physics, biology, aeronautics, electricity, farming, art, and law

Information part II: a composite score based on another 15 diverse information scales, including such subjects as military knowledge, accounting, Bible, colors, photography, games, hunting, and fishing

[1]This research was contributed by Dr. Russell Langley, Caulfield Institute of Technology, Victoria, Australia, to whom the authors are grateful.

Table 12-3   Correlations for the Mathematics Learning Study
(Data for 271 Girls above the Diagonal; Data for 234 Boys below the Diagonal)

Variates	1	2	3	4	5	6	7
1 Information part I	1.00	.840	.595	.439	.566	.710	.722
2 Information part II	.861	1.00	.533	.432	.549	.711	.584
3 Mechanical reasoning	.602	.504	1.00	.511	.335	.578	.535
4 Abstract reasoning	.544	.515	.537	1.00	.376	.545	.444
5 English composite	.634	.611	.336	.494	1.00	.534	.604
6 Reading comprehension	.752	.791	.443	.537	.605	1.00	.584
7 Mathematics composite	.777	.658	.513	.542	.679	.669	1.00

R indicators
Mechanical reasoning: the usual items involving pulleys, gears, etc.

Abstract reasoning: series extension items of the "What number comes next?" sort

V indicators
English: a composite score based on scales for spelling, capitalization, punctuation, word usage, and expression

Reading: a test of comprehension of printed paragraphs from a variety of literary, historical, practical, and technical sources

Table 12-4   Langley's Sex-replicated Factorial Models for 505 Subjects

	g_F	(g_M)	R_F	(R_M)	V_F	(V_M)	$h_F{}^2$	$(h_M{}^2)$	d_F	(d_M)
g indicators										
Information part I	.97	(.97)	.02	(.03)	.00	(−.01)	.94	(.94)	.25	(.24)
Information part II	.95	(.96)	−.02	(−.04)	.00	(.01)	.90	(.92)	.31	(.28)
R indicators										
Mechanical reasoning	.59	(.58)	.64	(.57)	−.07	(−.14)	.76	(.68)	.49	(.57)
Abstract reasoning	.45	(.55)	.75	(.75)	.07	(.09)	.77	(.88)	.48	(.35)
V indicators										
English composite	.58	(.65)	.08	(.10)	.81	(.73)	.99	(.97)	.09	(.18)
Reading comprehension	.74	(.80)	.25	(.08)	.17	(.24)	.64	(.70)	.60	(.55)
Key criterion										
Mathematics composite	.69	(.75)	.19	(.16)	.23	(.24)	.56	(.65)	.66	(.60)

Paired factor structures (spanning g_F through (V_M))

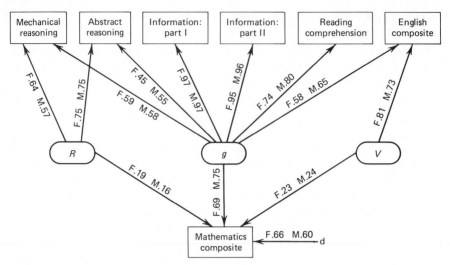

Figure 12-2 Diagram for Langley's sex-replicated models for TALENT subjects.

The key criterion was a mathematics composite score based on tests for the elements of the high school-college–preparatory mathematics curriculum which was more or less standard in 1960. Not all the 505 students were college-preparatory curriculum students, however. The tests, the subjects, and the full story of Project TALENT are documented in Lohnes (1966).

The correlations for both samples are presented in Table 12-3. The fact that all the correlations among the seven tests were positive suggested that a general intellectual development factor would be most useful. Note that the mathematics criterion correlated positively and relatively uniformly with all six predictors. The inspiration for Langley's hypothesized factors was the Vernon (1965) hierarchical model, which placed a g (for general intelligence) factor at the apex and two group factors at the base of a pyramid. One group factor was called k:m by Vernon, and was indicated by practical, mechanical, spatial, and physical knowledge tests. Langley's R factor corresponded to Vernon's k:m factor. Vernon called his other group factor v:ed, to which Langley's V factor corresponded. Vernon specified verbal, numerical, and educational tests as indicators of this group factor. It is important to realize that Vernon insisted that every mental test contributed to the g factor as well as to one of the two group factors.

Langley's computed models, as shown in Table 12-4 and Figure 12-2, were dominated by the g factor, which emerged as a general factor even though it was specified as a group factor. The real surprise in Langley's models was that the V factor was credited with more influence on the mathematics criterion than was the R factor, contrary to what one might have expected, and despite the circumstance that R was factored before V.

One reason the model did not account for more of the mathematics variance was that it did not specify a curriculum factor as a cause. Whatever their aptitudes, only the students who actually undertook preparatory mathematics courses had much opportunity to acquire the tested mathematics knowledge and skills.

The similarities of the models for the two sexes greatly outweighed the differences, suggesting that the same structural model of aptitudes for mathematics learning could be applied to adolescents of both sexes in America in 1960.

STABILITY OF ALIENATION

Using data borrowed from Wheaton et al. (1977), the *LISREL IV User's Guide* (Jöreskog and Sörbom, 1978, pp. 22–30) provided a model for repeated measurements (in 1967 and 1971) on two indicators of alienation. Besides the repeated measurements on the two indicators, called anomia and powerlessness, the 932 subjects from rural Illinois were also measured on two indicators of socioeconomic status (SES), namely Duncan's SEI and education. On the assumption of correlated errors between like forms of the alienation indicators on the two occasions, a model in terms of three disattenuated and correlated factors for the covariances showed a path coefficient of $-.58$ from SES to 1967 alienation,

Table 12-5   Factorial Model for Stability of Alienation

	Correlations					
	X_1	X_2	X_3	X_4	X_5	X_6
X_1 = education	1.000					
X_2 = SEI	.540	1.000				
X_3 = 1967 anomia	−.360	−.300	1.000			
X_4 = 1967 powerlessness	−.410	−.290	.660	1.000		
X_5 = 1971 anomia	−.350	−.290	.560	.470	1.000	
X_6 = 1971 powerlessness	−.370	−.280	.440	.520	.670	1.000

Model				
	Structure			
Variate	SES	Alienation	d	h^2
X_1	.911	−.034	.411	.831
X_2	.839	.045	.543	.706
X_3	−.380	.805	.455	.793
X_4	−.407	.836	.369	.864
X_5	−.368	.444	.817	.332
X_6	−.376	.408	.832	.308

Predicted changes in criteria (rows) for unit changes in predictors (columns)			
	X_1	X_2	X_3	X_4
---	---	---	---	---
X_5	−.076	−.054	.203	.212
X_6	−.092	−.070	.185	.193

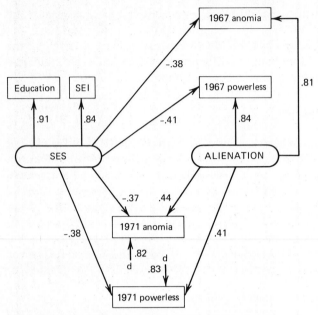

Figure 12-3 Diagram of model for stability of alienation.

and path coefficients of .61 from 1967 alienation to 1971 alienation and of $-.23$ from SES to 1971 alienation. The authors offered no interpretation of the model, but it would seem to suggest that alienation was moderately stable over the 4-year period and that alienation was moderately influenced by SES in 1967, but only modestly influenced by SES in 1971. The change in influence of SES on alienation is a puzzle.

A FaM model for the data in terms of two real (i.e., error-incorporating) and uncorrelated factors for the correlations (rather than the covariances) is presented in Table 12-5 and Figure 12-3. This model suggests that the SES factor and the 1967 alienation factor had modest and similar influence on the 1971 anomia

Table 12-6   Correlations for Peer Influence on Aspirations (N = 329)

Variate	2	3	4	5	6	7	8	9	10
1 Subject's parental aspiration	.049	.184	.115	.019	.078	.214	.274	.112	.084
2 Subject's socioeconomic status	1.000	.222	.093	.271	.230	.324	.405	.305	.279
3 Subject's intelligence		1.000	.102	.186	.336	.411	.404	.290	.260
4 Best friend's parental aspiration			1.000	−.044	.209	.076	.070	.278	.199
5 Best friend's socioeconomic status				1.000	.295	.293	.241	.411	.361
6 Best friend's intelligence					1.000	.300	.286	.519	.501
7 Subject's occupational aspiration						1.000	.625	.327	.422
8 Subject's educational aspiration							1.000	.367	.327
9 Best friend's occupational aspiration								1.000	.640
10 Best friend's educational aspiration									1.000

and powerlessness performances. It also suggests that SES had essentially the same modest influence on the 1967 and 1971 alienation indicators, thus avoiding the puzzle posed by the LISREL model. The $R^2 = U$ values for the multiple regressions of the two 1971 indicators on the four 1967 predictors are .352 and .314, which can be compared to the FaM communalities of .332 and .308.

PEER INFLUENCE ON ASPIRATION

The *LISREL IV Users' Guide* (Jöreskog and Sörbom, 1978) offers a reanalysis of data on family and peer influences on aspirations, originally reported by Duncan et al. (1968). These correlational data, reported in Table 12-6, have been re-analyzed once again by means of factorial modeling. For the present analysis, two factors were hypothesized to account for the variances in the four aspiration variates. The factors and their specifying variates were:

I Family and self
   1   Subject's parental aspiration
   2   Subject's socioeconomic status
   3   Subject's intelligence
II Peer
   4   Best friend's parental aspiration
   5   Best friend's socioeconomic status
   6   Best friend's intelligence

The four criteria were:

   7   Subject's occupational aspiration
   8   Subject's educational aspiration
   9   Best friend's occupational aspiration
   10   Best friend's educational aspiration

Table 12-7   Factorial Model for Peer Influence on Aspiration

	Variables			
Variate	Family and self	Peer	d	h^2
1 Subject's parental aspiration	.329	−.048	.943	.111
2 Subject's socioeconomic status	.772	−.012	.636	.596
3 Subject's intelligence	.764	.029	.645	.584
4 Best friend's parental aspiration	.141	.364	.921	.152
5 Best friend's socioeconomic status	.284	.593	.754	.432
6 Best friend's intelligence	.358	.792	.494	.756
7 Subject's occupational aspiration	.487	.175	.856	.268
8 Subject's educational aspiration	.546	.109	.831	.310
9 Best friend's occupational aspiration	.385	.504	.773	.402
10 Best friend's educational aspiration	.345	.460	.818	.330

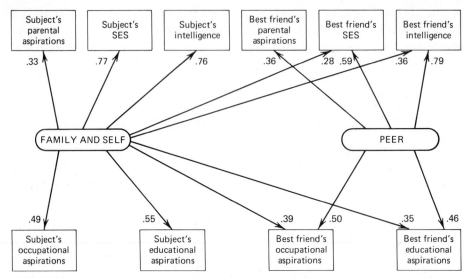

Figure 12-4   Diagram of model for peer influence on aspirations.

A special feature of the setup for computing a model for the data was that the educational aspirations of the 329 best friends (one for each subject) was the variate designated as the key criterion, even though the research hypothesis was focused on the explanation of variances in the two subject's aspirations variates. It was thought that this choice of a key criterion would prevent capitalization on chance in the extraction of the first factor, family and self, and thus lead to conservative estimates of the influence of that causal variable on the two subject's aspirations variates.

Table 12-7 reports the resulting factorial model, and Figure 12-4 depicts it. The family and self variable accounted for 23.7 percent of the variance in subject's occupational aspiration, and the peer variable accounted for only another 3.1 percent of that variance. The family and self variable accounted for 29.8 percent of the variance in subject's educational aspiration, and the peer variable accounted for only another 1.2 percent of that variance. Thus the model contradicted the hypothesis of strong peer influence on aspirations. (However, the model showed stronger influence of the subject's family and self variable on the best friend's aspirations. How do you interpret this result?)

Q: Modify the model by including variates 9 and 10 in the specification of the peer variable, and using only variates 7 and 8 as criteria. Report your results, comparing them with ours.

A MODEL FOR WELL-BEING[2]

The data for this study of variables which may be contributing causes to a young adult's sense of well-being were drawn from a survey conducted in July and

[2]This research was conceived, conducted, and written by Mary Jane Salmon, to whom we are grateful for permission to publish it.

August of 1971 by A. Campbell, P. E. Converse, and W. L. Rodgers of the Institute for Social Research. The data were distributed by the social science archive of the University of Michigan. Of the 2164 persons interviewed in this massive nationwide probability sample designed to provide information about perceptions of the quality of American life, 216 were between the ages of 18 and 22, and these 216 subjects were the source of the correlation matrix for this modeling study.

Five factors were hypothesized to have exerted causal influence on the distribution of reports of well-being from these young adults. The five factors and their specification variates were:

I Personal efficacy
   1 Confidence in life working out (CONFID)
   2 Frightened or worried about anything (WORRY)
   3 Plan life or leave to luck (PLAN-LUCK)
   4 Able to carry out plans (CARRYOUT)
   5 Capable of running own life (RUNLIFE)
   6 Worry about a nervous breakdown (NERVOUS)
   7 Satisfy ambitions (AMBITIONS)
   8 Fair opportunity to make most of self (OPPORTUN)
II Friends
   9 How many good friends (GOODFREND)
   10 Interest in meeting new friends (NEWFREND)
   11 Satisfaction with friendships (SATFREND)
III Leisure
   12 Types of hobbies (HOBBY)
   13 Leisure activities (ACTIVITY)
   14 Satisfaction with spare time (SPARETIME)
IV Health
   15 Health problems (HEALTHPR)
   16 Summary of health problems and restrictions (SUMHEALTH)
   17 Satisfaction with health (SATHEALTH)
V Family
   18 Closer to parents than most (CLOSPAR)
   19 Closer to siblings than most (CLOSSIB)

The key (and sole) criterion for the analysis was an index of well-being created by the original investigators (Campbell et al., 1975) as the average of the subject's responses to two items:

   20 Key criterion: index of well-being, based on:
      A How satisfied are you with your life as a whole?
      B How do you feel about your present life?
         a interesting—boring
         b enjoyable—miserable
         c worthwhile—useless
         d friendly—lonely
         e full—empty

Table 12-8 Correlations for the Well-being Study (N = 216)

Variate	1	2	3	4	5	6	7	8	9	10	11	12	13	14	15	16	17	18	19	20
1 CONFID	1.00																			
2 WORRY	-.23	1.00																		
3 PLAN-LUCK	.12	-.02	1.00																	
4 CARRYOUT	.11	.01	.20	1.00																
5 RUNLIFE	.20	-.16	.08	.10	1.00															
6 NERVOUS	-.09	.08	.04	-.04	-.18	1.00														
7 AMBITIONS	.17	-.08	.11	.21	.06	-.13	1.00													
8 OPPORTUN	.19	-.06	.03	.10	-.01	-.18	.29	1.00												
9 GOODFREND	.04	-.04	.03	.09	.06	-.17	.19	.18	1.00											
10 NEWFREND	-.04	-.02	-.11	-.14	.14	.05	-.07	-.03	.24	1.00										
11 SATFREND	.06	-.11	.01	.09	.01	-.15	.14	.21	.45	.21	1.00									
12 HOBBY	-.08	-.05	-.10	-.22	-.12	.03	-.16	.03	-.03	-.18	-.02	1.00								
13 ACTIVITY	-.09	-.06	-.09	-.24	-.16	.03	-.18	.02	-.07	-.18	-.08	.85	1.00							
14 SPARETIME	.14	-.16	-.03	.16	.07	-.17	.20	.16	.17	-.01	.23	-.07	-.10	1.00						
15 HEALTHPR	-.15	.04	-.07	-.14	.06	.08	-.14	-.12	-.05	.08	.06	-.10	-.16	-.01	1.00					
16 SUMHEALTH	-.13	.03	-.06	-.13	.03	.07	-.12	-.08	-.03	.04	.04	-.07	-.13	-.02	.96	1.00				
17 SATHEALTH	.05	-.07	.04	.04	-.14	-.02	.00	-.03	.05	.00	.14	.00	-.01	.11	-.27	-.29	1.00			
18 CLOSPAR	-.01	-.04	.00	-.02	.19	.05	.03	-.02	.09	.03	-.03	-.13	-.05	.12	.08	.08	-.06	1.00		
19 CLOSSIB	.01	-.09	.05	-.01	.02	.04	-.11	.00	-.16	-.31	-.10	.09	.13	.06	-.01	-.01	-.03	.10	1.00	
20 WELLBEING	.10	-.08	.07	.16	.08	-.06	.18	.11	.05	-.19	.10	-.01	-.03	.38	.10	.10	-.07	.18	.15	1.00

Table 12-9 Factorial Model for Study of Well-being

| | Variables | | | | | | |
Variate	Personal efficacy	Friends	Leisure	Health	Family	d	h²
1 CONFID	.52	−.02	−.01	−.06	−.01	.85	.27
2 WORRY	−.34	.04	−.06	.00	−.08	.94	.13
3 PLAN-LUCK	.33	.07	−.13	−.02	.03	.93	.13
4 CARRYOUT	.57	.08	.00	−.04	−.04	.82	.33
5 RUNLIFE	.37	−.20	−.03	.15	.17	.88	.23
6 NERVOUS	−.32	−.05	−.08	.02	.08	.94	.12
7 AMBITIONS	.68	.00	.00	.00	−.05	.73	.47
8 OPPORTUN	.52	.01	.02	.01	−.02	.86	.27
9 GOODFREND	.22	−.17	.12	−.02	.00	.95	.09
10 NEWFREND	−.09	−.96	.05	.01	−.03	.27	.93
11 SATFREND	.21	.04	.18	.03	−.11	.96	.09
12 HOBBY	−.20	.21	−.04	−.10	−.06	.95	.10
13 ACTIVITY	−.22	.19	−.06	−.15	.03	.94	.11
14 SPARETIME	.28	.03	.96	.00	.00	.02	1.00
15 HEALTHPR	−.20	−.03	.05	.91	−.02	.37	.86
16 SUMHEALTH	−.17	.00	.03	.92	−.01	.36	.87
17 SATHEALTH	.01	.03	.11	−.60	−.03	.79	.38
18 CLOSPAR	.03	−.05	.12	.09	.85	.50	.75
19 CLOSSIB	−.02	.30	.06	.01	.57	.77	.41
20 WELLBEING	.24	.18	.32	.16	.15	.87	.24

> **f** hopeful—discouraging
> **g** rewarding—disappointing
> **h** brings out the best in me—doesn't give me a chance

Table 12-8 reports the correlations for the 20 variates. Table 12-9 and Figure 12-5 report the factorial model for those correlations. The five factors accounted for 24 percent of the variance in the criterion of sense of well-being, which leaves a great deal of variance unaccounted for. Leisure and personal efficacy were shown to be the two factors with the greatest apparent influence on sense of well-being, with friends, health, and family following in that order. Overall, the specifications for the variables seemed to be successful for personal efficacy, health, and family, and less successful but not disastrous for friends and leisure. Figure 12-5 has been drawn to highlight the most salient variates in the specification of each variable.

A CONFIRMATORY FACTOR ANALYSIS

Using data borrowed from Holzinger and Swineford (1939), the *LISREL IV Users' Guide* (Jöreskog and Sörbom, 1978, pp. 39–42) tested a model involving three cognitive ability factors specified by two tests each as the explanation of three additional cognitive tests. The hypothesis was that each of the three criterion tests would be explained by one, only one, and a different one of the

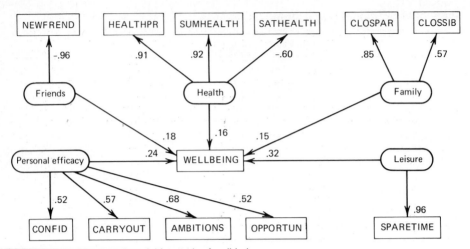

Figure 12-5 Diagram of model for study of well-being.

Table 12-10 Factorial Model for a Confirmatory Factor Analysis

(a) Correlations

	X_1	X_2	X_3	X_4	X_5	X_6	X_7	X_8	X_9
X_1 = visual perception	1.000	.417	.160	.195	.168	.248	.326	.228	.066
X_2 = cubes		1.000	.287	.347	.239	.373	.449	.328	.075
X_3 = paragraph comprehension			1.000	.685	.198	.356	.309	.719	.254
X_4 = sentence completion				1.000	.121	.272	.317	.715	.179
X_5 = addition					1.000	.528	.308	.104	.587
X_6 = counting dots						1.000	.487	.314	.418
X_7 = lozenges							1.000	.342	.104
X_8 = word meaning								1.000	.209
X_9 = straight-curved capitals									1.000

(b) Factorial model

Variate	Structure			d	h^2
	VIS	VKN	PSA		
X_1	.82	−.08	−.04	.57	.68
X_2	.86	.07	.03	.50	.75
X_3	.27	.91	.04	.31	.91
X_4	.33	.82	−.06	.47	.78
X_5	.24	.11	.90	.35	.88
X_6	.37	.24	.68	.58	.67
X_7	.47	.20	.25	.82	.32
X_8	.33	.71	−.04	.62	.62
X_9	.08	.23	.57	.79	.38

Table 12-10 Factorial Model for a Confirmatory Factor Analysis (continued)

				(c) Factor scoring coefficients					
Factor	X_1	X_2	X_3	X_4	X_5	X_6	X_7	X_8	X_9
Visual reasoning (VIS)	.556	.631	0	0	0	0	0	0	0
Verbal knowledge (VKN)	−.186	−.212	.691	.453	0	0	0	0	0
Perceptual speed (PSA) and accuracy	−.163	−.185	−.136	−.089	.761	.465	0	0	0

three factors. The correlation matrix for the nine measurements based on 145 subjects is given in Table 12-10(a). A factorial model for the nine measurements as given in Table 12-10(b) seems to confirm the hypothesis in a loose sort of way. The one obvious contradiction is that the second criterion test, word meaning, has a modest loading of .33 on the first factor, whereas it is supposed to load only on the second factor. Perhaps the more serious difficulty is that the communalities (h^2) for two of the three criterion tests are very low, suggesting that there may be a need for some other explanation of their variances. Table 12-10(c) reports the factor scoring coefficients for the three uncorrelated factors. Note the pattern in these coefficients. Each factor has substantial coefficients for the two tests which specified it, but in order to be uncorrelated with the first factor, the second factor also has to have nonzero coefficients for the two variates which specified the first factor. In order to be uncorrelated with the first and second factors, the third factor must have nonzero coefficients for the two variates which specified the first factor and the two variates which specified the second factor.

Figure 12-6 is a path diagram of the model, with structural coefficients smaller than .31 in absolute value omitted (since the deleted paths would explain less than 10 percent of the variance in a variate). In this cleaned-up presentation, the model seems to confirm the hypothesis fairly well.

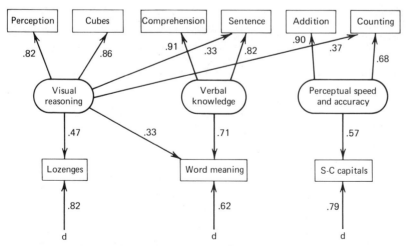

Figure 12-6 Diagram of model for the confirmatory factor analysis.

PERSISTENCE IN ADULT BASIC EDUCATION[3]

This report is an analysis of data collected as part of an adult basic education–problem-solving project funded by the New York State Education Department, Bureau of Special Continuing Education, and conducted at the research and development complex, State University of New York at Buffalo. The data were collected from 30 participants in an adult basic education program in a western New York city. The project ran from February through May 1978. A problem-solving pretest was administered to the subjects in February, after which they received 12 weeks of instruction in a problem-solving model, and were then posttested with an alternate form of the problem-solving test. Demographic information was taken from data sheets completed by the students. Reading level was obtained from student records and had been collected by means of the California Achievement Test. The criterion variate, persistence, was created as a dichotomous variate reflecting whether or not the student was still enrolled and attending adult basic education classes when a follow-up visit was made to the site in October, 5 months after the project ended.

Three factors were hypothesized to have exerted causal influence on the variance in the persistence criterion. These factors and their specifying variates were:

 I Aptitude
    1   Reading level
    2   Problem-solving pretest
 II Status
    3   Sex (female = 0, male = 1)
    4   Race (black = 0, white = 1)
    5   Age (in years)
    6   Marital status (married = 0, single = 1)
    7   Children (no = 0, yes = 1)
    8   Employed (no = 0, yes = 1)
 III Schooling
    9   Previous schooling (years of school completed in the traditional sequence)
    10 Time in program (years, or fractions thereof, in adult basic education classes)
Criteria
    11 Problem-solving posttest (extra criterion)
    12 Persistence (not enrolled in October 1978 = 0; enrolled in October 1978 = 1) (key criterion)

Table 12-11 reports the correlations for the 12 variates. Table 12-12 and Figure 12-7 present the FaM solution for the correlations. The three hypothesized causes accounted for 17.3 percent of the variance in the key criterion of persistence in adult basic education classes. Status was the useful cause, contribut-

[3]This study was planned, conducted, and reported by Doreen Reed Chassin, to whom the authors are grateful for permission to publish it.

Table 12-11 Correlations for Persistence in Adult Basic Education

Variates	1	2	3	4	5	6	7	8	9	10	11	12
1 Reading	1.00											
2 Problem pretest	-.006	1.00										
3 Sex (f = 0)	.123	.361	1.00									
4 Race (b = 0)	-.217	-.083	-.117	1.00								
5 Age	-.067	-.001	-.128	.208	1.00							
6 Marital (m = 0)	-.092	.116	.154	-.378	-.231	1.00						
7 Children (no = 0)	.126	.092	-.106	-.203	.574	-.489	1.00					
8 Employed (no = 0)	.291	-.059	.347	-.203	.267	.098	.139	1.00				
9 Schooling	.199	.077	-.152	-.372	-.702	.394	-.404	-.182	1.00			
10 Years in ABE	-.227	-.295	-.052	.256	.359	-.147	-.049	-.022	-.301	1.00		
11 Problem posttest	-.112	.463	.251	-.129	.063	.121	.187	-.136	-.081	.045	1.00	
12 Persistence	-.040	-.153	.089	.055	.149	.144	.085	-.056	-.153	.180	.257	1.00

Table 12-12   Factorial Model for Persistence in Adult Education

| | Factor structure | | | | |
Variates	Aptitude	Status	Schooling	Communality	Disturbance
1 Reading level	.245	−.154	.021	.084	.957
2 Problem-solving pretest	.968	.040	−.005	.939	.248
3 Sex	.381	.414	.006	.317	.837
4 Race	−.135	−.061	−.262	.091	.954
5 Age	−.018	.643	−.252	.478	.723
6 Marital status	.089	.323	.461	.325	.822
7 Children	.121	.318	−.326	.222	.882
8 Employed	.016	.263	−.103	.080	.959
9 Previous schooling	.124	−.522	.669	.736	.514
10 Time in program	−.343	.232	.416	.345	.810
11 Problem-solving posttest	.421	.252	.087	.248	.867
12 Persistence	−.159	.373	.093	.173	.909

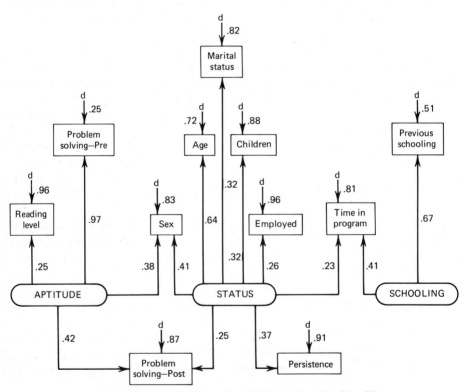

Figure 12-7   Diagram of model for persistence in adult basic education ($N = 30$).

ing 13.9 percent of persistence variance. The model accounted for 24.8 percent of the variance in the other criterion, the problem-solving posttest, with aptitude and status doing the work. As the large disturbances indicate, much of the variance in the measurement system is not accounted for by the model. Rather than looking for policy implications in this model, the results suggest that researchers should look beyond traditional variables and variates in the search for fruitful theoretical propositions about adult basic education.

EVALUATION OF A HEAD START SUMMER PROGRAM

Magidson (1977) critiqued a published analysis (Barnow, 1973) of data on 303 white 6-year-old first graders who were subjects in an evaluation of a Head Start summer program. Of this sample, 148 children had attended Head Start and 155 were "control" children. Head Start was a federally funded intervention intended to help disadvantaged children overcome their educational deficits. The control children were supposed to be similarly disadvantaged, but as often happens in such studies, they were in fact somewhat more advantaged than the treated children. Barnow had used a method called analysis of covariance to attempt a statistical equating of the two groups, in order to make a fair test of the effectiveness of the summer Head Start program possible. The covariance method has been the most popular data analysis procedure for studies which compare treatment programs with each other or with a control group, although we do not advocate its use. Barnow's covariance analysis led him to conclude that the impact of the program was slightly negative, which was devastating news for the federal sponsors of Head Start. Magidson believed that Barnow's choice of data analysis procedure was incorrect and had led to an incorrect evaluation of the intervention program.

Magidson applied a method called LISREL, named by its inventors (Jöreskog and van Thillo, 1973), in a reanalysis which suggested a slightly positive impact for the program. If correct, Magidson's conclusion would be far more sanguine and welcome news to the federal sponsor (who must now wish Magidson had been the evaluator of choice in the first instance). We do not recommend LISREL as a data analysis procedure, either, and we believe that Barnow's slightly negative evaluation is more reasonable. We will show that our FaM procedure yields almost exactly the same estimate of the program effect as Barnow's covariance analysis, and will say why we distrust Magidson's LISREL report.

The data available on the 303 children consisted of four variates which were indicators of a socioeconomic status factor (SES):

X_1 = mother's education
X_2 = father's education
X_3 = father's occupation
X_4 = family income

Table 12-13   Factorial Model for Head Start Summer Program

(a) Correlations

	X_1	X_2	X_3	X_4	X_5	X_6	X_7
X_1 = mother's education	1.000						
X_2 = father's education	.468	1.000					
X_3 = father's occupation	.241	.285	1.000				
X_4 = family income	.297	.209	.407	1.000			
X_5 = treatment	−.118	−.084	−.220	−.179	1.000		
X_6 = ITPA posttest	.259	.246	.217	.116	−.097	1.000	
X_7 = MRT posttest	.275	.215	.255	.190	−.094	.652	1.000

(b) Model

Variate	Structure		d	h^2
	SES	Treatment		
X_1	.752	.044	.658	.567
X_2	.695	.066	.716	.487
X_3	.701	−.072	.710	.496
X_4	.640	−.043	.767	.412
X_5	−.214	.977	.000	1.000
X_6	.307	−.032	.951	.095
X_7	.340	−.022	.940	.116

(c) Predicted changes in criteria (rows) for unit changes in predictors (columns)

	X_1	X_2	X_3	X_4	X_5
X_6	.105	.097	.098	.089	−.031
X_7	.117	.109	.108	.099	−.020

plus the dummy variate for treatment group:

$X_5 = 1$ if in Head Start group ($X_5 = 0$ if in control group)

and two posttests as criteria:

X_6 = Illinois Test of Psycholinguistic Abilities (ITPA)
X_7 = Metropolitan Readiness Test (MRT)

Table 12-13(a) contains the correlations. Notice that treatment correlated negatively with everything else, indicating that the treated group was disadvantaged in SES and did less well on the posttests than the control group. However, the average correlation of treatment with the four SES indicators was − .150, while the average correlation of treatment with the two criterion tests was − .096, a comparison which suggests that the treated group suffered less by comparison with the control group on the posttests than it did on the SES indicators. Without any model for the data, the program sponsors might well have been satisfied with this comparison, since it seems to show that the program closed the gap between the groups somewhat although not completely. No model for these data can possibly support an evaluation of the intervention program because of the fatal specification error represented by the absence of pretests of cognitive abilities. This statement about the simple correlations is no more naïve than an interpretation of any model for these data as an evaluation.

Magidson's LISREL computations provided him with separate models for the two criteria. He made some rather elaborate assumptions about correlated and uncorrelated error portions of the SES indicators and fitted a disattenuated (i.e., corrected for unreliability) causal factor to the SES domain. We object to this manipulation because we believe it introduced a variable which had no operational definition (i.e., which was unscorable on the data). Be that as it may, Magidson then allowed his treatment variable to be simply the dummy variate for treatment, with the result (disastrous from our viewpoint) that his two causal variables emerged correlated with each other. In his model for the ITPA posttest, the SES factor correlated $-.39$ with the treatment factor, and in the model for the MRT posttest the correlation was $-.41$. His estimated structural equations for the two posttests were

$$\text{ITPA} = .56 \text{ SES} + .12 \text{ TREATMENT} + d_{\text{ITPA}}$$
$$\text{MRT} = .57 \text{ SES} + .14 \text{ TREATMENT} + d_{\text{MRT}}$$
(all measures standardized)

All we can say is that models which deal in correlated causes do not attribute variance unambiguously. The partition of criterion variance which the LISREL models made available followed the rule for a squared multiple correlation based on two predictors:

$$\rho_{XS,T}^2 = \beta_S^2 + \beta_T^2 + 2\beta_S\beta_T\rho_{ST}$$

Magidson's numbers were

for ITPA: $.28 = (.56)^2 + (.12)^2 + 2(.56)\,(.12)\,(-.39)$
$= .3136 + .0144 - .0524$

for MRT: $.28 = (.57)^2 + (.14)^2 + 2(.57)\,(.14)\,(-.41)$
$= .3249 + .0196 - .0654$

Thus Magidson's models accounted for about 28 percent of the variance in each of the criteria, and this was partitioned so that about 31 percent was contributed by the SES factor, about 2 percent by the treatment variate, and about 6 percent by the joint action or the confounding of the correlated SES factor and treatment variate.

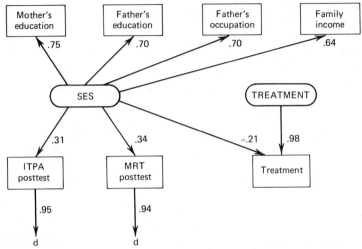

Figure 12-8 Diagram of model for the Head Start summer study.

The FaM solution is shown by Table 12-13(b) and Figure 12-8. The best interpretation of it is that differences among the 303 children in family SES caused about 10 percent of the variance in posttest scores on both tests, and that whether or not a child participated in the summer Head Start program had no influence on the criterion variance. The predicted changes in criteria for unit changes in a particular manipulatable variate supply the interesting suggestion that mother's education would be the policy variate of choice.

Incidentally, Barnow's covariance analysis reported − .04 as the correlation between treatment and SES-adjusted ITPA, which compares with the FaM loading of − .03, and he gave − .02 for treatment and SES-adjusted MRT, which is the same as the FaM loading of − .02. For these data, the FaM has accounted for almost the same amounts of criterion variance as does multiple regression, and in about the same partitions as created by covariance. The R^2 for ITPA regressed on the five predictors is .107, whereas the FaM h^2 for ITPA is .095. The R^2 for MRT is .120, and the FaM h^2 is .116. Without using differential calculus, FaM has pretty much found the multiple regressions. Magidson's larger ρ^2s are theoretical, not descriptive, and we do not trust them.

Magidson concluded that the summer Head Start program made a modest positive contribution toward remediation of the cognitive deficits of its clients. Barnow's covariance analysis and our FaM suggest that the program cannot be shown to have been effective on the basis of these data. Once again, we urge that the biggest flaw of the study is the lack of pretests of cognitive abilities.

SEX AS A DETERMINANT OF LEADERSHIP STYLE[4]

This study investigated the effectiveness of four theoretical constructs—personal identity, career pattern, sex, and school setting—on the administrative

[4]The authors are grateful to Dr. Nancy S. Miller for permission to publish this brief skim of results from her excellent dissertation, submitted to SUNY at Buffalo in May 1979.

Table 12-14   Factorial Model for Leadership Characteristics

	Variables				
Variates	Personal identity	Career pattern	Sex	School setting	h^2
Personal identity					
Age	.21	−.34	.28	.13	.25
Race	.36	.05	−.29	.02	.22
Marital status	−.24	−.11	−.36	.00	.16
No./dependents	−.20	−.08	−.56	.06	.36
Birth order					
Oldest	−.64	.07	.10	−.06	.42
Youngest	.52	−.10	.05	−.07	.28
Only	−.42	−.06	−.01	.10	.19
Middle	.52	.07	−.15	.05	.30
Career pattern					
Years/teaching	.08	.37	.29	.06	.23
Years/administration	.14	−.69	.01	.03	.49
Years/current post	.05	−.55	−.04	.08	.30
Education	.02	−.64	.04	−.03	.42
Commitment	−.14	.41	−.11	−.01	.20
Sex	.21	.25	.95	.00	1.00
School setting					
Percent/white students	.04	−.08	−.08	.29	.10
Percent/black students	−.04	.09	.06	−.24	.07
Percent free/red. lunches	.08	−.28	.01	.20	.12
School location	.08	−.04	.08	−.42	.19
School size	−.09	−.11	−.01	−.69	.50
No./teachers	−.12	−.07	−.01	−.73	.55
Percent/female teachers	.09	−.07	.05	.45	.22
Criterion					
Partic. Dec.-Mk (ideal)	−.02	.11	.03	.02	.01
Partic. Dec.-Mk (actual)	−.11	−.05	.17	−.11	.06
Conflict reconciliation	−.01	−.05	.00	−.03	.00
LPC	.14	.09	.00	.23	.08

leadership style of school principals. The primary interest was in obtaining a test of the hypothesis that sex of administrator had a great deal to do with the variance among administrators in leadership style, and this hypothesis was disconfirmed by the data analysis.

The data were collected from 185 principals by means of a mailed questionnaire. The specification variates for each of the variables are identified in Table 12-14, which also lists the four leadership style criterion variates and reports the FaM achieved. Figure 12-9 diagrams only the relations between the four causal variables and the four criterion variates, in order to dramatize (1) the overall weakness of the model and (2) the failure of the sex variable to explain any appreciable variance in the leadership style variates. It is probably reassuring rather than distressing to have this evidence of lack of sex linkage to leadership

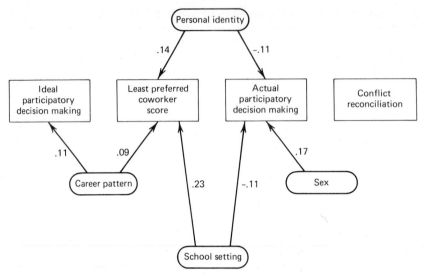

Figure 12-9   Diagram of model for leadership characteristics.

style. Here is a case where a model for research data challenges the ethos of the times.

A special feature of the factorial model reported in Table 12-14 is the communality of 1.00 for the sex variate. This is an unusual but legitimate case in which a variable had to be specified by a single variate, thus guaranteeing that variate an $h^2 = 1.00$ value. Note, however, that a small part of the sex variate variance was extracted by the two factors, personal identity and career pattern, which were extracted before sex was factored.

QUALITY OF NURSING CARE[5]

In the course of a major research project carried out in a Veterans Administration Medical Center, Ventura and Hageman (1978) collected data from 209 patients by means of the QPACS (Quality of Patient Care Scale) battery of six tests (Wandelt and Ager, 1974). The vendors of QPACS provide a total score for the battery which is a linear function of the six scale scores. This total score was used as the key criterion for a MODEL run designed to test the proposition that two uncorrelated factors would provide a suitable scoring scheme to replace the six scale scores in the research program. It was hypothesized that a general nursing care factor could be specified by three QPACS variates:

1   Psychosocial: individual
2   Psychosocial: group
3   Communication

[5] Richard N. Fox created this analysis using data provided by Dr. Marlene R. Ventura. We are grateful to them for permitting us to use it.

Table 12-15   Correlations and Factorial Model for QPACS (N = 209)

				Correlations			
Variates	1	2	3	4	5	6	7
1 Psychosocial: individual	1.00	.54	.39	.59	.71	.62	.86
2 Psychosocial: group		1.00	.14	.38	.52	.39	.60
3 Communication			1.00	.35	.42	.55	.57
4 Physical				1.00	.63	.64	.77
5 General					1.00	.68	.88
6 Professional implications						1.00	.82
7 Total score							1.00

	Factorial model			
	Structure			
QPACS variates	General N.C.	Physical N.C.	d	h^2
1 Psychosocial: individual	.90	.06	.44	.81
2 Psychosocial: group	.73	−.11	.68	.54
3 Communication	.63	.02	.78	.40
4 Physical	.60	.65	.47	.78
5 General	.74	.48	.47	.78
6 Professional implications	.69	.54	.49	.76
7 Vendor's total score	.91	.38	.18	.97

Factor scoring coefficients (apply to z scores for six QPACS scales)

	X_1	X_2	X_3	X_4	X_5	X_6
I General nursing care	.548	.383	.363	0	0	0
II Physical nursing care	−.658	−.459	−.436	.647	.587	.550

and a physical nursing care factor could be specified by the remaining three QPACS variates:

  4 Physical
  5 General
  6 Professional implications

These two factors were expected to extract and utilize more of the measurement variance collected by the six QPACS scales than that extracted by the vendor's total score.

  Table 12-15 reports the correlation matrix and the resulting FaM, and Figure 12-10 depicts the model. The first factor did turn out to be a general one, in that all six QPACS scales were substantially involved in it. This general factor extracted 52.1 percent of the battery variance, which can be compared to the 57.7 percent of battery variance extracted by the vendor's total score for these subjects. The

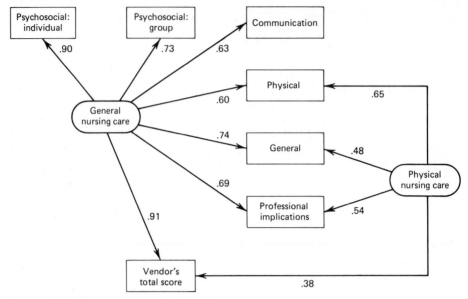

Figure 12-10   Diagram of model for QPACS.

new general nursing care factor correlated .91 with the vendor's total score, which suggests that the two variables are very similar.

The new second factor extracted an additional 16.0 percent of the battery variance, so that the two new factors together utilized 68.1 percent of the battery variance. This is significantly more than the 57.7 percent utilized by the vendor's total score. This physical nursing care factor (which is quite arbitrarily named, as factors always are) involved only the three scales by which it was specified, and appeared to be a potentially useful second variable based on the QPACS scales.

The conclusions drawn from this analysis were that a reduction in the number of variables to represent the QPACS variance was feasible, and that the two variables of the FaM solution might be a superior reduction to the vendor's total score.

Incidentally, whenever all the intercorrelations among the variates in a correlation matrix are positive, it is certain that a general factor is available which is positively correlated with every one of the variates. Look at the example of Chapter 11 and other examples in this chapter for evidence of this phenomenon. Take note that only the three variates which entered the MODEL specification of the general nursing care factor have nonzero scoring coefficients for that factor, but all six QPACS scales require nonzero scoring coefficients for the physical nursing care factor in order that the second factor may be totally uncorrelated with the first factor.

REFERENCES

Barnow, B. S.: *The effects of Head Start and socioeconomic status on cognitive develop-ment of disadvantaged children.* Unpublished doctoral dissertation, University of Wisconsin at Madison, 1973.

Campbell, A., P. E. Converse, and W. L. Rodgers: *The quality of American life*. Ann Arbor, Mich.: Institute for Social Research, Social Science Archive, 1975.

Duncan, O. D., A. O. Haller, and A. Portes: Peer influence on aspirations: A reinterpretation. *American Journal of Sociology*, 1968, *74*, 119–137.

Holzinger, K. J., and F. A. Swineford: *A study in factor analysis: The stability of a bifactor solution*. University of Chicago: Supplementary Educational Monographs No. 48, 1939.

Jöreskog, Karl G., and M. van Thillo: *LISREL: A general computer program for estimating a linear structural equation system involving multiple indicators of unmeasured variables (Research Report 73-5)*. Uppsala, Sweden: University of Uppsala, 1973.

_____, and Dag Sörbom: *LISREL IV user's guide: Analysis of linear structural relationships by the method of maximum likelihood*. Chicago, Ill.: National Educational Resources, 1978.

Lohnes, Paul R.: *Measuring adolescent personality*. Pittsburgh: American Institutes for Research and University of Pittsburgh, 1966.

_____, and William W. Cooley: *Introduction to statistical procedures: With computer exercises*. New York: Wiley, 1968.

Magidson, J.: Toward a causal model approach for adjusting for preexisting differences in the nonequivalent control group situation: A general alternative to ANCOVA. *Evaluation Quarterly*, 1977, *1*, 399–420.

Ventura, Marlene R., and Paul Hageman: *Testing for the reliability, validity, and sensitivity of quality of nursing care measures*. Final Report to Department of Medicine and Surgery, Health Services Research and Development Services. Washington, D.C.: Veterans Administration, 1978.

Vernon, P. E.: Ability factors and environmental influences. *American Psychologist*, 1965, *20*, 723–733.

Wandelt, Mabel A., and Joel W. Ager: *Quality patient care scale*. New York: Appleton-Century-Crofts, 1974.

Wheaton, B., B. Muthén, D. Alwin, and G. Summers: Assessing reliability and stability in panel models. In D. R. Heise (Ed.), *Sociological methodology 1977*. San Francisco: Jossey-Bass, 1977, pp. 84–136.

Chapter 13

How Is Research Disseminated?

THE WRITTEN REPORT

It is difficult to write a research report. Although nurses always have writing implements at hand and frequently scribble notes during the course of the day's work, they seldom find it necessary to write extended passages. Thus they may have lacked meaningful writing practice since their high school or early college days. In school, both students and teachers may have been more concerned with basic writing skills than with content. The necessity of writing a research report, however, emphasizes that you cannot merely write writing (Johnson, 1962), but must write about something—nurse-patient interaction, medication regimens, treatment plans, and so on. This something to be written about may involve complex ideas that are not yet perceived with total clarity even by the writer. Thus an unskilled or out-of-practice writer is faced both with the task of sorting out her thoughts and with putting them on paper in sufficiently good style to inspire, or at least to avoid offending, those persons she hopes will want to read her product.

It is not easy to make the two wild horses of writing style and subject matter work together in harness, and it must be done by the subject matter expert rather than by a writing expert. Sometimes the nurse-writer says, "I have a friend who is an English teacher, and he is going to look my paper over for me when I get it together." While all advice and aid are to the good, the writer should remember that the English teacher can correct only flagrant errors. Beyond that he can consult and attempt to identify what the writer intended to say. Finally, the subject matter expert must decide whether she has said what she meant.

Loose Logic

How effectively did the authors of the following sentences say what they intended to say?

The dying stage in our lives and the subject of death have long been taboo in our society.

In response as to whether exercise is part of a diet regime, seven replied affirmatively.

He calls this state of tension stress, which he says is a condition or a state and ties it to disease.

A large majority of these patients (43 percent) could give a return demonstration.

The one participant in the older age group that did not practice breast self-examination was due to a history of cystic mastitis and being unable to determine if the mass is new.

Variables that imply further investigation are: emergency hospitalizations, repeated hospitalizations due to chronic illness, undesirable experiences from previous hospitalizations, and the preparation of parents.

Various studies have been conducted in a search to conclude that exercise can be a model of preventative medicine.

Increasing the number of persons required to report will hopefully (1) increase the number of reports, and (2) identify the abuse before it becomes serious.

Many of the errors made by struggling authors are not the sort of errors made in school exercises in which you selected from alternatives, one wrong and one right. We are concerned not only with wrong and right, but with a variety of ways that are not equally effective even though they may be technically correct. Once you have thought about these choices, you can evaluate what is best for the piece you are writing.

Redundancy

Whether the examples given above are diagnosed as failure to write adequately or failure to complete a thought, they all should have been rewritten. The following examples can be characterized as redundant and also should have been revised:

The newsletter meets a current need today.

Society is prepared to move forward to the next stage of societal development.

Information available to the general public regarding the management of prisons is not generally available to the lay person.

This increased awareness, following publication of Dr. Kubler-Ross' book, has evidenced itself in medical literature, but also in psychological and social science journals as well.

The theories of motivation developed by Maslow in 1943 influenced future trends in such studies.

We recommend that future studies be done . . .

And yet it is still generally a taboo subject in our society.

We looked at peak demands for certain times.

These pollutants are often found in many factories.

Do we overemphasize the importance of careful use of language? Hardly. Language may be our most important possession. Pei put its importance into place with one neat question: "If you will scoff at language study . . . how save in terms of language will you scoff?" English, with all its peculiarities, is the only language most American nurses will ever possess, and we ought to lend some attention to its precision—perhaps even pride of the sort displayed by the smug remark of the Frenchman Rivarol, who declared, "Whatever is not clear is not French."

How much should we concern ourselves with the old rules of style? We are told that a language changes in the process of being used, that it is a living, growing thing (Weaver, 1962). But we should not confuse mere deterioration with mutation or growth. We are not free to use language in any way we please if we also want to be understood and to hand on the rich heritage of standard English to future generations. That precision of the language deserves conscious protection is a view that finds continual expression in both popular and scientific publications (Chase, 1976; Dunne, 1978; Sheils, 1975; Weaver, 1962). This view has been newly emphasized in government, too, finding expression in the publications of the Departments of Energy, Housing and Urban Development, Health, Education and Welfare, and the Federal Trade Commission (Reinhold, 1977).

Common Errors of Usage

The surest way to improve personal writing style is to refer often to stylebooks and follow their advice. What is a stylebook? According to *American Heritage* (1969), style is a customary manner of presenting printed material, including usage, punctuation, spelling, typography, and arrangement. Thus, authors' manuals, dictionaries, grammar books, textbooks on writing theses and dissertations, as well as those books titled stylebooks all qualify. The reporter of research should not restrict herself to one reference or one kind of resource book on style, even though she must select and identify one authority to follow in instances when experts fail to agree. Regardless of whether someone else has imposed a stylebook on you or you have selected it yourself, you should let it help you and follow it meticulously. Ultimately a question may arise that your authority does not give definite direction on. Then you must decide on the basis of what your reader would find easiest to follow. These are the two essentials of a referencing system: it must be consistent and easy for the reader to follow.

Nurses make the same kinds of writing errors that other Americans make. What are the common errors of usage? A *Newsweek* article (Sheils, 1975) listed eight common usage errors that were identified by teachers at Phillips Academy in Andover, Massachusetts. They were: sentence fragments, misplaced modifiers, faulty agreement of subject and verb, faulty agreement of noun and pronoun, vague pronoun reference, mixed metaphor, faulty parallelism, and shift of person. Our experiences with nurses suggest that they, too, make these errors, some more frequently than others. We have divided the errors into categories of occurrence (frequent, moderate, and seldom) and selected some examples from nursing papers to illustrate them. Examples of frequent errors follow.

Faulty agreement of noun and pronoun:

> In chronic bronchitis a person has thick mucus built up inside their air passageways (a person, his or her; persons or people, their).

> Have you ever considered how much money a person blows up in smoke because of their habit?

> Each subject will be invited to examine the questionnaire and asked if they will consent to filling it out.

> Each subject over 25 had their height and build plotted against the Metropolitan Life table.

> What is the relationship between the nurse's knowledge of the mechanism of discharge planning in their institution and recognition of nurse functions in discharge planning?

Faulty parallelism:

> Other techniques such as drying the skin and application of moisturizers also contribute (applying).

> The purpose of this Act was to encourage more complete reporting of suspected child abuse and maltreatment as well as establishing a child protection service (to establish).

> The chest is hyperresonant on percussion, and auscultation of the lung fields reveals diminished breath sounds, high-pitched wheezes and rhonchi.

> Reasons people drink coffee are enjoyment, taste, psychologically gives you energy, stimulation, dependency, and habit.

Procainamide exerts a depressing action on the heart, slowing the rate, slowing the conduction, reducing the myocardial contractility, and prolonged refractory period.

Some of the expanded role tasks or functions of nurse practitioners that are considered are: obtaining a complete health history, performing a complete physical examination, ordering laboratory tests, making an initial diagnosis, performing minor surgery, using local infiltrating anesthetics, and prescription practices (prescribing).

Lest the reader think that nurses are the only ones who commit this particular sin of syntax, permit us to quote this example from a letter written by an academic dean at, let us hasten to add, an institution with which neither of us has ever been associated:

Ms. _____ possesses the very desirable personal characteristics of: perseverance, a hard worker, analytical in thought, and is highly motivated professionally.

Faulty agreement of subject and verb:

Data reveals that . . .

After the data was tallied . . .

Somewhat less often, but still quite frequently, the reader of research papers sees misplaced elements:

An individual experiencing a severe, acute illness upon entering the hospital goes through at least three phases of care.

Report immediately significant changes.

Parents of children who will be starting school for the first time in September must be immunized against whooping cough, tetanus, and mumps.

Eighty-three percent reported they were able to utilize all the skills for which they were prepared in their present positions. (Use of skills in their present position was the issue.)

One of the purposes of a volunteer hot line is to try to locate a person who can speak Spanish within the institution. (The aim was to locate a person within the institution.)

Most terminally ill patients want relief from distressing symptoms of disease and sustained expert care.

In our experience, sentence fragments are relatively rare, but they do occur. Strunk and White (1972) say they result from the punctuation error of using a period instead of a comma:

These being asthma, chronic bronchitis, and emphysema.

The inevitable consequence being breakdown in aseptic technique.

These being mainly the control and disposal of wastes and by-products and in the intensity of the industrial operations.

The Andover teachers found more instances of shift of person and vague pronoun reference than we have found, but we propose another category to include both these errors. We like to call it "the phantom," since it always hints at some actor who has vanished without being clearly identified. Our favorite example (Lewis, 1976) is:

Hopefully, the dog went home.

One has a mental vision of dog with an anticipatory grin on his face as he trots homeward, or, failing that, of a kindly but unidentified person—a phantom—who is hoping that the animal came to no harm. Can such phantoms flit through nursing research papers? Indeed they can:

Hopefully, it won't be long until many more nurses seek higher academic degrees. (Who does the hoping?)

When scrutinizing where participants consumed their first alcoholic beverage, only four consumed it away from home. (Who did the scrutinizing?)

Due to difficulty getting interviews with doctors, doctors responded via questionnaire. (Who had the difficulty?)

Visual impairments noted that 60 percent of residents wore glasses.

When mixing insulins, they should have the same concentrations.

Participants' names are not required to participate in this study.

As a final example of the phantom, consider this statement from the bulletin of a hospital that is proud of the food trays it sends to patients:

Slip-ups are rare, Brown said, because missing items are tagged before they leave the hospital kitchen.

Real detective work is necessary to sort that one out. Unidentified persons are putting tags on items that are not there. What a breakthrough if we could catch them!

The previous passages have illustrated a sin of omission in neglecting to identify an actor clearly. We have noted a distressing opposite tendency to overpersonify nursing. Nursing is a profession performed by nurses. It will not or cannot do anything that nurses do not do. Yet some writers speak often of what nursing must do, and we question whether the writers would in every case be willing to say that nurses must, or even that nurses should, let alone "I should." For example:

> Nursing must anticipate its increasing responsibilities and take the necessary action for discharge planning prior to the enforcement of the federal mandates. Nursing can do this better if it understands the history, purpose, and to some extent the mechanism, of the utilization review process.

> Nursing has recognized the need for crisis intervention in special care areas.

Professional jargon is ugly (if not ludicrous) to outsiders and is therefore damaging to our professional image. Examples appear frequently:

> Positive responses were related to the number of inservices attended.

> The patient was post-op for cancer of the colon.

To round out the Phillips list we provide the following quote as an example of a mixed metaphor (we cannot regret that we have failed to encounter a "good" nursing example):

> The police commissioner said, "I assure you if there is any substance to the report, heads will roll. But we can't jump before we see if there is water in the pool."

Flawed Comparisons, Run-on Sentences, Faults in Quoting

Three additional errors that are likely to be found several times in any batch of research papers are confused comparisons, misuse of quotes, and run-on sentences. Consider this faulty comparison:

> Women who smoke and take the pill are twelve times as likely to have a fatal heart attack than women who do neither.

The sentence should employ the *as likely as* or *more likely than* construction. In the next example, the writer began a *so . . . as* comparison, only to get off the track:

> Herman and Dempsey maintain that definitions and acceptance of the nurse practitioner's role is not so much dependent on her abilities, but more on the attitudes of physicians and nurses with whom she works.

The run-on sentence should perhaps be called the run-away sentence. It seems likely that most writers understand that a sentence can have too many improperly subordinated clauses, but they get carried away with their thoughts:

> Half (15 of 30) of the nursing graduate students did not think that nurse practitioners should use prescriptions presigned by a physician, while 7 approved of this practice while the remaining 8 were undecided.

Sometimes readers are bounced around like passengers in a crashing auto, until they cannot remember what hit them first:

> The objectives of baccalaureate nursing programs are often broad and general, thus difficult to specifically understand the degree of depth of knowledge and skill expected, and being general, are difficult to measure reliably.

Many errors occur in quotations. Often the second mark of a pair of quotation marks is left off, thus forcing the readers to guess exactly where the quotation ended. Sometimes a series of quotes appears without integration into the writer's discussion or without transition from one quote to the next. Although someone else's words may be used to illustrate your points, they should not be counted on to make your points for you. In addition, a point can be obscured rather than illuminated by a quote involving a number of "hooks" that may have been appropriate to the original writer's purpose, but not all of which are apropos to yours. (We will return to hooks in our discussion of paragraphs.) The least pardonable error of quotation, though, is mixing direct and indirect quotes. Consider this example from the sports page:

> Asked if he felt the return to college recruiting would be a big departure from his years with the pros, the coach said, "It would still take both coaching and talent. We intend to recruit the best players possible."

Even without hearing the coach's remarks, we feel safe in guessing that the material between the quotation marks is not exactly what he said. Probably the first part is the reporter's paraphrase of something that was said. Our guess is that it would be more accurate to present the coach's remark this way:

> Asked if he felt the return to college recruiting would be a big departure from his years with the pros, the coach said it would still take both coaching and talent, adding, "We intend to recruit the best players possible."

Here is a nursing example of a mixed direct and indirect quote:

> He said that "he got a flu shot every year but it seemed to do no good."

The passage should be indirectly quoted, i.e., without the quotation marks. Alternatively, the direct quote could be used, probably like this:

> He said, "I get a flu shot every year but it seems to do no good."

Passive Constructions

Use of the passive voice is a handy ploy when the writer, for one reason or another, must avoid placing responsibility for an action or statement. Thus we have become accustomed to hearing or seeing in the news statements such as, "A disclosure by informed sources yesterday revealed that . . . ." If the active construction were used—"Informed sources revealed yesterday that . . ."—it would serve to emphasize the missing information more than the reporter would like. Reporters of research have the same need to discuss actions or statements without revealing or perhaps without knowing where they originated. This has led to a sometimes stereotyped research style that frequently employs passives. For example:

> Replication of this study may be done using a larger sample and a longer time period.

The passive is justified because we do not know who may be doing the replicating. Using replicating as a verb, however, gets rid of an awkward "done," always an improvement:

> The study may be replicated . . .

This leads to a handy rule of thumb. When you review your first draft, look to see where you can remove various forms of the verb *to be (is, was, were)* and its sidekicks *do, done, going.* You can replace most of them with livelier, working verbs that improve readability.

Weak:

> How are we in the health field going to teach adequately?

Better:

> How can health workers teach adequately?

> Passives were made to hide the phantom, but sometimes the fugitive takes into hiding part of the clear logic you would like to display. For example:

> Twenty-three questionnaires were returned for analysis and four were returned unanswered because the situation did not apply to them.

or

> Criteria need to be developed for evaluation.

One sees that crops can need water, but must question the needs criteria can have. Likewise,

Responses need to be supportive.

Passives can contribute to sequences of past participles which cause heaviness and reading difficulty:

While only two of the nurses surveyed smoked, all fourteen nurses in the sample crossed their legs while sitting.

Table 13-1   Guide to Words Leading to Errors and Imprecision in Research Writing

Use only in exact, statistical meaning:
   analysis
   correlation
   factor
   mean, mode, median
   population
   sample
   subject

Avoid these overused forms:
   determined
   do, done
   feels, felt
   hopefully
   utilize
   vast majority
   very
   was comprised of

Distinguish carefully:
   adapt, adopt
   affect, effect
   aid, aide
   alternative, choice
   apt, liable, likely
   cite, quote
   continual, continuous
   elicit, illicit, solicit
   few, less
   its, it's
   method, methodology
   oral, verbal
   relation, correlation
   their, there
   with regard to, as regards
   who, that

Source: Developed from the authors' experience, with reliance on Dunne, 1978; Lewis, 1976; Newman, 1974; Sheils, 1975; Strunk and White, 1972; and various dictionaries.

Since no studies reviewed questioned nurses on their willingness to utilize a nurse practitioner, comparison with the findings of this study on that question was impossible.

In the first example it would be slightly less ponderous to say, "While only two of the surveyed nurses smoked . . . ." The second example could be made active by saying, "Since the investigators found no studies that questioned nurses on their willingness to use a nurse practitioner . . . ."

We have tried to provide some help in constructing readable sentences. We have no intention of providing a list of rules which you can find in the stylebooks mentioned earlier. One handy but underused source of aid is the dictionary. If we were to look up simple words such as *to, by, for, when, among, regard,* and follow the usage suggestions more often, the clarity and grace of our language would be much enhanced. We hope you will use a variety of resources, because we do not advocate slavish adherence to one set of authoritarian rules. Such rules can lead to ridiculous impasses. One such impasse concerns use of a preposition to end a sentence. The injunction against such usage was satirized by school children who transformed it into, "Never use a preposition to end a sentence with," thereby doing it. Winston Churchill made the same satirical point by commenting that this was the sort of nonsense up with which he would not put.

Word Choice

Except in Table 13-1, we will say little concerning individual words. We urge you to look up the words in the table and consider thoughtfully the meaning, possible synonyms, examples of use—in short, all the information a good dictionary can give you with regard to your own habits of use or overuse. Loose use of the words we have identified tips us off early that the particular research paper we have in hand may not have been written with loving care.

We invite the reader to examine the accompanying sentences whose handicapped or critical condition is clued by imprecise use of the words we have identified.

The sentences:

He is unable to meet adequately the disturbances in his environment and therefore his needs are apt to remain unmet.

In general the more education a nurse had the less often she was apt to deal with dying patients.

All participants were knowledgeable about women apt to be placed in the high risk group for developing breast cancer.

Table 7. Correlation between source of knowledge regarding role of nurse practitioner and willingness to utilize nurse practitioner as primary health care provider. (The table showed crossbreaks.)

Because there was no objective criteria substantiating self-assessments, the questionnaire can only result in a description of the graduates' perspective.

The nurse who works daily in the critical care area can determine the areas where he or she feels intellectually, technically or psychologically weak.

Backscheider feels that today people are increasingly conscious of their responsibility to care for their health. The patient's role in health care, Backscheider feels, may have varying degrees of complexity.

The responses were tabulated to find the percentage of the sample that answered in the same mode.

The sample population for this study was comprised of 29 registered professional nurses.

Fourteen graduate nursing students became the sample population.

Written and verbal permission was obtained from each client's surgeon.

Sometimes a writer likes a word so well she overuses it, or even more confusingly, uses more than one meaning of it in the same sentence. In the following examples watch *concern, feel, information:*

Much concern exists concerning the increasing mortality of institutionalized persons.

Dodge's report of a study of client's perceptions of their cognitive needs attempts to provide clues of the kinds of information that medical and surgical recipients of information feel is important to be given.

The overuse of *information* is not the only weakness in the preceding sentence, of course, but it is the last straw.

While you are deleting weak words and introducing variety, why not have the fun of injecting an occasional "hard" word? Dale, a word expert, said (1957) that readers enjoy learning rare words when they are introduced in a context that suggests the meaning. Careful diction enhances learning for both writer and reader.

Paragraphs

We have tried to give help in lessening errors in sentence construction and word use. Even more important to the paper as a whole are paragraphs. They are the units of construction. If you move or change a word or a sentence, the structure will continue to stand, but if you fail to use strong paragraphs in a reasonable order, the creation will never rise to support itself in the first place.

We present four suggestions (borrowed from Kierzek and Gibson, 1960) for creating strong paragraphs:

1 Try presenting your material from the general to the particular. State the

general idea, then give reasons, examples, details, or illustrations.

2 Try the order of enumeration. In your topic sentence state that your idea may be seen from two points of view, or has three aspects, that four reasons have been identified, and so on.

3 Try the time order. While chronology may be a weak overall organizer for a paper or a literature review, it often benefits a paragraph.

4 Try the inductive order. Guide the readers' thoughts so that they are prepared for a summarizing topic sentence.

What these suggestions provide in common is internal form within the paragraph. A warning is in order, however, with regard to order of enumeration. If a stem is used, it must fit equally smoothly with each item that follows in the enumeration. That is, the reader should be able to read the stem with any item independently of the items that precede it. Misuse of a stem or pivot can sometimes be seen even in short sentences:

> Then, and even now, certain erroneous beliefs about menstrual disability are commonly accepted.

It is also the case that each paragraph must be connected to others. How can this be accomplished?

Barzun and Graff (1970) point out that all subjects have not one but half a dozen or a dozen handles to grasp. Your aim is to seize the one that allows you to couple smoothly into a related idea in the next paragraph. They illustrate the subject as a circle with radiating arms. These arms can radiate only a limited distance, as they must remain within the province of the subject. Such structures can be turned, however, so that similar handles or radiations from adjacent paragraphs can be linked. For a fuller (and more charming) exposition of this notion, we urge you to read their book.

Outlining has often been suggested as an ideal way to achieve good overall organization. We concur, providing we all agree that outlining can be used in various ways and at various stages. That is, the well-trained writer can use it as a preliminary blueprint that is carefuly delineated on paper. Or self-controlled writers can use it as did the nearly blind historian Prescott, who, Nevins said (1962), could clearly hold as many as 60 well-organized pages in his head before committing any of them to paper. Others, less disciplined, may find outlines more valuable as verification. In other words, once your creation is on paper, you can outline it to test whether it has an organization that holds together. If you cannot make a formal outline following the traditional

I Main topic
    A Subdivision of main topic
        1 Branch of subdivision
            a Detail of branch of subdivision

form, you may be able to do something much simpler and possibly equally helpful. In the margin, write a word or phrase that indicates the real topic of each paragraph. When these topics repeat themselves in various sections, a plan for reorganization will begin to emerge. The next step is to cut and paste, "turning" paragraphs and writing new transition sentences as necessary, until you recognize a good flow of thought from beginning to end.

REPORTING THE RESEARCH

The report takes a variety of forms depending on the audience it is being prepared for. Are you writing for an audience of health care consumers? For health workers of all levels? For health professionals only? For all nurses? For nurses in specialized practice? We are writing for nurses of various educational preparations whom we view as intelligent and interested in ideas, particularly those related to research activity.

If you are writing a thesis or dissertation, your university or department will provide some rules or guidelines, but these necessarily allow some leeway for differences in scholarly backgrounds and for experimentation with new forms. You have paid some attention to nursing journals and perhaps been more confused than aided. What you must keep in mind is that many journal articles are "reports of reports." That is, editors have been unable to provide space for publishing entire monographs. By publishing excerpts that center on the more interesting aspects of a study, space is conserved so that more reports can be printed.

Very experienced and prolific researchers may move almost directly from data printouts to journal articles, but certain situations demand a more complete and formal research monograph. What does a complete monograph look like? A variety of models are used in nursing research. There may be an even greater variety than in most fields because of the varied educational backgrounds of nursing researchers. We cannot advise you to use one model over another, but in Table 13-2 we have provided a comprehensive—some would say a fulsome—scheme that includes most of the items we have ever seen included in research reports both published and unpublished. We offer it as a general reminder and locater, but each nurse should use good taste and advice to trim it to the requirements of her situation.

Now we offer some advice concerning certain sections of the report we have not previously touched upon.

Abstract

Abstracts vary in length from approximately 200 to 600 words. Follow any guidelines you may have from an institution or editor, but if you have a choice make it shorter rather than longer. Do not waste words and space by repeating information from the title, spelling out numbers (use Arabic numerals, even at the beginning of sentences in the abstract), or by saying, "The author concludes . . . ." Who else would be speaking here? (APA, 1974). Do include brief statements of the problem, method, results, and conclusions. If you have room, indicate the number and kind of subjects, and explain more about the design and statistical results. If the abstract is of a review or discussion article, state the

**Table 13-2   Reminder Scheme for
Items That May Be Included in a
Research Monograph**

Abstract
Title
Table of Contents
List of tables
List of figures

Chapter 1 heading
Background of the problem/Justification for a
   nursing study/Objectives/Purpose

(Review of related literature here or as
   Chapter 2)

Statement of the problem
Hypothesis(es)/Subproblem(s)
Assumptions
Operational definitions
Theoretical population
Delimitations/Negotiating sites
Sample of subjects/Safeguards to subjects
Data-collection instruments and procedures
Plan for data analysis
Time schedule
Limitations encountered at proposal stage

Chapter 2 heading
Theoretical-conceptual framework
Related research done and needed

Chapter 3 heading
Problem
Tables
Discussion of tables and noteworthy findings

Chapter 4 heading
Interpretations
Support or nonsupport of hypotheses
Additional limitations encountered
Conclusions/Generalizations
Implications for nursing
Recommendations for policy
Recommendations for further research

References
Appendixes
   Permission to conduct study
   Observations/Raw data
   Instrument(s)
   Human subjects clearance

topics covered, the central thesis, and theoretical background. A knowledgeable reader should be able to comprehend the abstract without reference to the main document. If the abstract is likely to be reproduced on a separate page from the document, be sure to include a full bibliographic reference (*American National,* 1971).

Although it appears early, perhaps even before the title, the abstract is usually the last thing written. Sometimes an abstract of the proposal may be required in a university program or for a funder. Follow the same general guidelines, and make no attempt to be original.

Title

The most important consideration for a title in this age of computerized information retrieval is that it should be accurately indexable. Most computer searches use cross-indexing. Thus, you should try to use phrases or words in your title that can be used as labels in a cross-indexing system. For example, "Instruction of Clients Concerning Medication Regimes" is a far better title than "The Problem of Medications." The *International Nursing Index* (INI) has published a nursing thesaurus which lists commonly used nursing terms that are also used as cross-references to the subject headings in INI. Most INI headings (after a trial period) are included in *MeSH* (medical subject headings), which provides the cross-reference labels for *Index Medicus.* Thus it may be a good idea to browse in the thesaurus or *MeSH* for words or phrases to include in your title. Deliberate over your title, since it need not be written until the rest of your manuscript has been written and polished.

Table of Contents, Lists of Tables and Figures

If you have guidelines from an institution or publisher, follow them. If not, strive for parallelism in length of entries, grammatical constructions, etc. Follow examples in a book you like.

Chapter Headings

Number of chapters or whether to have any at all is an arbitrary matter. The scheme sketched here may be used, altered, or abandoned altogether. If you have such divisions, then Chapter 1 should ideally have some title other than "Introduction."

Background, Justification, Objectives, Purpose

This section answers the question "Why?" It should bring the reader from a larger context (i.e., American life, the health care system, the nursing profession) and clarify why the problem is a nursing problem. Chinn and Jacobs (1978) point out that the solid central core of any science represents its historical past, but this core changes in a cumulative manner. Thus, a study totally new and unrelated to past concerns of nursing will not be a nursing study. You can have an original idea, but you must show how it relates to the central core. (See also Chapters 2 and 3.)

Statement of the Problem

This is easily the most important sentence in your report. Do not be shy about it. Give it a formal heading of its own and state it strongly. Do not be satisfied with a weak question such as, "Is there a relationship . . . ?" Of course there is. Everything on earth is related in some way. It is better to ask, "What is the relationship . . . ? What is the effect . . . ?" You have consciously kept the problem in the front of your mind during the entire research process; do not be afraid to remind the reader of it at strategic points, such as at the end of the literature review or at the beginning of the data discussion.

Hypothesis(es)

State positively in the present tense what you expect to find. As Downs and Newman (1977) put it, the hypothesis answers the question posed by the problem. We encourage the statement of probable causes and abjure the null hypothesis, as Cronbach (1975) suggested. We do not intend to test it and therefore have no need for the null. (For assumptions see Chapter 3.)

Operational Definitions

The phenomena you study must be defined so you can count or measure them. If possible, you should use established definitions for your variates and variables. If you cannot find such definitions in the literature, you will have to make your own, but too many self-operationalized definitions will detract from the credibility of your research.

Theoretical Population

Describe the theoretical population your sample is derived from. In your data analysis you can lump together hospital nurses and community health nurses if you have described a theoretical population of nurses and drawn the sample appropriately. Lack of clarity about the theoretical population is the most drastic limitation of all on the generalization.

Delimitations, Negotiating the Site(s)

Hodgman (1978) listed six questions that should be asked concerning clinical agencies. These should be asked (with different emphases) by both the researcher and the nursing administrator who grants permission for the study:

1 Can the clinical agency provide the data?
2 Are the projected data-collection dates reasonable?
3 Will the study interfere with ongoing or projected research within the agency?
4 Does the study duplicate current or projected research within the agency?
5 Does any aspect of the study conflict with institutional or departmental philosophy, objectives, or policy?
6 Must the study be approved by the institutional review boards?

Time Schedule

This requires only a sentence or two, but it becomes increasingly important to the reader as a study ages.

Limitations Encountered at Proposal Stage

These must be identified thoughtfully with relation to everything you know about validity and generalization. They should be stated honestly but not too humbly, e.g., leave out apologies about your inexperience.

Theoretical and Conceptual Framework, Review of Related Literature

This is the weakest section of most research reports, according to experts (Hardy, 1978). We have had our say in the first section of Chapter 3. Now we offer this quote from *College and University Bulletin:*

> *Manuscript Style*—There is a skill involved in writing a literature review or state-of-the-art report. This type of publication is much more than a string of paragraphs that summarize individual pieces of literature, all being held together by a common theme. It is a form of research, and the data base is the literature. The objective is not to develop new data, but to review existing data and to combine it into a conceptual whole. While it is necessary to document the sources of the information, the main concern is to review major events, methods, theories, philosophical positions, research findings, practices, programs, policies and the like, analyze their importance, and develop conclusions concerning present and future impact (Fife, 1978).

Tables and Discussion of Tables

Stylebooks (especially the APA manual) contain invaluable technical advice on the preparation of tables. Since it is mandatory that every research writer choose and use a stylebook, we will not repeat all the advice here, but will reinforce several points:

1 Do not include columns of data that can be calculated easily from other columns. That is, do not use both numbers of responses and percentage of responses. In general, reserve % to compare samples of different sizes. When % is used, put it only at heads of columns.

2 Go easy on lines. When in doubt, pencil them in lightly and let an editor or other advisor help you decide where they should be used.

3 Reduce the table size sufficiently so that it can be read without turning the monograph or journal sideways. (For only a dime or so, a photocopy service can reduce a table to a size that fits neatly on a page with appropriate margins.)

4 Avoid useless words such as "category." Avoid duplication in caption and headings.

5 Try to make items in a column conceptually comparable. For example, how can a reader interpret a column headed "Areas of nursing practice" that has the following entries: adult health, medical-surgical, community health, primary care, surgery, pediatrics, respiratory, cardiac? All these classifications may be seen in practice, but the reporter of research must use scientific (mutually exclusive) categories.

    6 Call graphs and illustrations *figures*. Only tables should be called tables.

    7 Line up decimals and round all entries to the same number of places beyond the decimal.

    8 Use a zero or row of periods (rather than a blank) where a value is missing.

    9 Continue your willingness to rewrite. If several forms of a table are possible, sketch them and select the most effective.

Summary of Study

The final chapter or sections should put the entire project into perspective for the reader. Many readers are likely to read only this part of the report, so it is useful if it can stand alone or nearly so. Probably you will not use all the topics suggested in Table 13-2. Possibly you will subsume several under a *Summary* heading, but it may help your thinking and writing to consider each heading to see whether it suggests points not already suggested by other headings.

Interpretations, Discussion

Here you can use your experience in professional practice and in performing the study to evaluate information and speculate about the causes of findings that surprised you. You cannot claim retrospectively that your data test hypotheses that you did not postulate before you collected the data, but you can and should speculate about the future.

Hypotheses Supported, Not Supported

This can be a brief general statement because you have already reported your analysis in considerable detail.

Additional Limitations Recognized during Research

Describe the difficulties you ran into or at least suggest what kind they were. If nursing research is to mature, we must share data and experiences, encourage replications and extensions. It is not necessary to be overly modest or run yourself down, but it is desirable to advise other researchers of difficulties they are likely to encounter.

Conclusions, Generalizations, Implications for Nursing, Policy Recommendations

You may not need all of these sections, but all are permissible and worth considering. However your statements may be organized, the reader should be able to see how your study is related to the literature you reviewed as well as to your empirical investigation and your hypotheses. If you make policy recommendations, you should make it clear what group you are addressing.

Recommendations for Further Research

This section should discuss logical extensions and replications of the study.

PUBLISHING AN ARTICLE

Possibly no one will want to publish the monograph you have just completed, but chances are that you may be able to interest a journal editor in a condensed version. Your best approach is to pick out some likely journals and review recent issues. If it seems to you that a given journal may be ready for an article on your topic, write a letter inquiring whether the editor is interested in publishing such an article. Incorporate an abstract of the article you might provide. This approach is better than sending an article on approval because the inquiry letter does not commit you. You can correspond with more than one editor if you wish, while it is ethically questionable to submit an article to more than one journal at a time. Chances are you know someone with more publishing experience than yourself whom you can ask for suggestions about appropriate places to send your inquiries.

If you receive encouragement from an editor, it should not take long to produce an article since you have your carefully written, completed monograph to refer to. The editor may offer to publish your work as a letter to the editor or as an abstract, and you will have to weigh the advantages of a given journal and an immediate contract to publish against the possibility of a longer article in some other journal.

Once you make an agreement to publish, follow through by seriously considering the editor's suggestions and meeting deadlines. The editor may have sent you the journal's instructions to authors, or they may be printed periodically in the journal. In either case, you should make your references conform to the citation style the journal uses and should tailor the length of your report to the editor's specification. When you send the article, send a cover letter with it so it will be routed correctly when it reaches the paper-laden editorial office.

The technique described here is appropriate for placing other kinds of articles, too, but remember that it may be risky to promise an article before it is at least partially developed. Writing your research monograph should have taught you that it can be a long way from conception to completion. Seeing your words in print is a unique thrill, and we urge each of you to try to capture that peak experience for yourself if you have not already done so.

REFERENCES

American national standard for writing abstracts. New York: American National Standards Institute, 1971.

(APA) Publication manual of the American Psychological Association (2d ed.). Washington, D.C.: American Psychological Association, 1974.

Barnlund, Dean C.: A transactional model of communication. In Johnnye Akin, Alvin Goldberg, Gail Myers, and Joseph Stewart, *Language behavior.* The Hague, The Netherlands: Mouton, in press.

Barzun, Jacques, and Henry F. Graff: *The modern researcher.* New York: Harcourt, Brace, Jovanovich, 1957, 1970.

Cargill, Oscar, William Charvat, and Donald D. Walsh: *The publication of academic writing.* New York: Modern Language Association, 1966.

Chase, Mary Ellen: Why teach English? *NRTA Journal,* 1976 (September–October).

Chater, Shirley: *Understanding research in nursing.* Geneva: World Health Organization, 1975.

Chinn, Peggy L., and Maeona K. Jacobs: A model for theory development in nursing. *Advances in Nursing Science,* 1978, *1*(1).

Cronbach, Lee J.: Beyond the two disciplines of scientific psychology. *American Psychologist,* 1975 (February).

Dale, Edgar, 1957: Quoted in J. Wilson McKenney, *Publish—don't perish.* Bloomington, Ind.: Phi Delta Kappa, 1973.

Downs, Florence S., and Margaret A. Newman: *A sourcebook of nursing research* (2d ed.). Philadelphia: F. A. Davis, 1977.

Dunne, Philip: Just between you and I. *Newsweek,* 1978 (February 13).

Fife, Jonathan D.: Call for proposals. *AAHE Bulletin* (American Association for Higher Education), 1978, *31*(4).

Hardy, Margaret: Perspectives on nursing theory. *Advances in Nursing Science,* 1978, *1*(1).

Hodgman, Eileen C.: Student research in service agencies. *Nursing Outlook,* 1978, *26*(9).

Jennings, Gary: *Personalities of language.* New York: Thomas Y. Crowell, 1965.

Johnson, Wendell: You can't write writing. In S. I. Hayakawa, *The use and misuse of language.* New York: Fawcett, 1943, 1962.

Kierzek, John M., and Walker Gibson: *The Macmillan handbook of English.* New York: Macmillan, 1939, 1960.

Lancaster, Arnold (Ed.): Guidelines to research in nursing. *Nursing Times,* 1975, *71*(occasional paper).

Lewis, Ralph F.: Letter from the editor and publisher. *Harvard Business Review,* 1976 (May–June).

Mallam, William D.: A focus on footnotes. *Journal of Higher Education,* 1960, *31*(2), 99–102.

McKenney, J. Wilson: *Publish—don't perish.* Bloomington, Ind.: Phi Delta Kappa, 1973.

Nevins, Allan: *The gateway to history.* Garden City, N.Y.: Doubleday, 1938, 1962.

Newman, Edwin: *Strictly speaking.* New York: Warner, 1974.

Reinhold, Robert: Simplicity of words born again in capital. *Buffalo Courier-Express Dimensions,* 1977 (December 18).

Research Notes. Office of the Vice President for Research, State University of New York at Buffalo, 1979, *6*(8).

Rhinelander, Philip H.: Furtive and frivolous functions of footnotes. *Phi Delta Kappan,* 1963, *44,* 458.

Sheils, Merrill: Why Johnny can't write. *Newsweek,* 1975 (December 8).

Strauss, Samuel: Guidelines for analysis of research reports. *Journal of Educational Research,* 1969, *63* (December), 165.

Strunk, William, and E. B. White: The elements of style. New York: Macmillan, 1935, 1959, 1972.

Turabian, Kate L.: *A manual for writers of term papers, theses, and dissertations* (4th ed.). Chicago: University of Chicago, 1955.

Weaver, Warren: Communicative accuracy. *Science,* 1958 (March 7), *127,* 499.

_____: Stability and change. *Science,* 1962, *137* (2535).

Chapter 14

Can Research Recreate the Profession of Nursing?

To what extent does our hard core of beliefs and values about nursing, the living heart of our theory of nursing, need to be recreated? How much discontent with what we now know about nursing should we feel? To the extent that we are smug about present knowledge, beliefs, and values, we may see little need for research as a basis for recreating our profession.

Your authors do not think that there is an emergency in the profession. It is far from being a disaster area. Nurses can be proud of the existing theory and knowledge foundations of their profession. A nursing education is a profoundly intellectual experience in America, at least where it is at its best, and graduate study in nursing exemplifies the finest ideals and traditions of graduate education in American universities. If you have been studying our book as a course assignment in your graduate program, or if you have been reading it as a self-inflicted refreshment of your previous graduate training in research methods, you are aware of the scope and rigor of theoretical studies required of nurses who would qualify as leading professionals by attainment of a graduate degree.

Nursing practice has the authority of sound nursing theory, and it is therefore truly a professional practice.

But . . .

The health services delivery system in our civilization is anything but perfect. Everyone wants to see it improved. Most of us acknowledge that it requires widespread and substantial improvements, even if we ourselves enjoy superlative services. Many of us sense that important changes are needed *at the systems level* to provide the distributive justice our highest political morality mandates.

Systems-level changes in health services delivery will inevitably entail changes in the nature and conditions of nursing. We do not think that the nursing profession can rest on its laurels. It will have to move with the times as systemic reforms are attempted around it. More positively, nurses *can* provide leadership in the reformation of the health services system. We trust that they *will*.

One could accept the need for change and growth in nursing but reject nursing research as a guide to nursing development. Undoubtedly a vast and diversified array of researchers who are not nurses and who are not doing "nursing research" are producing quantities of new knowledge which is important to nurses, which impinges on nursing practice, and which contributes to the reconstruction of the profession of nursing. Why, then, should nurses do a thing called nursing research?

How nice for us if we have induced in you a sense that doing nursing research could be so enjoyable that you ought to try to find the time and resources to do it just for the fun of it. Realistically, however, research is work, and with so much other work for nurses, why should they look for more?

Well, there are issues in nursing which no one but a nurse is apt to research. These include aspects of patient care provided by nurses, or

doing nursing for patients

but also

recruitment and retention of nurses
nursing education
administration of nursing
systemic relations of nursing

You will have your own additions to this list and will wonder how we missed them.

Another argument flows from the attitudinal consequences of leading the life of a researcher. There are attitudes toward authority, tradition, custom, law, and habit which the research life sponsors and which have to be represented within the nursing profession. There is a predisposition to question established truths, to wonder how good they are, to wonder how far they stretch, to ask, "How do we know that?" which is needed in the profession and is encouraged by research experience. There is a humility among working researchers because they confront the limitations of existing knowledge and are aware of all the dark around the existing light. Prudence is born in the fires of uncertainty that burn in the furnaces of statistical models for nursing realities. We are saying that trying to do scientific research on nursing issues is good medicine for nurses.

This may seem cynical, but another argument is that research is prestigious. Research is in the saddle and riding us, as it were. Doctors, politicians, legislators, judges, professors, journalists, and all the other collaborators and critics of nurses can be impressed with a research posture we display before them, and in this sense doing research is good protective coloration. Appearances do count in our world. Research results have propaganda value. They are political ammunition. Research is a platform a reformer can stand on to be seen and heard. Florence Nightingale understood this. Tragically, Ignaz Semmelweis did not.

A special argument for research in nursing follows from the relationship research has come to have to program evaluation in our time. Florence Nightingale did a great deal to create this relationship, and was thus a pioneer policy scientist. Nurses do design, promote, establish, and staff *programs* of various sorts (e.g., nursing education programs), and thus they do encounter demands for program evaluations. Program evaluation is a study in its own right (one of us has coauthored a book about it), and a worthy subject for a course or even a sequence of courses in graduate school. Yet all that you have learned in this research methods course is relevant to program evaluation, and some of it is indispensable. We admit that we resolved some of the hard choices about what to put in this syllabus and what to leave out by the principle that what bore on evaluation was worthier than what did not. We did this because we expect that as leaders in nursing you are likely to be required to participate in program evaluations, and we wanted to give you some tools.

Speaking of program evaluation reminds us that we wanted to mention that important nursing research is likely to be *programmatic*. That is, the contribution to the recreation of nursing is much more likely to flow from an extensive, coordinated series of research studies stretched out in time and fanning outward in sites and in general complexity (and cost) from a rather simple, parochial (and relatively inexpensive), original inquiry, than it is to spring full-blown from a single crucial research act. The crucial experiment, the blockbuster study, is not likely in nursing because of the social, institutional, collaborative nature of the nursing game. Manipulate one variable in nursing and waves of effect roll out in all directions. Inquiry has to follow those waves outward. Soon another wave system from another policy manipulation is intersected in any given direction, and on the full map of what is happening huge numbers of such interactions are found. "It all depends" becomes a cliché. The researcher has to hang on, get around, extend her map, persevere. Almost any first step leads to a long journey of exploration. This is what happened to Semmelweis. It is what is likely to happen to you.

DESIGN AND ANALYSIS OF EXPERIMENTS

In this introduction to nursing research we have been highly selective, visualizing a student taking a one-semester graduate course with our text as her guide, in the context of a very busy semester of graduate studies and with little or no background in quantitative research methods. We have ruthlessly ignored the traditional syllabus for this course, which we believe to have been far too ambitious, and have eliminated the "nice to know" topics for the sake of emphasis on what we consider "must know" topics. On the strength of the course you are now completing you can do competent research. However, the full training of a researcher cannot be accomplished in a one-semester course. If you have enjoyed this work and can imagine a career commitment to nursing research for yourself, it is time to talk about what else you should study. Two statistical subjects you will probably want to tackle are (1) the design and analysis of experiments and (2) the multiple regression method. We want to give you a preview of these subjects to whet your appetite. The catalog of your graduate school will reveal that there are several departments on campus offering instruction on these matters.

Since Sir Ronald Fisher did the great pioneering work on the subject, for which he was properly knighted, the design and analysis of experiments has become a highly technical, largely embroidered specialty. The logic of the subject is so elegant and entertaining that people who have no intention of ever doing an experiment elect to study it. There are scientific fields as diverse as agriculture and psychology which cannot be fully understood without an appreciation of the tremendous role the design and analysis of experiments has played and does play in their development. Much of medical research is conducted according to the canons of this subject. It is one of the great intellectual achievements of the twentieth century and will stand as such forever. Our own conviction is that true experiments are not possible or desirable in nursing research, for the most part, but some people feel differently about this. Anyway, we concede that sometimes a true experiment is an appropriate design for a nursing research project, and beyond that we do see real value in knowing about the logic of experimentation even if one does not do experiments. That logic sheds useful light on all other research designs used in nursing research.

Since Fisher, the design *and* analysis of experiments has been a unitary subject, in that the selection of a design for an experiment has totally committed the researcher to a specific method of experimental data analysis and to a specific rule for deciding whether the treatment experimented with has the expected effect, or any effect. It's as though a machine is selected by the researcher from among a variety of possible machines cataloged as experimental designs, and once the selected machine is turned on, everything else follows mechanically as the preprogrammed operations of the selected machine. This may be fine if everything goes according to the plan, but if accidents throw a monkey wrench into the machine, the researcher can be left with an empty bag. Basically, we expect that if an experiment can be designed so that nothing will go wrong, the chances are that experiment will involve such artificialities as will invalidate it as a source of knowledge about real-world nursing issues.

Random assignment of two or more treatment conditions to research subjects (or objects) is the sine qua non of experimental design. When there are only two treatment conditions to be randomly assigned, they may be named the *experimental* and *control* conditions. Often the research subjects can be classified on other variables besides the treatment variable (e.g., sex, age, certification status, years of experience, type of illness), giving rise to other *factors of the design*. These design factors are additional independent variables. It is also often the case that measurements can be collected on the subjects for variates which are known to be causally related to the outcome, or criterion, measure, and which therefore ought to have their influence on the criterion partialled out by the analysis. Such causally implicated measurements are called *covariates*. If the criterion variate is a measurement, the method of analyzing the data is called analysis of variance. If the criterion is a taxonomic (i.e., classification) variate (such as 1 = dead, 2 = dying, 3 = recovering, 4 = well), the method of analysis is called *multivariate contingency analysis*. Either method can have the additional feature called *analysis of covariance* if there are covariates in the design. Usually the analysis of variance is the statistical method taught in design and analysis of experiments courses, just because Fisher conceived it so and established that tradition.

You will have heard or read of null hypotheses, t tests, F ratios, χ^2 (chi-square), planned comparisons, type I and type II errors, and estimates of effects. These are technical devices of the analysis of variance. Just the frequency with which they occur in research literature justifies studying the subject. We have fought off the temptation to give you thumbnail sketches of these technicalities because we do not think these are must-knows, we do not see anything wrong with an honest admission of ignorance in confrontations with them, and we do see grave dangers in trying to interpret them on the basis of slight knowledge. If a researcher has brought off a true experiment, you can probably trust her statistics. In all likelihood they were popped out of a competent computer program that was carefully constructed to do the analysis appropriate for her design. Such programs exist as "canned" or library routines in all computer centers. You can concentrate on the proportions of criterion variance attributed to each independent factor, including the treatment factor, and to each covariate, if any, by her results. You have learned that this is the crucial question about any quantitative research findings. What is the meaning of those attributions of variance for theory and practice? What are the limits of generalizability for those attributions? Careful reading of the report will often leave you frustrated because the author has gotten so wrapped up in the technical details of analysis of variance that she has neglected to answer the most important questions of all. Often, too, careful reading will reveal that the experiment was not brought off or that the design was ruptured by accidents, and then any such analysis of variance included in the report is window dressing anyway. That usually does not stop people from publishing such things. *Caveat emptor* applies.

People who are experts in the analysis of variance delight in answering questions about its technical details. There's an almost erotic pleasure in doing so. Don't be afraid to ask. (Hint: Ask two or several experts the same questions to get the full fun out of this.)

MULTIPLE REGRESSION

Multiple regression is the statistician's way of doing the analyses we taught you in Chapters 9 and 11 by methods we called multivariate correlation and factorial modeling. The big difference between the multiple regression procedures and the procedures we taught you is that the former use differential calculus of linear systems and the latter do not. It is not that we do not know differential calculus and the multiple regression methods based on it. We know them too well. One of us has coauthored two technical textbooks about them (Cooley and Lohnes, 1962; Cooley and Lohnes, 1971), as well as a nontechnical exposition of them which you might find helpful (Cooley and Lohnes, 1976, chapter 6). We have chosen to teach you a set of multivariate methods based on simpler, weaker mathematics only because we are convinced that the calculus-based methods of multiple regression too often overpower the data which are available in nursing research studies. However, some nursing studies do produce data worthy of the powerful analytic strokes of multiple regression, and anyway there is a great deal to be learned from study of the subject even if one chooses simpler analytic techniques for one's research data. The analysis of variance is totally a subset of multiple regression lore in its mathematics (but not in its mystique), so we would set a higher priority on your studying multiple regression than on *anova* (a popular acronym for you can guess what). If you can locate a graduate course that uses Cohen and Cohen (1975) as its text, you cannot go wrong. You could self-study Cohen and Cohen to great advantage right now, even if you misunderstood parts of it.

Multiple regression fits the regression weights (the b's) of an equation like this:

$$\hat{X}_p = b_0 + b_1 X_1 + b_2 X_2 + \cdots + b_{p-1} X_{p-1} \tag{1}$$

where $\hat{X}_p$ is a predicted score on the criterion variate and the X_1 to X_{p-1} are the predictor variates. By means of differential calculus the b's are chosen so that the correlation between X_p and $\hat{X}_p$ is maximized (made as large as possible). This correlation is called a multiple correlation and is designated R. The usefulness statistic U which we taught you in Chapter 9 is actually the R^2 of multiple regression, but we did not show you how to get the b weights because we saw advantages to teaching you to get the a weights in Chapter 11 instead. Notice the formal resemblance between the structural equation for the key criterion in the FaM method, given in Chapter 11, Detailing Causal Models, as

$$X_p = a_{p1} F_1 + a_{p2} F_2 + \cdots + a_{pn} F_n + d_p W_p \tag{2}$$

and the multiple regression equation shown above. In fact, if the disturbance term d_p is dropped from the structural equation, a prediction equation for the FaM emerges as

$$\hat{X}_p = a_{p1} F_1 + a_{p2} F_2 + \cdots + a_{pn} F_n \tag{3}$$

which is technically the multiple regression of the key criterion on the n factors of the model. However, the squared multiple correlation for Equation (3) is the communality $h_p{}^2$ and will usually be less than the R^2 for Equation (1), precisely because FaM does not use calculus to fit the a_{pj}. Experience has shown us that usually little is lost when our method is used (in that $h_p{}^2$ is usually quite close to R^2), and we think much is gained. We have warned you that statisticians will think differently. We would much rather that you studied statistics than that you trusted statisticians. That we have asked you to trust our recommendations may seem arrogant, but of course we think our convictions are well-founded. Even the statisticians will be happy if it turns out that we have enticed you into the waters of quantitative analysis, made a minnow swimmer of you, and persuaded you to aspire to become a shark in later courses. Meanwhile, if critics look at your research and inquire why you are not using multiple regression, tell them that you are using a good multivariate correlation analysis you learned from Ackerman and Lohnes, that it is much like multiple regression, and that it has its own virtues and charms. Among these are the requirements that you be very thoughtful and explicit about the model you are fitting and that you state very clearly the relationships between variables and variates, and that the analysis does not overfit the data. You might quietly compute $U = R^2$ by the method of Chapter 9, Multiple Correlations, and compare it with $h_p{}^2$ of the FaM. If, as we hope, the two are close, you might say so. Do not be upset, however, if R^2 is much larger than $h_p{}^2$. There are cases where multiple regression is known to produce terribly overinflated R^2 values. Read Cohen and Cohen (1975, pp. 106–107) about correction of R^2 for shrinkage.

RESEARCH WHICH IS NOT STATISTICAL

Nowhere is it written that all nursing research must be statistical. Nursing research should produce useful answers to important questions which confront the nursing profession. Sometimes a useful answer can be synthesized by intelligent juxtapositioning of elements of knowledge dug out of library resources. This requires at least three types of ability. First, the researcher must know how to dig in the library. If we recognize that "library" here stands for all the nation's archives, full information-retrieval skills can be very complex and impressive. Second, the researcher must be able to read research documents critically. She must be able to weigh the evidence and the arguments recovered from archives. We have not spoken much about critiquing, but we believe that the standards for research we have exposited provide at least a partial basic critiquing capability. Third, the researcher must be able to write her new synthesis effectively. We have emphasized writing skills.

Intensive case studies can provide answers to some questions. There are methodologies for case studies for which we have the greatest respect, even as we have placed them beyond the scope of this text. Contemporary American anthropology has been particularly inventive of systems of inquiry called ethnography and the participant-observer method, which we commend to you. Paul

Diesing's *Patterns of Discovery in the Social Sciences* (1971) is an excellent overview of such methods. We are interested in historical studies and the biographical method. One of us based her dissertation on historical and biographical studies (Ackerman, 1975), and that work has inspired the other of us to make definite plans to study Florence Nightingale in search of an answer to the live issue of how intellectual women can become actively involved in statistics as a way of knowing and problem solving.

How does a woman whose primary motive is altruistic service become a passionate, persistent, inventive statistician? Obviously such a woman can be a role model for other women, but is there anything in the psychology of her experience with statistics that could be applied in the education of women to encourage commitment to mathematical thinking? Florence Nightingale was one such woman. No thorough analysis of her experience with statistics has ever been made. Indeed this great woman is one of the least understood heroines of all history, perhaps precisely because her intellectual achievements were concentrated on the application of quantitative methods to political and social issues which men like to consider their territory. For whatever reasons, a false myth of Florence Nightingale has concealed the most fascinating and potentially useful truths about her. The study which is planned would attempt to recover those truths and relate them to pedagogical strategies.

Our criticism of statistical inference and differential calculus is based on the belief that a good idea is shown to be good by the success with which it travels to new situations, rather than by its perinatal circumstances. There are many ways to improve nursing theory. Perhaps the most inescapable role of the statistical methods we have taught you is in the demonstration of the applicability of theory to a large number of situations. The origins of the knowledge that is tested in the crucible of statistical studies may have been in the furnaces of historical studies, biographical and autobiographical studies, case studies, ethnographies, or just the blast furnace of hard, sustained, systematic thought. Human intelligence is the great source of knowledge. The record of human affairs writ in a thousand ways in thousands of places is the foremost aid to intelligence. Measurement and statistics are important aids, too, but they are not the only ways to truth.

CRITIQUING MEASUREMENT AND STATISTICAL RESEARCH

Many of you are too busy nursing, or teaching nursing, or administering nursing, or involved in other vital tasks to become actively involved in nursing research. Your concern is to be able to read nursing research reports critically, rather than to be able to plan, execute, and report research. Well and good. We assert that the understandings needed to critique research reports are not very different from those needed to generate them. The author of a research report needs to critique her report in much the same way that you, as an informed reader, will critique it. Here are some questions that will be answerable in positive ways when one has read a good report of good research.

1 Why was this research done? What theoretical or practical problems did it address?

2 What was already known about the problems? Was a thorough, focused review of the literature provided? Were conclusions drawn from it? Were those conclusions about the a priori state of knowledge sound ones?

3 What assumptions and evaluations were involved in the theoretical framework for this research? Were these made explicit and justified? Were they sound, in your judgment? Can you propose an alternative framework for this research? Does your framework lead to a quite different understanding of this research, of its importance, of its findings?

4 In your list of priorities for nursing research, how important or useful was this research? Should it have been done? How much attention does it deserve? Whose attention does it deserve?

5 Were the research variables adequately representative of the theoretical constructs in terms of which the problems were framed? Were any crucial variables missing from the research? Were the variables adequately specified by the measurement variates used in the research? Were any variates wasteful because they were not related clearly to variables by specification statements?

6 Were the criterion variates appropriate? Were all the relevant aspects of output or productivity brought under observation? Were the criteria prioritized?

7 Were the settings, sites, and subjects adequately described? Were the rights of human subjects adequately protected? Were the settings and subjects representative enough to delimit a reasonable population and to promise an unbiased assessment of that population? What role did missing data play in estimates obtained?

8 Was a clear, convincing causal model for the phenomena under study hypothesized? Was the model adequately fitted by the data analysis? Was the hypothetical model adequately tested by the outcomes on the data?

9 Were the limits of generalizability discussed forthrightly and reasonably? What do you think the limits for the generalizations produced actually are? How far would you trust the results to apply? In exactly what ways should nursing theory or nursing practice be modified in the light of these results?

10 What research should be done next in the light of these results? What replications or variations of this work are required? What new directions for research are inspired?

AU REVOIR

You have listened to us and presumably learned from us. Unfortunately, we have not heard from you or learned from you (unless we have cited your publications). It doesn't have to stay that way. We include our addresses here with the sincere wish that you will write to us, sharing with us your problems, corrections, and suggestions, and especially your own research experiences and results. We don't think of this as a finished book. You can help us to make the next edition better. You can also try to get us to put your research into the next edition. We don't think of ourselves as finished persons or finished editors, either. You might like to help us to grow, even if you think our book deserves no future. Thank you for reading us, and do let us hear from you.

Winona B. Ackerman
School of Nursing
East Carolina University
Greenville, North Carolina 27834

Paul R. Lohnes
Department of Educational Psychology
State University of New York at Buffalo
379 Baldy Hall
Amherst, New York 14260

REFERENCES

Ackerman, Winona: *Women's search for roles*. Unpublished doctoral dissertation, SUNY at Buffalo, 1975.
Cohen, Jacob, and Patricia Cohen: *Applied multiple regression/correlation analysis for the behavioral sciences*. New York: Lawrence Erlbaum/Wiley, 1975.
Cooley, William W., and Paul R. Lohnes: *Multivariate procedures for the behavioral sciences*. New York: Wiley, 1962.
_____ and _____: *Multivariate data analysis*. New York: Wiley, 1971.
_____ and _____: *Evaluation research in education*. New York: Irvington/Halsted/Wiley, 1976.
Diesing, Paul: *Patterns of discovery in the social sciences*. Chicago: Aldine/Atherton, 1971.

FORTRAN Code for the MODEL Program

```
MODEL
      PROGRAM MODEL (INPUT, OUTPUT, DATAPE, TAPE5 = INPUT, TAPE6 = OUTPUT,
   C   TAPE 1 = DATAPE)
C
C      MODEL CORRELATIONS. P. R. LOHNES, SUNY AT BUFFALO, , 1978*)
C
C      INPUT
C
C      1) SETUP VALUES
C          COLS  4 - 5   M = NUMBER OF VARIATES (LITTLE P IN TEXT)
C          COLS  6 - 10  N = NUMBER OF SUBJECTS
C          COLS 14 - 15  NAF = NUMBER OF FACTORS (LITTLE N IN TEXT)
C          COLUMN 20  K1 = 0 TO COMPUTE FROM SCORES
C                             1 TO READ IN UPPER-TRIANGULAR R MATRIX
C          COLUMN 25  K2 = 0 IF NO REMAKE OF R IS REQUIRED
C                             1 TO REMAKE R MATRIX (I.E., TO EDIT R)
C          COLUMN 30  M1 = NUMBER OF VARIATES IN REMAKE R
C                             (M1 = 0 IF K2 = 0)
C          COLUMN 35  K3 = 0 TO READ DATA FROM DATAPE FILE
C                             = 1 TO READ DATA FROM INPUT FILE
C      2) FORMAT WITHIN BRACKETS (FOR SCORES IF K1 = 0,
C          FOR R MATRIX IF K1 = 1)
C      3) DATA FILE (SCORES OR R MATRIX)
C      4) ORIGINAL POSITION NUMBERS, IN THE FORMAT, OF VARIATES TO BE
C          INCLUDED IN THE REMAKE R, IN THEIR NEW ORDER AND IN TWO-
C          COLUMN FIELDS (OMIT IF K2 = 0)
C      5) NUMBER OF VARIATES WHICH ARE KEY INDICATORS OF EACH FACTOR,
C          IN FIVE COLUMN FIELDS.
C
C          IT IS ESSENTIAL THAT CAUSES BE PROPERLY ORDERED FOR FACTORING.
```

```
C       ORIGINAL OR REMAKE R MATRIX MUST HAVE VARIATES ORDERED AS FOLLOWS
C       1) KEY INDICATORS OF FIRST CAUSAL FACTOR
C       2) KEY INDICATORS OF SECOND CAUSAL FACTOR
C       3) ETCETERA THROUGH LAST CAUSAL FACTOR (NUMBER NAF)
C       4) ADDITIONAL INDEPENDENT VARIATES, IF ANY
C       5) EXTRA DEPENDENT VARIATES, IF ANY
C       6) KEY CRITERION AS LAST VARIATE IN R
C
        DIMENSION FMT(16), R(20,20), RI(20,20), A(20,20), B(20,20),
      C S(20), T(20), U(20), V(20), W(20), X(20), Y(20), Z(20),
      C MV(20), D(20,20)
        WRITE (6,2)
2       FORMAT (*1 MODEL CORRELATIONAL DATA, PROGRAMMED BY P. R. LOHNES*)
        READ(5,3) M, N, NAF, K1, K2, M1, K3
3       FORMAT (16I5)
        WRITE (6,4) M, N, NAF
4       FORMAT (*0 *I3,* VARIATES, *I6,* SUBJECTS, *I3,* VARIABLES*)
        EM = M
        EN = N
        READ (5,5) FMT
5       FORMAT (16A5)
        NX = 1
        IF (K3.NE.0) NX = 5
        IF (K1) 6, 6, 25
6       DO 7 J = 1, M
        Y(J) = 0.
        DO 7 K = 1, M
7       A(J,K) = 0.
        DO 9 L = 1, N
        READ (NX,FMT) (X(J), J = 1, M)
        DO 9 J = 1, M
        Y(J) = Y(J) + X(J)
        DO 9 K = J, M
9       A(J,K) = A(J,K) + X(J) * X(K)
        DO 10 J = 1, M
        U(J) = Y(J) / EN
        DO 10 K = J, M
10      A(J,K) = (A(J,K) − Y(J) * Y(K)/ EN) / EN
        DO 13 J = 1, M
13      Z(J) = SQRT (A(J,J))
        DO 16 J = 1, M
        DO 16 K = J, M
16      R(J,K) = A(J,K) / (Z(J) * Z(K))
        WRITE (6,17)
17      FORMAT(*0VARIATE   MEAN   S. D.*)
        DO 20 J = 1, M
20      WRITE (6,21) J, U(J), Z(J)
21      FORMAT(* *I3,2F10.2)
        GO TO 73
25      DO 26 J = 1, M
26      READ (NX,FMT) (R(J,K), K = J, M)
73      DO 27 J = 1, M
        DO 27 K = J, M
27      R(K,J) = R(J,K)
        WRITE (6,28)
28      FORMAT(*0CORRELATION MATRIX*)
        DO 29 J = 1, M
```

```
29        WRITE (6,30) J, (R(J,K), K = 1, J)
30        FORMAT (*0ROW*I3,20F6.3/(8X,20F6.3))
          IF (K2) 47, 47, 31
31        READ (5,32) (MV(J), J = 1, M1)
32        FORMAT(40I2)
          DO 33 J = 1, M1
          JT = MV(J)
          DO 33 K = J, M1
          KT = MV(K)
          IF (JT.LT.KT) GO TO 34
          A(J,K) = R(JT,KT)
          GO TO 33
34        A(J,K) = R(KT,JT)
33        CONTINUE
          M = M1
          DO 35 J = 1, M
          DO 35 K = J, M
35        A(K,J) = A(J,K)
          DO 36 J = 1, M
          DO 36 K = 1, M
36        R(J,K) = A(J,K)
          WRITE (6,37) M
37        FORMAT(*0REMAKE CORRELATION MATRIX, ORDER = *I3)
          WRITE (6,38) (MV(J), J = 1, M)
38        FORMAT(*0 NEW ORDER FOR VARIATES IS *20I4)
          DO 43 J = 1, M
43        WRITE (6,30) J, (R(J,K), K = 1, J)
47        DO 11 J = 1, M
          DO 11 K = 1, M
11        D(J,K) = R(J,K)
          READ (5,3) (MV(J), J = 1, NAF)
C
          KC = 0
          MC1 = 1
          MC2 = 0
          DO 12 NF = 1, NAF
          KC = KC + 1
          DO 54 J = 1, M
54        V(J) = 0.
          MC2 = MC2 + MV(KC)
          DO 55 J = MC1, MC2
55        V(J) = R(J,M)
          MC1 = MC1 + MV(KC)
          WRITE (6,14) NF
14        FORMAT(*0 HYPOTHESIS VECTOR *I3)
          WRITE (6,15) (V(J), J = 1, M)
15        FORMAT(* *10F7.3)
          DO 18 J = 1, M
          U(J) = 0.
          DO 18 K = 1, M
18        U(J) = U(J) + V(K) * R(K,J)
          C = 0.
          DO 19 J = 1, M
19        C = C + U(J) * V(J)
          C = SQRT(C)
          DO 22 J = 1, M
          U(J) = V(J)/C
```

```
22      B(J,NF) = U(J)
        DO 23 J = 1, M
        A(J,NF) = 0.
        DO 23 K = 1, M
23      A(J,NF) = A(J,NF) + R(J,K) * U(K)
        DO 24 J = 1, M
        DO 24 K = 1, M
24      R(J,K) = R(J,K) − A(J,NF) * A(K,NF)
        IF (NAF − KC) 61, 61, 63
61      WRITE (6,62) R(M,M)
62      FORMAT(*0 FINAL UNEXPLAINED VARIANCE IN CRITERION = *F6.4)
        GO TO 12
63      WRITE (6,64) KC, R(M,M)
64      FORMAT(*0 RESIDUAL CRITERION VARIANCE AFTER *I3,* STAGES = *F6.4)
12      CONTINUE
C       R IS NOW A RESIDUAL MATRIX WITH NAF FACTORS OUT, AND
C       IS RANK (M-NAF). FACTORS ARE IN FIRST NAF
C       COLUMNS OF A (STRUCTURE COEFFICIENTS).
42      FORMAT(*0FACTOR*I3,* PROP. VAR.*F5.3,* CUM. PROP.*F6.3)
        DO 1 J = 1, M
        V(J) = 0.
        DO 8 K = 1, NAF
8       V(J) = V(J) + A(J,K) * A(J,K)
1       U(J) = SQRT(1. − V(J))
        WRITE (6,44)
44      FORMAT(*0TEST COMMUNALITY DISTURBANCE FACTOR STRUCTURE*)
        DO 45 J = 1, M
45      WRITE (6,46) J, V(J), U(J), (A(J,K), K = 1, NAF)
46      FORMAT(* *I3,2(6X,F5.3),8X,10F7.3/(32X,10F7.3))
        C = 0.
        DO 66 J = 1, NAF
        V(J) = A(M,J) * A(M,J)
        C = C + V(J)
66      U(J) = C
        WRITE (6,67)
67      FORMAT(*0 CONTRIBUTIONS OF DOMAINS TO KEY CRITERION VARIANCE*)
        DO 68 J = 1, NAF
68      WRITE (6,42) J, V(J), U(J)
        WRITE (6,39)
39      FORMAT(*0FINAL RESIDUAL MATRIX*)
        DO 49 J = 1, M
49      WRITE (6,30) J, (R(J,K), K = 1, J)
        DO 51 J = 1, M
        DO 51 K = 1, M
51      R(J,K) = 0.
        DO 52 L = 1, NAF
        DO 52 J = 1, M
        DO 52 K = 1, M
52      R(J,K) = R(J,K) + A(J,L) * A(K,L)
        WRITE (6,53)
53      FORMAT(*0TOTAL THEORY PARTITION OF R FOR ALL FACTORS*)
        DO 56 J = 1, M
56      WRITE (6,30) J, (R(J,K), K = 1, J)
        DO 57 J = 1, M
        DO 57 K = 1, NAF
```

```
57      R(J,K) = B(J,K)
        DO 40 L = 2, NAF
        LL1 = L - 1
        MVT = 0
        DO 41 J = 1, LL1
        MVT = MVT + MV(J)
        MVU = 0
        DO 58 J1 = 1, LL1
58      MVU = MVU + MV(J1)
        MVK = MVU + 1
        MVL = MVU + MV(L)
        T(J) = 0.0
        DO 48 K = MVK, MVL
48      T(J) = T(J) + B(K,L) * A(K,J)
        DO 50 K = 1, MVT
50      R(K,L) = R(K,L) - T(J) * R(K,J)
41      CONTINUE
40      CONTINUE
        WRITE (6,65)
65      FORMAT(*0FACTOR-SCORING COEFFICIENTS*)
        DO 69 J = 1, M
69      WRITE (6,30) J, (R(J,K), K = 1, NAF)
        WRITE (6,71)
71      FORMAT(*0PREDICTED CHANGES IN CRITERIA (ROWS) FOR UNIT CHANGES*)
        WRITE (6,74)
74      FORMAT(* IN A PARTICULAR MANIPULABLE PREDICTOR (COLUMN)*)
        M1 = M - MC2
        DO 72 J = 1, M1
        JT = J + MC2
        DO 70 K = 1, MC2
        Z(K) = 0.
        DO 70 L = 1, NAF
70      Z(K) = Z(K) + A(JT,L) * R(K,L)
72      WRITE (6,30) J, (Z(KT), KT = 1, MC2)
        DO 101 J = 1, NAF
        DO 101 K = 1, M
        A(J,K) = 0.0
        DO 101 L = 1, M
101     A(J,K) = A(J,K) + R(L,J) * D(L,K)
        DO 102 J = 1, NAF
        DO 102 K = 1, NAF
        RI(J,K) = 0.0
        DO 102 L = 1, M
102     RI(J,K) = RI(J,K) + A(J,L) * R(L,K)
        WRITE (6,103)
103     FORMAT(*0VARIANCE-COVARIANCE MATRIX FOR FACTORS*)
        DO 104 J = 1, NAF
104     WRITE (6,30) J, (RI(J,K), K = 1, NAF)
        CALL EXIT
        END
*WEOR
```

Project TALENT Data for 147 Nursing Aspirants

Selected Variates for 147 Nurse Aspirants on Project TALENT 1971 Follow-up of 1479 Women Who Were in the Eleventh Grade in 1960

No.	Columns	Contents
ID	1–3	Subject identification in this file
1	5	Certainty of occupational choice in 1960
2	7–9	Information test score in 1960
3	11–13	English test score in 1960
4	15–16	Reading comprehension test score in 1960
5	18–19	Visualization in three dimensions in 1960
6	21–22	Abstract reasoning test score in 1960
7	24–25	Mathematics test score in 1960
8	27–28	Interest in biological science and medicine in 1960
9	30–31	Interest in social service in 1960
10	33–35	Socioeconomic environment index in 1960
11	37	High school curriculum in 1960 (1 = academic, 0 = other)
12	39–40	High school grades in 1960
13	42	Job code nurse in 1971? (1 = yes, 0 = no)
14	44	Registered nurse in 1971? (1 = yes, 0 = no)

Note: Missing data are indicated by a zero, but there are no missing data for the dichotomous variates (i.e., variates 11, 13, 14).

```
 1 3 226 107 35 12 12 30 38 27  99 1 28 1 1
 2 0 185  92 26  5  9 33 38 38 106 1 27 0 0
 3 3 288  99 46 12 11 41 24 30 108 1 27 0 0
 4 3 290 107 45 10 13 43 24 19 101 1 45 0 0
 5 2 161  97 29  9  7 16 35 30 115 0 43 1 0
 6 4 256  97 42  9  8 34 33 33 119 1 24 0 0
 7 0 164  89 20  5  8 21 40 37 110 1 15 0 0
 8 3 279  98 46 12  8 30 26 28 108 1 35 0 0
 9 1 172  83 28  8  8 21 33 26  98 1 25 0 0
10 1 263  98 38 10 11 31 25 22  93 0 25 0 1
11 1 177  82 26  6  6 15 26 31  92 0 24 0 0
12 0 221  90 41  9 11 33 29 28  99 1 23 0 0
13 1 111  73 18  8  4  9 20 19 103 1 36 0 0
14 1 196  92 42  9 12 27 28 22 101 1 31 0 0
15 2 180  91 35  2  4 15 36 21 107 1 12 0 0
16 0 197  90 22 13 13 25 35 20 115 0 18 0 0
17 2   0  78 41  6  9 18  0  0 109 1 27 1 1
18 3 225   0  0  0  0  0 33 30  88 1 27 0 0
19 3 234  89 38 10 12 28 10 28 101 1 25 0 0
20 1 223  94 28 12 12 22 33 32  99 0 36 0 0
21 3 238  87 36 11 10 34 35 36 103 1 17 0 0
22 3 223  90 38 11 13 34 21 33  95 1 20 1 1
23 0 230  95 43  8 12 19 33 30 106 1 32 1 1
24 0 137  88 16  8  7 10 21 17  89 0 27 0 0
25 3 300 106 44 11 13 40 29 18  90 1 47 1 1
26 3 203  75 27  8  7 24 34 28  82 0 23 0 0
27 2 277 101 47 12 12 41 31 28  96 1 33 1 1
28 3 183  96 36  6  5 20 11 27  80 1 28 0 0
29 2 193  96 32 10 11 31 25 34  94 0 21 0 0
30 4 218  94 37  9 10 22 15 21 100 1 44 0 0
31 3 199  87 37 10  7 18 10 21  91 0 22 0 0
32 5 154  77 22  3 10 11 21 28 109 0 19 0 0
33 2 202  88 34 12 14 23 29 16 112 1 25 0 1
34 1   0   0 42  6 12  0  0  0 107 1 28 1 1
35 2   0   0  0  0  0  0  0  0 112 1 20 0 0
36 1 173  94 30  8 11 27 30 38 110 1 21 0 0
37 1 207  88 40 12 11 26 28 28 101 1 18 0 0
38 5 223  80 44  8 12 34 25 38  92 1 42 0 0
39 0 289  98 32 12 13 23 33 22  99 1 31 1 1
40 3 255  95 28  9  7 25 28 26 100 1 23 0 0
41 0 206  96 43 13 11 27 39 28 105 1 20 0 0
42 0 235  98 37  9  9 33 28 24 100 1 33 0 0
43 3 185  89 34 12  8 24 34 29  97 0 42 0 0
44 3 169  77 31  6 10 12 24 29  93 0 16 0 0
45 4 208  90 33  4 11 18 20 25  98 0 14 0 0
46 4 220  86 38 14 10 34 11 27  95 1 20 0 0
47 3 189  86 35  7  6 16 31 29  98 0 22 0 0
48 2 242  88 42  9 10 26 26 21  98 1 28 0 0
49 3 246 108 39 11 12 41 29 26 109 1 35 0 0
```

50	4	256	97	48	12	11	34	18	24	97	1	38	0	0
51	6	120	69	9	8	6	10	10	23	91	0	25	0	0
52	0	280	93	42	7	11	28	36	20	109	1	28	0	1
53	1	273	105	43	11	12	37	28	29	110	1	39	0	0
54	5	0	103	41	11	11	39	0	0	96	1	35	0	0
55	2	165	91	37	4	9	11	29	26	83	0	29	0	0
56	0	145	71	8	3	9	15	20	19	102	0	13	0	0
57	3	323	104	44	10	10	45	39	31	102	0	42	0	0
58	2	257	87	43	5	10	13	35	18	98	0	42	0	1
59	3	227	84	38	10	10	38	24	34	82	1	42	0	1
60	3	251	101	45	4	10	29	25	28	90	0	45	1	1
61	3	132	64	22	6	4	13	21	15	89	0	7	0	0
62	1	262	84	39	13	11	27	35	36	109	1	25	1	1
63	3	195	99	30	4	11	21	26	33	110	1	28	0	1
64	3	266	95	42	12	10	23	35	33	104	1	29	0	0
65	3	235	88	41	9	11	32	34	32	101	1	36	0	0
66	0	82	69	10	6	4	12	11	11	83	0	9	0	0
67	4	140	59	20	5	8	13	15	25	87	0	11	0	0
68	3	244	88	43	13	13	36	30	21	95	0	40	1	1
69	2	259	97	42	6	9	24	23	31	116	1	30	0	1
70	3	196	91	31	8	11	27	24	36	116	0	23	0	0
71	3	140	67	17	10	11	14	6	11	91	0	12	0	0
72	3	189	81	28	7	0	16	11	22	107	0	15	0	0
73	2	247	90	37	15	12	35	29	32	111	1	28	0	0
74	2	280	105	45	13	14	43	21	28	109	1	28	0	0
75	3	275	92	41	12	9	32	39	36	114	1	30	0	1
76	6	165	80	34	6	5	18	3	11	98	0	10	0	0
77	1	258	89	38	15	10	22	39	32	119	1	50	1	1
78	0	260	97	41	14	14	27	33	25	98	1	31	0	0
79	6	249	91	44	13	12	25	13	15	116	1	22	0	0
80	4	149	70	26	10	9	14	36	26	89	0	10	0	0
81	0	158	83	32	13	13	15	20	28	99	0	25	0	0
82	3	175	97	28	13	12	27	31	23	94	1	22	0	0
83	5	263	86	45	11	6	21	26	29	103	0	17	0	0
84	1	233	97	38	7	11	28	33	28	90	0	43	0	0
85	3	197	85	31	6	12	21	33	32	95	0	20	0	0
86	4	178	84	27	9	8	16	9	30	104	0	18	0	0
87	4	242	96	39	9	12	17	20	33	90	1	20	0	0
88	3	206	88	29	11	11	32	9	36	100	0	26	0	0
89	0	163	68	21	7	5	18	33	29	89	0	32	0	0
90	2	190	0	0	0	0	0	40	38	100	0	28	0	0
91	5	233	85	26	7	8	15	29	25	107	1	10	0	0
92	0	252	88	43	13	11	32	34	20	101	0	24	0	0
93	3	194	91	25	12	10	14	39	26	100	1	30	0	1
94	4	153	84	34	7	12	14	14	18	103	0	14	0	0
95	5	188	88	37	9	12	27	6	32	86	0	30	0	0
96	4	155	85	27	6	3	19	18	23	101	0	41	0	0
97	3	222	104	32	12	13	22	16	28	106	1	25	0	0
98	2	223	90	26	6	3	12	30	31	95	1	12	0	0

```
 99 2 182  85 28  9 11 13 15 15 105 0 32 0 0
100 0  82  67 12  4  2  8 21 32  80 1 15 0 0
101 0  94  56  8  4  5 11 11 25  78 0 27 0 0
102 5   0   0  0  0  0  0  0  0  94 1 48 0 0
103 0 143  60 12  7  3 12 25 21  83 1 34 0 0
104 1 196  72 27 10  7 11 33 28  88 1 34 0 0
105 6 174  93 36  6  8 24  6 22 100 0 22 0 0
106 6 202  87 41  3  5 16 20 31  95 0 24 0 0
107 1 182  89 28  8 11 19 29 39  97 1 35 0 0
108 3 171  75 28  5  7 23 31 28  99 0 15 0 0
109 1 147  80 25  6  4 11 19 18 104 1 34 0 0
110 3 203  80 35  8  7 18 21 23 113 1 18 0 0
111 3 252  91 39  6 10 25 29 28 101 0 41 1 1
112 0  87  54 11  6  4 11 20 22  75 0 23 0 0
113 0 172  86 29 11 10 12 34 27 105 1 18 0 0
114 1 196  82 31  8  6 17 33 27  87 0 37 0 0
115 3 292  96 44  8 11 26 35 24 117 1 29 0 0
116 0 100  77 24  4  6 18  4 19  83 0 16 0 0
117 0 215   0  0  0  0  0 40 18  95 0  0 0 0
118 0 158  71 19  7 10 14 18 24  92 0 19 0 0
119 2 197  95 34  7  9 18 25 25 104 1 27 0 1
120 3 259  92 41 14 14 30 35 33 111 1 23 0 1
121 1 242 102 46 14 13 36 28 38 104 0 35 0 0
122 3 171  99 30 11 10 18 16 32 100 0 24 0 0
123 3 130  53 13  9  4 10 39 16  86 0 13 0 0
124 1 195  89 33  7 10 19 20 29  91 0 35 0 0
125 3 253  95 40  9 10 28 38 14  99 1 40 0 0
126 0 223  96 43 12 11 34 23 28 108 1 24 1 1
127 6 155  84 21  5  4 11 23 26 102 0 15 0 0
128 3 266  90 46 10  8 36 39 33 107 1 47 0 0
129 1   0 102 47  5 10 19 24 29 107 1 15 0 0
130 2 138  78 18  1  4  1 31 34  97 0 26 0 0
131 3 274  95 45 10  8  2 30 23 100 1 30 0 0
132 3 145  74 16  5  8 13 14 16 103 0 17 0 0
133 0 154  82 27 13 10 16 15 26 103 0  0 0 0
134 0 247  89 46 11 12 22 29 27  85 0  0 0 0
135 4 239  86 37  8 11 27 29 21 114 1 12 0 0
136 2 230  97 42  6 10 18 30 27 105 1 18 0 1
137 2 264  96 44 12 12 36 36 23 101 1 38 1 1
138 3 239  96 40  6 11 33 25 29 104 1 20 0 0
139 3 190  90 40  9  9 18 34 29 103 0 25 1 1
140 0 207  84 41  5 11 16 26 17  94 0  0 0 0
141 2 235  98 46 14 14 40 17 21  95 0 50 0 0
142 0 243 100 44  6 10 20 29 22 100 1 28 0 0
143 4 205  97 33 10 11 27 30 25 101 0 20 0 0
144 3 246  95 37  5  6 16 36 38 103 1 35 0 0
145 3 228  96 42  8 12 28 29 25 111 1 33 0 0
146 3 246 102 41 11 12 38 30 22 106 1 25 1 1
147 3 248  88 35 11  9 25 34 35 112 1 37 0 0
```

Index

Index